Role Development for the Nurse Practitioner

Second Edition

Edited by

Julie G. Stewart, DNP, MPH, MSN, FNP-BC, FAANP
Associate Professor & Director of the FNP and DNP Programs
Sacred Heart University
Fairfield, Connecticut

Susan M. DeNisco, DNP, APRN, FNP-BC, CNE, CNL
Professor, Doctor of Nursing Practice Program
Sacred Heart University
Fairfield, Connecticut

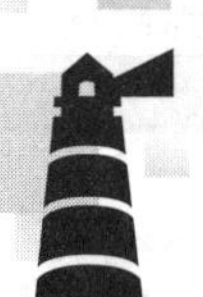

JONES & BARTLETT
LEARNING

World Headquarters
Jones & Bartlett Learning
5 Wall Street
Burlington, MA 01803
978-443-5000
info@jblearning.com
www.jblearning.com

Jones & Bartlett Learning books and products are available through most bookstores and online booksellers. To contact Jones & Bartlett Learning directly, call 800-832-0034, fax 978-443-8000, or visit our website, www.jblearning.com.

Substantial discounts on bulk quantities of Jones & Bartlett Learning publications are available to corporations, professional associations, and other qualified organizations. For details and specific discount information, contact the special sales department at Jones & Bartlett Learning via the above contact information or send an email to specialsales@jblearning.com.

Production Credits
VP, Product Management: David D. Cella
Director of Product Management: Amanda Martin
Product Manager: Rebecca Stephenson
Product Assistant: Christina Freitas
Senior Vendor Manager: Sara Kelly
Senior Marketing Manager: Jennifer Scherzay
Product Fulfillment Manager: Wendy Kilborn
Composition and Project Management: S4Carlisle Publishing Services
Cover Design: Kristin E. Parker
Rights & Media Specialist: Wes DeShano
Media Development Editor: Troy Liston
Cover Image (Title Page, Part Opener, Chapter Opener): © ARTappler/iStock/Getty Images Plus/Getty
Diagonal textures: © briddy_/iStock/Getty Images Plus/Getty
Printing and Binding: Edwards Brothers Malloy
Cover Printing: Edwards Brothers Malloy

Library of Congress Cataloging-in-Publication Data
Names: Stewart, Julie G., editor. | DeNisco, Susan M., editor.
Title: Role development for the nurse practitioner / [edited by] Julie G. Stewart and Susan M. DeNisco.
Description: Second edition. | Burlington, MA : Jones & Bartlett Learning, [2019] | Includes bibliographical references and index.
Identifiers: LCCN 2017040236 | ISBN 9781284130133
Subjects: | MESH: Nurse Practitioners | Nurse's Role
Classification: LCC RT82.8 | NLM WY 128 | DDC 610.7306/92--dc23 LC record available at https://lccn.loc.gov/2017040236

6048

Printed in the United States of America
22 21 20 19 18 10 9 8 7 6 5 4 3 2

I am fortunate to have loving and supportive children, Kirstin, Karine, and Tyler, who all have wonderful spouses and children. My grandchildren, always increasing in numbers but as of today include Kyle, Kaia, Kaden, Kolton, Juliana, Lucien, Mackenzie, Elida, and Warren—they are the most amazing loves of my life.

To Jack, who has been supportive of my professional career and passion about the role of nurse practitioners. I also offer my sincere gratitude to my colleagues who are a joy to work with and true scholars who I admire more than they realize. Finally, and importantly, my dear friend and colleague without whom I would never have made it to this point in my profession. Sue DeNisco, thank you for supporting and encouraging me through the good times and the not-so-good times, and for being my professional partner in everything I do.

Julie G. Stewart (MorMor)

Life is full of changes; therefore, I want to dedicate this book to my mother who was my first editor during my early writing days. By passing on her love of learning, gift of writing, and resilient spirit, I have had the fortitude to sit at the computer for exorbitant periods of time. I miss her every day but know that she is sitting at my shoulder.

It goes without saying that my children, Alison, Michael, Spencer, Sarah, Brooke, and granddaughter Lenore, are major sources of pride and invigorate my spirit. They are all amazing human beings with unique gifts and talents to share. There is never a dull moment!

I have been very fortunate in both my clinical and academic career to have interfaced with amazing nurse colleagues who have been students, friends, fellow clinicians, mentors, and mentees. Julie G. Stewart is a nurse educator, nurse practitioner, and nurse leader whom I call "the triple threat." Her passion for life, sense of humor, and vision for the future of nursing keep me at her side.

And lastly, Rick, you continue to amaze me with your patience, kindness, and support. I know how much you have sacrificed to have a wife that is a self-proclaimed workaholic. I love you always and forever.

Susan M. DeNisco (Mom, Yia Yia)

© ARTappler/iStock/Getty Images Plus/Getty

Contents

Foreword

This unique and timely book was inspired and developed by two doctor of nursing practice alumni from one of the most prestigious DNP programs in the country. Collectively, with more than 7 decades as nurse practitioners in primary care practice and education, the authors took on the task of summarizing the key aspects of their roles, including preparing for NP certification and licensure as well as often overlooked areas such as consultation, collaboration, billing, and reimbursement. Critically important clinical information on cultural aspects of practice, the intersection of primary and mental health care, and the NP–patient relationship is also highlighted. Chapters on mentoring and professionalism, the hallmark activities of any high-level occupation, are included.

Throughout the text, case vignettes and interviews with nurse practitioners are used to highlight key information and inspire critical thinking. The information outlined in this publication will provide the foundation needed to practice at the highest level of NP preparation in order to meet societal needs for quality, cost-effective, and outcome-driven health care. This book will serve as a resource for the NP at a variety of stages from student to expert clinician.

Margaret A. Fitzgerald, DNP, FNP-BC, NP-C, FAANP, CSP, FAAN, DCC
President, Fitzgerald Health Education Associates, Inc.

Preface

Educating colleagues, family, and friends about what a nurse practitioner is and does has been an important and frequently needed topic since the day I applied to graduate school, so this book was a natural outcome for me.

I vividly remember when I was 8 years old, I set up my "medical office" in a spare bedroom, opening my little plastic medical equipment bag to find my durable plastic stethoscope while wearing my nurse's cape. I called my first patient in, my patients being all the neighborhood children I could coerce into making "appointments." Unfortunately for me, my mother put a stop to the comprehensive physical exams that day, but I remained determined that one day I would take care of people.

Fast-forward to the intensive care unit where I relished in providing comprehensive care to critically ill patients and supported their loved ones. I loved being a critical care nurse. After numerous years in that arena, it was time for a change. The hospital had hired a nurse practitioner to run our employee health department. I found it fascinating that a nurse could be my doctor! So off I went to graduate school to become a family nurse practitioner. It was hard, I remember that clearly; however, I also remember very well the evening we started history-taking and physical assessment. This was my "AHA!" moment. I drove home thrilled that I had finally found my professional role.

Over the past 20 years after graduating from the FNP program, I have experienced the joys of successful patient–provider relationships and health outcomes, as well as the frustrations of being a healthcare provider in such tumultuous times. I am most proud of my ability to teach students in both the classroom and clinic. Watching each one develop into a competent primary care provider is a highlight in my career. I have been fortunate to work with my colleague, mentor, and dear friend to help you as you develop your role as a nurse practitioner.

Julie G. Stewart

As a new graduate nurse, I was very interested in working with medically underserved populations and was influenced by the work of Mary Breckenridge, a nurse–midwife who founded the Frontier Nursing Service. Off I went to my first professional nursing role as a surgical nurse in a small country hospital in eastern Kentucky. On weekends, a physician friend of mine and I traded the "horse" for a "Jeep" and visited many families that had few resources and no transportation out of the "hollers" to obtain medical care. Following the 2 years spent in Appalachia, I solidified my interest in primary care by working for the U.S. Public Health Service on the western slope of Colorado where I set up clinics for migrant Mexican farm workers. I was then hooked and decided that I could make the largest impact on vulnerable populations by becoming a family nurse practitioner. My 31 years as a primary care provider has afforded me the opportunity to provide direct patient care to both rural and urban populations in a wide variety of settings. Each patient I have been honored to care for has taught me so much and helped fuel my passion for "nurse practitioneering." A large part of my career has been spent on passing on my knowledge to the next generation of NPs. I have precepted many NP students over the years and enjoy seeing them blossom from neophyte, entry-level nurse practitioners to those that practice with competence and compassion.

In the words of Khalil Gibran, "Generosity is giving more than you can, and pride is taking less than you need."

Susan M. DeNisco

Contributors

Jean Boucher, PhD, RN, ANP-BC, AOCNP®
Associate Professor of Nursing & Medicine
UMass Medical School
Graduate School of Nursing
Worcester, MA

Holly B. Bradley, DNP, MS, ANP-BC, APRN
Clinical Assistant Professor
College of Nursing
Sacred Heart University
Fairfield, CT

Stephen C. Burrows, DPM, MBA, CPHIMS, FHIMSS
Program Director, Healthcare Informatics
Sacred Heart University
Fairfield, CT

Michelle A. Cole, DNP, MSN, RN, CNP
Director of Undergraduate Nursing and Assistant Professor
College of Nursing
Sacred Heart University
Fairfield, CT

Brandi Parker Cotton, PhD, MSN, APRN
Assistant Professor
Nursing Instructor, College of Nursing
University of Rhode Island
Kingston, RI
Gateway Healthcare, Inc.
Pawtucket, RI

Elizabeth Ercolano, DNSc, MSN, RN
Associate Research Scientist
Yale School of Nursing
Yale University
Orange, CT

Christina B. Gunther, MA
Director, Global Health Programs & Health Science Program
Instructor, Sacred Heart University
Fairfield, CT

Michelle Johnson, EdD, RN, CPNP-PC
Associate Professor and Chief Nurse Administrator
Department of Nursing
Hawaii Pacific University
Honolulu, HI

Julie A. Koch, PhD, MEd
Assistant Dean of Graduate Nursing and the DNP Program Director
College of Nursing and Health Professions
Valparaiso University
Valparaiso, IN

Kerry Milner, DNSc, RN
Associate Professor, Department of Nursing
Sacred Heart University
Fairfield, CT

Linda S. Morrow, DNP, MSN, MBA, CNOR, CPHQ
Assistant Professor and Program Director Patient Care Services Administration, Department of Nursing
Sacred Heart University
Fairfield, CT

Lynn Rapsilber, DNP, APRN, ANP-BC, FAANP
Owner: NP Business Consultants and NP Wellness Care
Torrington, CT

Marylou Siefert, DNSc, RN, AOCN®, APRN
Assistant Professor
College of Nursing
Sacred Heart University
Fairfield, CT

Tammy A. Testut, PhD, MSN, RN, NEA-BC
Clinical Assistant Professor
College of Nursing
Sacred Heart University
Fairfield, CT

© ARTappler/iStock/Getty Images Plus/Getty

Reviewers

Lucie J. Agosta, RNC, PhD
Adult/Family Nurse Practitioner
Assistant Professor & Coordinator, Family Nurse Practitioner Track
Southeastern Louisiana University
Baton Rouge, LA

Claudia Anderson Beckmann, PhD, APN-C
Associate Professor
Specialty Director Women's Health Nurse Practitioner
Rutgers University College of Nursing
Newark, NJ

Greg Brooks, DNP, APRN, FNP-C
Assistant Professor of Nursing
Director, Family Nurse Practitioner Program
Oklahoma City University, Kramer School of Nursing
Oklahoma City, OK

Gina Crawford, MS, APRN, FNP-C
Clinical Instructor of Nursing
Oklahoma City University, Kramer School of Nursing
Oklahoma City, OK

Freida Fuller, RN, DSN, FNP-BC
FNP Program Coordinator
Mercer University, Georgia Baptist College of Nursing
Atlanta, GA

Gwendolyn S. George, DNP, APRN, FNP-BC
Assistant Professor and DNP Program Coordinator
Loyola University
New Orleans, LA

S. Renée Gregg, MSN, FNP-C
Ball State University
Muncie, IN

Frances Johnson, DNP, APRN, NNP-BC
Professor of Nursing
Southern Adventist University
Collegedale, TN

Katherine Kenny, DNP, RN, ANP-BC, CCRN
DNP Program Director
Arizona State University
Phoenix, AZ

Laura LaRue, DNP, FNP-BC
Assistant Professor, FNP Coordinator
Radford University
Radford, VA

Eileen McCann, DNP, FNP-BC
Director of Family Nurse Practitioner Program and Assistant Professor
St. Xavier University
Chicago, IL

Cynthia Ricci McCloskey, DNS, APRN-BC, WHNP
Associate Professor and Graduate Program Director, Nursing
Wegmans School of Nursing
St. John Fisher College
Rochester, NY

Debra Miller-Saultz, DNP, FNP-BC
Assistant Professor of Nursing
College of New Rochelle
New Rochelle, NY

Patricia A. Nielsen, DNP, FNP-BC
Program Director of Nursing
Programs for School of Graduate and Continuing Studies
Olivet Nazarene University
Bourbonnais, IL

Debbie Nogueras, PhD, MSN, APRN-BC
Associate Professor and Coordinator of FNP and DNP Programs
Northern Arizona University
Flagstaff, AZ

Cindy Parsons, DNP, PMHNP-BC, FAANP
Associate Professor of Nursing
University of Tampa
Tampa, FL

Alberta Peters-Herron, DNP, FNP-BC, RN
Goldfarb School of Nursing
St. Louis, MO

Erin Shankel, MSN, RN, FNP-BC
Adjunct Professor
Belmont University School of Nursing
Nashville, TN
Nurse Practitioner
Allergy and Asthma Associates of Middle Tennessee
Franklin, TN

Jennifer Sipe, RN, MSN, ANP-BC
La Salle University School of Nursing and Health Sciences
Medical Office of Michael J. Palazzolo, MD
Philadelphia, PA

Dellarie L. Shilling, DNP, FNP-BC
Georgia Southern University School of Nursing
Statesboro, GA

Carole G. Traylor, DNP, CPNP, CAE
Assistant Professor
Beth-El College of Nursing and Health Sciences
University of Colorado
Colorado Springs, CO

Barbara Wilder, DSN, CRNP
Professor
Auburn University School of Nursing
Auburn, AL

Diane Wink, EdD, ARNP, FNP-BC, FAANP
Professor and Hugh F. and Jeannette G. McKean Endowed Chair in Nursing
University of Central Florida
Orlando, FL

PART 1

Scientific Underpinning of the Nurse Practitioner Role

CHAPTER 1

Historical Perspectives: The Art and Science of Nurse Practitionering

Julie G. Stewart

U.S. News and World Report (2017) lists nurse practitioner (NP) as the second top occupation for 2017. There were 23,000 new NP graduates in 2015 who joined the ranks of the nation's roughly 234,000 NPs, a number that has almost doubled within 10 years (American Academy of Nurse Practitioners [AANP], 2017).

In 2010, the Institute of Medicine (IOM) released a report that identified the need for nurses to be placed at the forefront of health care. The report strongly recommended that advanced practice registered nurses—including nurse practitioners—be allowed to practice to the full scope of their abilities and that barriers be removed to enable moving forward. We have come a long way since 2010, but there are still milestones to reach and barriers to break.

Nurse practitioners reached a tipping point as a profession (Buerhaus, 2010). Malcolm Gladwell states that the "tipping point is that magic moment when an idea, trend, or social behavior crosses a threshold, tips, and spreads like wildfire" (Gladwell, 2000, p. 12). Nurse practitioners have been given the opportunity to shine and to experience growth professionally. Nurse practitioners provide a solution to some of the issues affecting health care in America today. The need for NPs is growing as we consider the IOM's recommendation and the large population of aging baby boomers, which is anticipated to increase the use of the healthcare system (DHHS, 2011; Van Leuven, 2012). In addition, the Patient Protection and Affordable Care Act signed in 2010 instituted comprehensive health insurance reform and expanded healthcare insurance coverage to 32 million Americans (DHHS, 2011). Researchers have validated the cost, quality, and competence of NPs' role in providing primary care with outcomes that are similar to primary care physicians (Hamric, Spross, & Hanson, 2009; Laurant et al., 2005; Mundinger et al., 2000; Wilson et al., 2005). Medical economist and health futurist Jeffrey C. Bauer (2010) reviewed evidence-based data in an article to illustrate how NPs functioning independently can meet the cost-effective needs of healthcare reform while providing high-quality care for patients in multiple settings. Indeed, more than 1 billion patients visit NPs for health care annually (AANP, 2017).

At least 85% of NPs are educated to provide primary care, and two out of three are educated as family NPs (AANP, 2017); however, in some states, many NPs are not working in primary care possibly because of the state's restrictions on requiring collaborators and written agreements with physicians. Many states have recognized this barrier and have removed those requirements, and many insurance companies are including NPs in their provider networks. So, will we meet the near future needs for healthcare providers? The answer appears to be a resounding yes. In an age-cohort, regression-based model, RAND Health projected the future workforce of NPs will grow to 244,000 by the year 2025 (Auerbach, 2012), and as previously mentioned, we are already more than 234,000 strong. Clearly, there is a need to fully understand the role of the NP in order to advance professionalism and unity of the NP workforce. Seminar discussions regarding pertinent issues must be part of the education of student NPs and included in discussion among those already in practice.

Historical Perspective

The role of the nurse practitioner was developed as a way to provide primary care for the underserved. The role is typically described as having emerged during the 1960s, yet Lillian Wald's nurses of the late 1800s bear a striking resemblance to NPs of today. The nurses of Wald's Henry Street Settlement House in New York City provided primary care for poverty-stricken immigrants, and treated common illnesses and emergencies that did not require referral (Hamric et al., 2009). In 1965, the role of nurse practitioner was formally developed by Loretta Ford, EdD (nurse educator), and Henry Silver, MD (professor of medicine), both of whom were teaching at the University of Colorado (Sullivan-Marx, McGivern, Fairman, & Greenberg, 2010). This nurse practitioner program was developed not only to advance the nursing profession; it was also developed in response to the need for providers in rural, underserved areas. The program was initially funded by a $7,000 grant from the School of Medicine at the University of Colorado (Bruner, 2005; Weiland, 2008). The first program was a pediatric NP program based on the nursing model, yet the program advanced the clinical practice of these students by teaching them how to provide primary care and how to make medical diagnoses.

These early NP pioneers were focused on having a positive effect on advancing the profession, "making a difference," and gaining autonomy (Weiland, 2008, p. 346). However, due to the socioeconomic and political climate of the times, the NP was viewed to be a cost-effective way to provide healthcare providers for the underserved. During the 1970s, federal funding helped to establish many NP programs to address a shortage of primary care physicians, particularly in underserved areas. Idaho was the first state to endorse nurse practitioners' scope of practice to include diagnosis and treatment in 1971. NP programs doubled between 1992 and 1997. By the year 2000, there were 321 institutions that offered either a master's level or a postmaster's-level NP program (Health Resources and Services Administration [HRSA], 2004). By 2002, more than 30% of NPs were working with vulnerable populations, including the homeless, indigent, chronically ill, and elderly (Jenning, 2002). Today there are more than 400 institutions educating nurse practitioners, and 234,000 licensed nurse practitioners in the United States (AANP, 2017).

Nurse Practitioner Education and Title Clarification

In the 1960s, the role of the NP was not warmly welcomed by nurse educators; therefore, many educational programs to train nurses in the NP role were more often continuing education programs rather than university-housed programs (Pulcini, 2013). In the 1980s and 1990s, NP education moved into the university setting as master's-level programs, although confusion arose when there were efforts to interchange the clinical nurse specialist (CNS) and NP roles. Today there are well over 330 graduate-level NP programs, and many have gone to offering only a clinical doctorate—the doctor of nursing practice (DNP)—for NP education in response to the American Association of Colleges of Nursing's (AACN's) recommendation that advanced practice nurses be educated at that level by 2015.

In 2008, the *Consensus Model for APRN Regulation: Licensure, Accreditation, Certification & Education* was finalized through the collaborative efforts of the APRN Consensus Work Group and the National Council of State Boards of Nursing APRN Advisory Committee. To clarify who is an advanced practice registered nurse, the document included the following definition (APRN Consensus Work Group, National Council of State Boards of Nursing APRN Advisory Committee, 2008):

An advanced practice registered nurse (APRN) is a nurse:

1. Who has completed an accredited graduate-level education program preparing him or her for one of the four recognized APRN roles;
2. Who has passed a national certification examination that measures APRN, role and population-focused competencies, and who maintains continued competence as evidenced by recertification in the role and population through the national certification program;
3. Who has acquired advanced clinical knowledge and skills preparing him or her to provide direct care to patients, as well as a component of indirect care; however, the defining factor for *all* APRNs is that a significant component of the education and practice focuses on direct care of individuals;
4. Whose practice builds on the competencies of registered nurses (RNs) by demonstrating a greater depth and breadth of knowledge, a greater synthesis of data, increased complexity of skills and interventions, and greater role autonomy;
5. Who is educationally prepared to assume responsibility and accountability for health promotion and maintenance as well as the assessment, diagnosis, and management of patient problems, which includes the use and prescription of pharmacologic and nonpharmacologic interventions;
6. Who has clinical experience of sufficient depth and breadth to reflect the intended license; *and*
7. Who has obtained a license to practice as an APRN in one of the four APRN roles: certified registered nurse anesthetist (CRNA), certified nurse-midwife (CNM), clinical nurse specialist (CNS), or certified nurse practitioner (CNP).[1]

---

1 APRN Consensus Work Group and the National Council of State Boards of Nursing APRN Advisory Committee (2008). Consensus model for APRN regulation: Licensure, accreditation, certification & education. APRN Joint Dialogue Group Report, July 7, 2008.

Clearly, NPs are one of the four roles that fall under the umbrella definition for APRN; however, using the title "APRN" does not clearly define which role and educational background the professional has. Each APRN role differs from the others, and state regulatory agencies vary in requirements for licensing in each state, and in many cases, for each APRN role.

The Master's Essentials

The American Association of Colleges of Nursing (AACN) prepared the *Essentials for Master's Education in Nursing* (AACN, 2011). There are nine essentials that focus on outcomes and are for all master's-level programs. In addition, direct patient care provider (APRN) education must offer three separate courses on the "3 Ps," which are advanced pharmacology, advanced pathophysiology, and advanced physical assessment. The nine essentials are (AACN, 2011):

I. Background for practice from sciences and humanities
II. Organizational and systems leadership
III. Quality improvement and safety
IV. Translating and integrating scholarship into practice
V. Informatics and healthcare technologies
VI. Health policy and advocacy
VII. Interprofessional collaboration for improving patient and population health outcomes
VIII. Clinical prevention and population health for improving health
IX. Master's-level nursing practice

Essential IX, master's-level nursing practice, recognizes that nursing practice, at the master's level, is broadly defined as any form of nursing intervention that influences healthcare outcomes for individuals, populations, or systems. Master's-level nursing graduates must have an advanced level of understanding of nursing and relevant sciences as well as the ability to integrate this knowledge into practice. Nursing practice interventions include both direct and indirect care components (AACN, 2011).

Nurse Practitioner Core Competencies

In addition to the AACN, which strives to advance the education of nurses in general, the National Organization for Nurse Practitioner Faculties (NONPF) sets the standards for nurse practitioner programs. NONPF has stated there are core competencies for nurse practitioners in all tracks and specialties. These are listed here so the NP student can review and understand how coursework reflects these competencies (NONPF, 2017).

Scientific Foundation Competencies

1. Critically analyzes data and evidence for improving advanced nursing practice.
2. Integrates knowledge from the humanities and sciences within the context of nursing science.

3. Translates research and other forms of knowledge to improve practice processes and outcomes.
4. Develops new practice approaches based on the integration of research, theory, and practice knowledge.

Leadership Competencies

1. Assumes complex and advanced leadership roles to initiate and guide change.
2. Provides leadership to foster collaboration with multiple stakeholders (e.g., patients, community, integrated healthcare teams, and policy makers) to improve health care.
3. Demonstrates leadership that uses critical and reflective thinking.
4. Advocates for improved access, quality, and cost-effective health care.
5. Advances practice through the development and implementation of innovations incorporating principles of change.
6. Communicates practice knowledge effectively both orally and in writing.
7. Participates in professional organizations and activities that influence advanced practice nursing and/or health outcomes of a population focus.

Quality Competencies

1. Uses best available evidence to continuously improve quality of clinical practice.
2. Evaluates the relationships among access, cost, quality, and safety and their influence on health care.
3. Evaluates how organizational structure, care processes, financing, marketing, and policy decisions affect the quality of health care.
4. Applies skills in peer review to promote a culture of excellence.
5. Anticipates variations in practice and is proactive in implementing interventions to ensure quality.

Practice Inquiry Competencies

1. Provides leadership in the translation of new knowledge into practice.
2. Generates knowledge from clinical practice to improve practice and patient outcomes.
3. Applies clinical investigative skills to improve health outcomes.
4. Leads practice inquiry, individually or in partnership with others.
5. Disseminates evidence from inquiry to diverse audiences using multiple modalities.
6. Analyzes clinical guidelines for individualized application into practice.

Technology and Information Literacy Competencies

1. Integrates appropriate technologies for knowledge management to improve health care.
2. Translates technical and scientific health information appropriate for various users' needs.
   a. Assesses the patient's and caregiver's educational needs to provide effective, personalized health care.
   b. Coaches the patient and caregiver for positive behavioral change.

3. Demonstrates information literacy skills in complex decision making.
4. Contributes to the design of clinical information systems that promote safe, high-quality, and cost-effective care.
5. Uses technology systems that capture data on variables for the evaluation of nursing care.

Policy Competencies

1. Demonstrates an understanding of the interdependence of policy and practice.
2. Advocates for ethical policies that promote access, equity, quality, and cost.
3. Analyzes ethical, legal, and social factors influencing policy development.
4. Contributes in the development of health policy.
5. Analyzes the implications of health policy across disciplines.
6. Evaluates the impact of globalization on healthcare policy development.
7. Advocates for policies for safe and healthy practice environments.

Health Delivery System Competencies

1. Applies knowledge of organizational practices and complex systems to improve healthcare delivery.
2. Effects healthcare change using broad-based skills, including negotiating, consensus building, and partnering.
3. Minimizes risk to patients and providers at the individual and systems level.
4. Facilitates the development of healthcare systems that address the needs of culturally diverse populations, providers, and other stakeholders.
5. Evaluates the impact of healthcare delivery on patients, providers, other stakeholders, and the environment.
6. Analyzes organizational structure, functions, and resources to improve the delivery of care.
7. Collaborates in planning for transitions across the continuum of care.

Ethics Competencies

1. Integrates ethical principles in decision making.
2. Evaluates the ethical consequences of decisions.
3. Applies ethically sound solutions to complex issues related to individuals, populations, and systems of care.

Independent Practice Competencies

1. Functions as a licensed independent practitioner.
2. Demonstrates the highest level of accountability for professional practice.
3. Practices independently, managing previously diagnosed and undiagnosed patients.
   a. Provides the full spectrum of healthcare services to include health promotion, disease prevention, health protection, anticipatory guidance, counseling, disease management, palliative care, and end-of-life care.

   b. Uses advanced health assessment skills to differentiate between normal, variations of normal, and abnormal findings.
   c. Employs screening and diagnostic strategies in the development of diagnoses.
   d. Prescribes medications within scope of practice.
   e. Manages the health or illness status of patients and families over time.
4. Provides patient-centered care recognizing cultural diversity and the patient or designee as a full partner in decision making.
   a. Works to establish a relationship with the patient characterized by mutual respect, empathy, and collaboration.
   b. Creates a climate of patient-centered care to include confidentiality, privacy, comfort, emotional support, mutual trust, and respect.
   c. Incorporates the patient's cultural and spiritual preferences, values, and beliefs into health care.
   d. Preserves the patient's control over decision making by negotiating a mutually acceptable plan of care.
   e. Develops strategies to prevent one's own personal biases from interfering with delivery of quality care.
   f. Addresses cultural, spiritual, and ethnic influences that potentially create conflict among individuals, families, staff and caregivers.
5. Educates professional and lay caregivers to provide culturally and spiritually sensitive, appropriate care.
6. Collaborates with both professional and other caregivers to achieve optimal care outcomes.
7. Coordinates transitional care services in and across care settings.
8. Participates in the development, use, and evaluation of professional standards and evidence-based care.[2]

The comprehensive components of the competencies that must be met for role development are necessary and useful for developing curricula and for evaluating the NP student during the educational training period, as well as containing standards to which the practicing NP can be held accountable.

Doctor of Nursing Program (DNP)

In response to the confusion arising from the variety of doctoral degrees that nurses seeking to advance their education were obtaining, the AACN developed a task force to address the issue in 1999 (Zaccagnini & White, 2011). Until this point, nurses had obtained doctorates in education (EdD), PhDs in nursing or other disciplines, doctorates in nursing science (DNS/DNSc), and doctorates in nursing (ND). In 2004, the AACN formally approved the doctor of nursing practice (DNP) degree, which is focused on clinical practice in contrast to the research-focused doctoral degree

2 National Organization of Nurse Practitioner Faculties (NONPF). (2012). *Domains and core competencies of nurse practitioner practice.* Washington, DC: Author. Reprinted with permission of the National Organization of Nurse Practitioner Faculties.

obtained with a PhD. This degree is not only for NPs, but offers a clinical doctorate for all nurses who seek to improve healthcare delivery systems and patient outcomes. Although an original goal was to have the DNP as entry level for the NP by 2015, the complexities associated with the endeavor, particularly at the state licensure level, makes this unlikely to enforce in such a short time. However, AACN endorses the DNP as a goal for all APRNs (AACN, 2013). The DNP is recognized as the terminal practice degree (AACN, 2006).

Why the need for a DNP when numerous studies have validated the excellent and cost-effective care provided by MSN-level NPs (AANP, 2010a, 2010b)? Owing to the ever-increasing complexity of health care and healthcare delivery systems, it is optimal to have clinicians who are well educated in the areas of health policy, quality improvement, evidence-based practice, and outcomes evaluation. Currently, MSN-level programs for NPs require 42–50 credits—much more than other MSN tracks that typically are approximately 30 credits for completion. In addition, most NP programs require at least 500–600 clinical hours to graduate and take certification examinations. The DNP offers the NP student additional education and preparation to meet the needs of the complex healthcare system of the near future. In addition, NPs work collaboratively with numerous other doctorally prepared clinicians whose doctorate is clinically focused, including pharmacists (PharmD), physical therapists (DPT), physicians (MD), doctors of osteopathy (DO), naturopaths (ND), and others. To achieve educational parity, the clinical doctorate (DNP) is recommended for nurse practitioners.

There are currently 303 DNP programs enrolling students in the United States, and there are at least another 124 DNP programs being developed (AACN, 2017). More than 25,200 nurses were enrolled in a DNP program in 2015–2016 (AACN, 2017). At this time, there are differences in the existing programs, particularly as they relate to the scholarship of the terminal project, the title of which in itself has sparked numerous passionate debates among leaders in doctoral-level nursing education. The AACN published *The Essentials of Doctoral Education for Advanced Nursing Practice* (2006) to shape the education for the DNP to meet quality indicator criteria. These essentials were developed to build upon the baccalaureate and master's essentials and are aligned with recommendations from the Institute of Medicine's (IOM) multiple reports emphasizing quality in education, evidence-based practice, and nurses practicing to the full extent of their scope of practice (Zaccagnini & White, 2011).

The DNP essentials are listed below.

DNP Essentials

I. Scientific underpinnings for practice
II. Organizational and systems leadership for quality improvement and systems thinking
III. Clinical scholarship and analytical methods for evidence-based practice
IV. Information systems/technology and patient care technology for the improvement and transformation of health care
V. Healthcare policy for advocacy in health care
VI. Interprofessional collaboration for improving patient and population health outcomes

VII. Clinical prevention and population health for improving the nation's health

VIII. Advanced nursing practice (AACN, 2006)

In addition, the DNP essentials also contain language that reflects the need for the *3 Ps* and the expertise required for APNs, which is detailed below for ease of access during seminar discussions.

AACN published a White Paper—*The Doctor of Nurse Practice: Current Issues and Clarifying Recommendations* (2015)—which describes and clarifies the "characteristics of DNP graduate scholarship, the DNP project, efficient use of resources, program length, curriculum considerations, practice experiences, and collaborative partnership guidelines" (AACN, 2015, para 4). Of particular interest to the DNP educator and student are the components required for the DNP Scholarly Project which must:

a. Focus on a change that impacts healthcare outcomes either through direct or indirect care.

b. Have a systems (micro-, meso-, or macro-level) or population/aggregate focus.

c. Demonstrate implementation in the appropriate arena or area of practice.

d. Include a plan for sustainability (e.g., financial, systems or political realities, not only theoretical abstractions).

e. Include an evaluation of processes and/or outcomes (formative or summative). DNP Projects should be designed so that processes and/or outcomes will be evaluated to guide practice and policy. Clinical significance is as important in guiding practice as statistical significance is in evaluating research.

f. Provide a foundation for future practice scholarship. (AACN, 2015, p. 4)

Advanced Practice Nursing Focus

The DNP graduate prepared for an advanced practice role must demonstrate practice expertise, specialized knowledge, and expanded responsibility and accountability in the care and management of individuals and families. By virtue of this direct care focus, advanced practice nurses (APNs) develop additional competencies in direct practice and in the guidance and coaching of individuals and families through developmental, health–illness, and situational transitions (Hamric et al., 2009). The direct practice of APNs is characterized by the use of a holistic perspective; the formation of therapeutic partnerships to facilitate informed decision making, positive lifestyle change, and appropriate self-care; advanced practice thinking, judgment, and skillful performance; and use of diverse, evidence-based interventions in health and illness management (Brown, 2005).

APNs assess, manage, and evaluate patients at the most independent level of clinical nursing practice. They are expected to use advanced, highly refined assessment skills and employ a thorough understanding of pathophysiology and pharmacotherapeutics in making diagnostic and practice management decisions. **To ensure sufficient depth and focus, it is mandatory that a separate course be required for each of these three content areas: advanced health/physical assessment, advanced physiology/pathophysiology, and advanced pharmacology.** In addition to direct care, DNP graduates emphasizing care of individuals should be able to use their understanding of the practice context to document practice trends, identify potential systemic changes, and make improvements in the care of their particular patient populations in the systems within which they practice (AACN, 2006, p. 18).

The National Organization of Nurse Practitioner Faculties provides further clarification related to competencies for the NP educated to the DNP level (NONPF, 2006). These areas include independent practice, scientific foundations, leadership, quality, practice inquiry, technology & information literacy, policy, ethics, and health delivery systems.

Nurse Practitioners' Approach to Patient Care

Sometimes I am asked why I did not become a physician instead of an NP. My response is that becoming a nurse practitioner gave me the best of both worlds, nursing and medicine. I support my answer by stating that nursing continues to be the top trusted profession in the United States (Gallop Politics, 2016). I also point out that NPs have extremely high patient satisfaction scores. Nurse practitioners have a unique approach to health care. This is not to say that there are no physicians who are amazing—because I personally have worked with and been under the care of fantastic physicians—but a common theme I hear from my patient population is that "nurses listen to what I have to say." One study found that only 50% of the patients seen by physicians reported that they felt that the physician "always" listened carefully, compared to more than 80% of NP patients (Creech, Filter, & Bowman, 2011). In a study of more than 1.5 million veterans, satisfaction levels were highest in primary care clinics when the healthcare provider was an NP (Budzi, Lurie, Singh, & Hooker, 2010). The authors state that the interpersonal skills of NPs in patient teaching, counseling, and patient-centered care contribute to positive health outcomes and patient satisfaction. Encouragement to hire more NPs to increase access to cost-effective quality care for the largest healthcare system in the United States was a conclusion reached by these researchers.

Of course, it is important to review and analyze quantitative research regarding the cost-effectiveness and improved health outcomes when NPs are providing primary care, but it is also as important (in many cases, more important) to listen to what patients have to say about their experiences with NPs as healthcare providers.

STEPHANIE'S STORY

At the turn of my 25th birthday, life was going well for me. I had just completed my master's degree in elementary education and secured my first job as a head teacher in a local private school. I enjoyed my time during the day with my students, excited to employ the learning strategies I had discovered in graduate school. After school hours and on the weekends, I spent my time exercising outside, traipsing around New York City, and socializing with my friends and family. All of this changed the day I visited my gynecologist seeking treatment for a yeast infection.

Having no relief from an over-the-counter antifungal medication, I turned to my gynecologist—a highly regarded physician who studied at the Chicago School of Medicine. I found Dr. X to be warm, attentive, and funny; she did her best to make me feel comfortable despite the lay-on-your-back-feet-up-in-stirrups position. After confirming my self-diagnosis with a culture, Dr. X prescribed an antifungal suppository cream and sent me on my way home.

At the end of treatment, I still had severe itching and called my gynecologist's office. After discussing my situation with the nurse, we both assumed that I was fighting off a tough strain. Dr. X prescribed a stronger medication for me, and although I was itchy throughout this course of treatment, I held hope that my symptoms would abate soon after.

Still plagued with itching, I visited Dr. X a week after I finished the latest medicine. She asked me to remind her if diabetes ran in my family. She asked me to have my primary care physician run some blood work to be certain that I had not developed type II. Throughout this, Dr. X and I still kept our humor about my condition. Although we were puzzled about why it lasted so long, we both assumed that it would clear up shortly.

Unfortunately, we were wrong. For 3 more months, Dr. X examined me at least twice each month as I was still experiencing relentless itching and redness. At each visit, she swabbed my vagina; ran a culture; asked if I was certain that I was not diabetic; and then prescribed me a cream, suppository, or pills. Dr. X explained that I would always test positive for yeast, as it is normal for a small amount to live in the vagina. However, she was surprised that the small amount of cells that I had caused me to be so itchy and red, that I must be sensitive to yeast.

Throughout my treatment with Dr. X, she maintained her warm demeanor; however, her nursing staff grew irritated with me. They became curt with me; sighing on the phone upon hearing my voice and rushing me through procedures at office visits. Through their lack of professionalism, they made it clear that I was not an important patient and that they were skeptical of my condition.

I began to feel worn down, broken. A simple infection had turned into a chronic illness, causing my gregarious nature to fade. I no longer wished to go out with friends. I pushed prospective boyfriends away so I would not have to contend with intimacy. I stopped exercising as body heat and sweat further aggravated my symptoms. I was tired of being sick.

Understanding my discomfort, which seemed to intensify after each round of medication, Dr. X decided to try something that was not a typical course of treatment: gentian violet. This antifungal dye was "painted" onto the outside of my vagina as well as inside the first third of the canal. As with the previous medications, my symptoms worsened. My skin felt raw and burned. And although I thought it impossible at this stage, the incessant itching intensified. Dr. X was all out of ideas and sent me to see a *Candida* specialist located 90 minutes away.

Dr. Y was an older man who entered the exam room while laughing with his nurse. Immediately he acted as though we had known each other for years. He was overly familiar, touching my arm, and doing his best to assure me that there wasn't a patient yet who presented a medical condition he couldn't fix. I quickly regretted taking Dr. X's recommendation to see him.

After Dr. Y questioned me about my condition, he asked me to lie back and then made sure to point out the strategically placed artwork in the room. Above my head on the ceiling, was a painting by Georgia O'Keefe. O'Keefe is famous for her floral still lifes that strongly resemble parts of the female anatomy. Dr. Y thought this was not only comical considering his line of work, but also believed the art helped distract his patients from why they were in the stirrups. Personally, I found this strange, and rather than diverting my attention away from the purpose of my visit, I was forced to stare at a visual reminder while lying down!

Dr. Y separately swabbed the inside of my mouth, vagina, and anus, all the while sharing double-entendre jokes with his nurse. Half-naked and vulnerable, I willed myself to go through with the exam thinking that if I could get through these lousy 10 minutes I could finally have an answer to my problem. Dr. Y sent the swabs off to a lab, and then wrote me a prescription for an antidepressant. He told me that sometimes when a person has an illness as long as I have, it really is no longer a medical condition as much as a psychological one. He told me to take the antidepressant for at least 6 weeks and that it should help get my mind off dwelling on my problem and that he wouldn't be surprised if my symptoms vanished by that time. The nurses at Dr. X's office made me feel as though they didn't believe that I had an actual medical issue, and now this "specialist" was saying the same thing.

Desperate for relief and willing to consider the possibility that my illness was "all in my head," I began the antidepressant. When Dr. X's office called to say that my tests were negative for *Candida*, I continued the antidepressant, now hoping that it was a psychological issue, meaning there would be an end eventually. Although my mood had improved a bit, the itching and redness did not. During this time, I had scheduled an appointment with my dermatologist to check a questionable mole. Prior to her exam, Dr. Z asked how I was doing, what was new with me. I opened my mouth to say "fine," but broke down in tears. I had been uncomfortable and frustrated for so long, that I couldn't control my emotions. I explained my ordeal to Dr. Z, which by this point had been going on for over 6 months, and she replied, "I think I know what you have."

Dr. Z. suspected that I had acquired eczema from being over-medicated. A biopsy of my labia proved her correct, and I started a course of steroid treatment that lasted for several months. The relief was immediate! While I was ecstatic that I was on my way back normal, I was also very angry. Initially, yes, I had a yeast infection. But at some point, the infection cleared and the itching and redness was from the medications. So having a small amount of yeast cells in the cultures should have been a clue to Dr. X that it was not an infection. Dr. Y could not correctly diagnose my condition either and could only focus on yeast. After my experiences with Drs. X and Y, I lost trust in their capabilities as diagnosticians. I stopped seeing Dr. X and missed a year between my annual exams.

Months after I ended my steroid treatment, I developed what I was certain was a yeast infection. Scared to return to a gynecologist, I called my neighbor, a nurse practitioner, for a recommendation. She referred me to a fellow nurse practitioner who was working at the local Planned Parenthood. The NP was a friendly woman, who patiently listened as I told her my recent medical history. She examined me, found a high number of yeast cells in the culture, and then prescribed me an oral antifungal so as not to cause the eczema to return. Having experienced recurring yeast infections, she asked if I was diabetic. Unlike Drs. X and Y, and the nurses at their offices, the NP didn't stop after my reply of no. She then asked if I had a lot of wheat and/or chocolate in my diet as some recent studies have shown a correlation between those foods and yeast infections. Not able to do a thorough evaluation of my diet on the spot, I told her that I didn't think so. She told me to think about it and to give her a call to let her know how I fared with the medication.

On my drive home from Planned Parenthood, I started thinking about what I ate that morning and noon for lunch and couldn't believe how unaware I had been earlier with the NP. My breakfast had consisted of fruit and almond butter on two wheat waffles. Lunch was ham and cheese on whole wheat bread. The more I thought about my eating habits, the more I realized that wheat was in heavy rotation in my daily diet, and chocolate did indeed play a role during my menstrual cycle. I drove past my house and directly to the supermarket to purchase both wheat-free waffles and bread.

In the 8 years since spending those enlightening 30 minutes with the NP, I have had only two yeast infections, both successfully treated with over-the-counter medications. The NP shared invaluable information with me, information that has changed my life. To this day, if one is available, I prefer to see an NP to a doctor. I have found that the NPs tend to think more outside the box to solve a problem. They seem to be more aware of current research and studies and are willing to share this with their patients.

Thanks to my NP, I no longer have a chronic illness.

What Nurse Practitioners Do

In an effort to articulate what a nurse practitioner actually does, it is easy to discuss the tasks involved with the daily work of the NP. These tasks involve reviewing laboratory tests, performing physical examinations, charting, writing prescriptions, and ordering radiological procedures, yet this approach describes the profession or duties of the NP, and not the actual art of nurse practitionering. Dr. Loretta Ford described *holistically oriented goals for self-care* as what sets NPs apart from physicians in primary care (Weiland, 2008).

Nurse practitionering (as a unique verb) incorporates the vital elements of nursing and philosophical theories, communication skills, diagnostic skills, coaching and educating, and most importantly, developing reciprocal relationships with patients. It is the foundation of nursing that forms the basis for taking a holistic approach to the interview, assessment, diagnosis, and mutually agreed upon goals for patient care, which help NPs to engage patients as full partners in aspects of their health care.

Florence Nightingale recognized the main difference between nursing and medicine by writing that while medicine focuses on disease, nursing focuses on illness and suffering with the goal(s) being to ease suffering and promote disease prevention (Nightingale, 2009). Physicians are trained in a different framework than NPs. In an interesting article, "The Total Package: A Skillful, Compassionate Doctor," the theme was stated thusly:

> Traditionally, medical school curricula have focused on the pathophysiology of disease while neglecting the very real impact of disease on the patient's social and psychological experience, that is, their illness experience. It is in this intersection that humanism plays a profound role. (Indiana University, 2009)

NPs, with their comprehensive, humanistic nursing background, formulate nurse practitionering in that intersection.

The role of the nurse practitioner has the foundation of nursing and has integrated segments of the medical model to become the unique profession of nurse practitioner; therefore, differences in the role and practice of nurses and nurse practitioners exist (Haugsdal & Scherb, 2003; Kleinman, 2004; Nicoteri & Andrews, 2003; Roberts,

Tabloski, & Bova, 1997). However, there remains confusion among the public and other members of the healthcare team, as well as among some NP students, as to what NP practice truly means.

It is not surprising that defining nurse practitionering is difficult when one considers that it has historically been difficult to define nursing (Chitty & Black, 2007). Certainly today we have comprehensive definitions of nursing developed by the American Nurses Association, the Royal College of Nursing, and the International Council of Nurses; however, it seems that Florence Nightingale wrote the first definition of a holistic approach to patient-centered care:

> I use the word *nursing* for want of a better. It has been limited to signify little more than the administration of medicines and the application of poultices. It ought to signify the proper use of fresh air, light, warmth, cleanliness, quiet, and the proper selection and administration of diet—all at the least expense of vital power to the patient. (Nightingale, 2009)

Nursing Theories for Nurse Practitioners

Many nursing philosophies, theories, and models exist today, and NPs can and should build upon these for their professional practice. For example, Henderson identified the 14 basic needs of the patient (**BOX 1-1**), which are common needs to all humankind.

Jean Watson's 10 Carative Processes (**BOX 1-2**) exemplify the changing relationship between patient and nurse attending to the unification of body, mind, and soul to achieve optimal health. Watson has spent many years as director of the Center for Human Caring at the University of Colorado in Denver. Watson's Theory of

BOX 1-1 The 14 Components of Virginia Henderson's Need Theory

1. Breathe normally.
2. Eat and drink adequately.
3. Eliminate body wastes.
4. Move and maintain desirable postures.
5. Sleep and rest.
6. Select suitable clothes—dress and undress.
7. Maintain body temperature within normal range by adjusting clothing and modifying environment.
8. Keep the body clean and well groomed, and protect the integument.
9. Avoid dangers in the environment and avoid injuring others.
10. Communicate with others in expressing emotions, needs, fears, or opinions.
11. Worship according to one's faith.
12. Work in such a way that there is a sense of accomplishment.
13. Play or participate in various forms of recreation.
14. Learn, discover, or satisfy the curiosity that leads to normal development and health, and use the available health facilities.

Reproduced from Henderson, V. A. (1991). *The nature of nursing: Reflections after 25 years*. New York, NY: National League for Nursing Press. pp. 22–43. Reprinted by permission of National League for Nursing.

BOX 1-2 Ten Caritas Processes™

1. Embrace altruistic values, and practice loving kindness with self and others.
2. Instill faith and hope, and honor others.
3. Be sensitive to self and others by nurturing individual beliefs and practices.
4. Develop helping, trusting, and caring relationships.
5. Promote and accept positive and negative feelings as you authentically listen to another's story.
6. Use creative scientific problem-solving methods for caring decision making.
7. Share teaching and learning that addresses the individual needs and comprehension styles.
8. Create a healing environment for the physical and spiritual self that respects human dignity.
9. Assist with basic physical, emotional, and spiritual human needs.
10. Open to mystery, and allow miracles to enter.

Reproduced from Ten Caritas Processes™, Jean Watson 2007; 2008 www.watsoncaringscience.org; Watson, J. (2008). *Nursing: The philosophy and science of caring*. New revised edition. Boulder, CO: University Press of Colorado. Reprinted by permission of Jean Watson.

Human Caring meets the criteria for Carper's four fundamental ways of knowing, and Watson defines the metaparadigm of person, environment, nursing, and health in her theoretical base.

Hildegard Peplau (1952) focused as well on the relationship between patient and nurse during which the nurse takes on the role of counselor, resource, teacher, technical expert, surrogate, and leader, as needed. Whether one is practicing professionally in the United States or elsewhere in our global arena, to be successful in clinical practice, the NP must use transcultural nursing theory, which was founded by Leininger (1995). The NP must use culturally sensitive and aware skills to develop relationships and to assess, diagnose, and treat patients.

King's framework (1981) uses personal, interpersonal, and social interacting systems to form a theory for nursing. Interestingly, when one reviews the Calgary Cambridge guide to the medical interview for physicians in training (Kurtz, Silverman, & Draper, 1998), many of the concepts are the same. The focus is on the concerns of the patient for both of these methods for interacting with patients. King's framework gives the NP the ability to see the patient holistically by including the family and community aspects. Both King's framework and the Calgary Cambridge guide focus on mutual goal setting—taking the time during each step of the interview, assessment, and planning stages to truly understand the patient's issues and perspectives. By frequently eliciting the patient's input, it is easier to develop mutual understanding and develop interventions and goals to reach a state of optimal health. The idea of forming a partnership with the patient is hardly new. Whitlock, Orleans, Pender, and Allan (2002) wrote about this concept in a U.S. Preventative Services Task Force recommendation, "Evaluating Primary Care Behavioral Counseling Interventions: An Evidence-Based Approach." Developing mutually respectful relationships with patients is more likely to prevent patients' resistance to advice on healthy living and behavior change suggestions by healthcare providers. Also detailed in this recommendation is an approach the National Cancer Institute developed to guide physician intervention in smoking cessation known as the "5 As": assess, advise, agree, assist, and arrange.

- **Assess:** Ask about and assess behavioral health risk(s) and factors affecting choice of behavior change goals/methods.
- **Advise:** Give clear, specific, and personalized behavior change advice, including information about personal health harms/benefits.
- **Agree:** Collaboratively select appropriate treatment goals and methods based on the patient's interest in and willingness to change the behavior.
- **Assist:** Using behavior change techniques (self-help and/or counseling), aid the patient in achieving agreed-upon goals by acquiring the skills, confidence, and social/environmental supports for behavior change, supplemented with adjunctive medical treatments when appropriate (e.g., pharmacotherapy for tobacco dependence, contraceptive drugs/devices).
- **Arrange:** Schedule follow-up contacts (in person or by telephone) to provide ongoing assistance/support and to adjust the treatment plan as needed, including referral to more intensive or specialized treatment (Whitlock et al., 2002).

All of the approaches mentioned in this chapter focus on the need for the healthcare provider to be open to patients' needs, to hear what they really have to say, to understand what they really believe is wrong or right, and to let them work with you to develop goals. The ability to be culturally sensitive—and to be flexible and willing to collaborate and compromise when needed and appropriate—will help to form the framework for a successful patient–NP relationship, and most importantly, assist patients to reach a state of optimum health. This is not to say that becoming expert in these skills is easy or that it can be accomplished in one course; however, the student NP should start practicing these skills starting as soon as the educational program begins.

Nurse Practitioners' Unique Role

In a survey seeking to identify barriers for nurse practitioners to use standardized nursing language (SNL) for documenting nursing practice, the researchers found that NP survey participants identified that their role was a blending of the nursing and medical models, and most were not aware of what SNL consisted of (Conrad, Hanson, Hasenau, & Stocker-Schneider, 2012). Jacqueline Fawcett (in Cody, 2013) exhorts us to sever our "romance" with medical science and non-nursing professions, and in particular, with NPs being compared to physicians providing primary care. Instead, she advises we integrate nursing science as nurse scholars. With this in mind while clarifying the professional practice of nurse practitioners, it is important to distinguish the profession from that of physicians and physician assistants.

A qualitative study by Carryer, Gardner, Dunn, and Gardner (2006) was undertaken in Australia and New Zealand where NPs were interviewed to illustrate the core role of NPs. Three components were described: dynamic practice, professional efficacy, and clinical leadership. Dynamic practice described the clinical skills and expertise the NP uses in direct patient care, including physical assessment and treatment. Professional efficacy was what the researchers titled the aspects of NP practice that are highly autonomous and accountable. This level of practice does not exclude the need for collaboration; however, the NP acts as an integral member of the multidisciplinary team. The participants also described the overlap in role boundaries that occurs with

NPs and physicians. Another aspect of professional efficacy was described as being an illustration of the NP–patient relationship. Being able to integrate the complex components of psychosocial aspects in addition to the concrete physical aspects means taking the time needed in a patient visit to do so—and to develop the therapeutic link for a significant relationship. Finally, the researchers described the advanced education and clinical experience that the NP brings to the advanced professional role. NPs understand the vital place that nurses need to occupy in healthcare delivery systems and how important it is to be a part of designing and implementing systems that can improve access to quality care. Therefore, NP leadership occurs in both the direct practice environment as well as within the context of the larger healthcare system. This final theme was not recognized at the same level by all participants. Many were still developing in this portion of role identity.

Nicoteri and Andrews (2003) sought to uncover any theory that was unique to NPs and associated attributes. This integrative review of the literature found that the role of the NP is influenced by many disciplines, especially medicine. The authors posited that an emergence of theory that is unique to NPs and grounded in nursing, medicine, and social science was discovered. The authors suggested developing the concept of "nurse practitionering" (p. 500). The concept of nurse practitionering as a unique phenomenon has been written about in only a few journal articles. The term itself is not one used in typical conversation between healthcare providers and patients, nor within the nursing community; thus, there may be confusion with the term. The goal for this endeavor is not to elevate or denigrate one profession or another, but to better understand the components of nurse practitionering.

Hagedorn (2004) posits that the difference between nurse practitioners and "biomedical practitioners" is related to nurse practitioners' humanistic approach to patient care. According to many theorists such as Jean Watson, Patricia Benner, and Boykin and Schoenhofer, nursing's essence is that of caring (Zaccagnini & White, 2011). The interpersonal focus of nursing within a caring and nurturing framework is the building block of all nursing theories (Brunton & Beaman, 2000; Chinn & Kramer, 1999; Green, 2004; Nicoteri & Andrews, 2003; Visintainer, 1986). If one accepts this as a core element of being a nurse, it would be difficult to imagine one losing this essence when acquiring advanced education that contains skills and competencies associated with the practice of medicine. In fact, NPs should be familiarizing themselves with nursing theories in order to use nursing theory to guide their practice. By doing so, one is practicing beyond the medical model, offering a unique approach to the relationship, assessment, and treatment plan.

In an effort to expand upon the concept of nurse practitionering, ninety NPs in Connecticut responded to an online survey about "nurse practitionering" and what they believed it encompassed. Fifty-nine (65.6%) respondents stated that nurse practitionering is a unique term that describes what they do, which is different than solely the practice of nursing or medicine. Because many activities of practice overlap and are subjective, participants were not given definitions of nursing activities versus medical activities. Regarding how much time they perceived is spent in solely nursing activities, 36.7% of participants felt it was low, between 0% and 25%. In contrast, 34.4% of NP participants felt that the amount of time spent performing medical activities was greater, being between 36% and 50%. These results are included in **TABLE 1-1**.

The respondents were requested to enter key terms and phrases that described what is encompassed when providing care to patients as a nurse practitioner. Participants were not given terms or phrases from which to choose; rather, this portion

TABLE 1-1 Percentage of Clinical Practice Time in Nursing and Medical Activities (N = 90)

Percent of Time	Nursing Activities	Medical Activities
0–25%	**36.7% (n = 33)***	13.3% (n = 12)
26–50%	30.0% (n = 27)	**34.4% (n = 31)***
51–75%	25.6% (n = 23)	32.2% (n = 29)
75–100%	7.8% (n = 7)	20.0% (n = 18)

*Bold denotes highest value.

of the survey was open-ended. Similar terms were grouped together where deemed appropriate. The most frequent key phrases in order of the number of times mentioned were nurture/care/empathy ($f = 31$), educate ($f = 30$), assess/diagnose/treat/prescribe ($f = 30$), holistic ($f = 22$), listener ($f = 17$), collaborate ($f = 13$), advocate ($f = 11$), and coach ($f = 5$). The majority of the key phrases and terms in this pilot study confirm that the core of nurse practitionering is based on the nursing model. Key phrases and terms relating to medical practice included diagnosing and treating/prescribing, which were as frequent as the caring (nursing) category, but the nursing elements were mentioned most often.

In an effort to expand upon the key phrases, invitations to participate in interviews to share their perceptions of "nurse practitionering" were sent to 150 NPs in Connecticut. A total of fourteen individual interviews were held with a convenience sample of experienced NPs willing to participate and share their perceptions. The fourteen participants of the interviews were all female, between the ages of 31 and 70 years, and currently practicing as nurse practitioners.

Authentic Listening

The NPs in this study were exemplars for authentic listening. According to Bryant (2009), listening well involves being present, interested, spending time, and showing respect. One NP explained:

> I think the biggest reason why people like to come here is they say, "You listen. The docs don't listen to me." It is probably what I do the most and, one of the nurses got very frustrated with me and said, "You nurse practitioners, when a patient comes in to see the doctor and their finger is the problem, the doctor just looks at the finger and the patient is out. You go and you guys talk about everything. You have to talk about everything!"

Another NP described the time she spends teaching patients:

> I prescribed the medications, I go out, I get the inhaler, you know, the sample inhaler and the sample spacer, and I go right back in and I tell the

patient, "This is what I am ordering, and this is how you use it," versus the pediatrician or the pulmonologist who says, "Here are your medications. I'll have the nurse come in to teach you how to use it."

Empathy

Empathy is the ability to relate to the patient's thoughts and feelings and develop an understanding of what the patient is experiencing (Baillie, 1996). The NPs in this study are genuinely concerned about the patient's psychosocial well-being, family matters, and future goals and aspirations:

> This woman this morning has lots of what I perceive as small complaints. She's a relatively healthy 28-year-old woman, and I asked her, "Tiffany, are you working?"
>
> She said, "No."
>
> I said, "When was the last time you worked?"
>
> She said, "Oh, 9 years ago, before my daughter was born." Then she said, "It's really hard to get a job."
>
> I asked, "Do you have your high school diploma?"
>
> She said, "No."
>
> So I recommended to her a local learning center program. I encouraged her, and that's where I think the nurse practitioner is different. It was me listening first, caring about what she was telling me, and then offering her something and trying to be an advocate for her.

Empathy enabled another NP to gain a deep understanding of what motivated the patient:

> She has a disabled child at home that needs total care. That's something that I know about her and her situation. That's an example of, I guess, advocating and coordinating and knowing that a lot of people don't have transportation. Like if I want to send them to radiology, I'll ask them, "What time of the day is good for you?" because a lot of these people are grandmothers raising grandkids, and they need to arrange their life. Some of them are pretty capable of making appointments for themselves, but others are not. They are scared to or they don't think that they're going to do it right. Maybe we are enabling them by doing it for them, but we will take the extra time and, you know, ask "What's the best day for you to go for that ultrasound? Morning or afternoon?"

Negotiating

Authentic listening and empathy enabled the NPs in this study to communicate more effectively and negotiate with patients when formulating treatment plans. An integrated literature review on communication styles of NPs and the impact on patients (Charlton, Dearing, Berry, & Johnson, 2008) found that NPs who are trained to use a patient-centered communication style are most likely to have patients with better understanding of their health and treatment options and who are more likely to follow the treatment plan, thereby having better health outcomes. This was found in

NPs in this study who involved patients in the decision-making process and actively negotiated with patients:

> One of the things here that we do well, I think, is negotiate with the patients. Part of when I see people I'm not going to be paternalistic and tell them you have to do this, this, and that. I have a woman I saw this morning; she came in for follow-up of her labs. She has hypertension, and the first time she had a hemoglobin A1C of 6, and she has a family history of diabetes, so we talked. She's not a dummy; she is a registered nurse. She just became a registered nurse, just got out of school, and I said "Let's talk about this new thing that's coming up. Do you have diabetes? Or are you prediabetic? Let's discuss it." So we negotiated what she was going to do next. I didn't want to say to her, "You have to start on more meds today." Her fasting sugars have been normal, the A1C was 6, and she is a woman that takes care of herself, pretty much. Now she may go on metformin in 3 months, but I know she doesn't like to take pills. She cares about a healthy lifestyle, so we negotiated: try lifestyle changes for 3 months and check the A1C in 3 months; if it goes up, then we'll talk about starting medication.

Going Above and Beyond

NPs describe going beyond what is expected or required of the role of primary care provider. The NPs in our study were motivated to do more for their patients and ensure that patients were satisfied with their care:

> My patient that came in this morning was status posthospitalization. When she was in the hospital, they did a big cardiac and neuro workup. I had sent her out by ambulance the week before, and they kept her for 4 days because they did a really good workup on her, but they didn't do a stress test, so she needed to have that done. And so, I coordinated today for her to have a stress test, and I picked a Spanish-speaking cardiologist for her because I thought she would be more comfortable with that. And then they also recommended that she see a therapist because she's on an antidepressant, so we talked about that today, and I coordinated that for her.

Another NP describes her ability to take on a difficult patient and help to gain his trust, thereby improving his adherence to the treatment plan, and reducing costs for overusing the emergency room:

> Treating marginalized patients with multiple comorbidities is challenging. This challenge is amplified by mental illness and substance abuse, combined with mistrust of the healthcare system. An example of this begins with the discharge of a difficult patient from a clinic for threatening front desk staff and a few nurses. He was belligerent, and when he felt he was not being respected, he threatened staff members, including his physician. He had been followed in the medical resident clinic for his chronic medical illnesses but was not addressing his anger management, cocaine abuse, obsessive compulsive disorder, and depression, and ultimately he was not adherent to medications or medical appointments either. The patient had been fired by multiple agencies in the town he lives in for the same behaviors, and at

> this point was about to be fired from the only medical provider left within walking distance. He does not own a car and could not afford to travel by bus. Final discharge from the clinic and care would render this man with no primary care locally, except the emergency room.
>
> A final attempt was made to have the patient receive his care with a nurse practitioner, as she could at least provide continuity, if he showed up for the appointment, and she was not afraid. But really, the NP provided more than the same face in the clinic each visit. The NP provided this man with a milieu of empathy and teamwork between patient and care provider. Her approach to practice sparked a level of trust of the practitioner. The patient recognized the NP's genuine interest in providing him individualized care and respect. She built upon this practitioner–patient relationship. The NP helped the patient realize his control of his healthcare commitment and his role in his health outcome. This empowerment and trust lead to successful engagement in following through for his routinely scheduled medical visits as well as medication adherence. When the patient was ready to address his mental health and addiction, he asked the NP to be his advocate.
>
> The NP's commitment to holistic patient-centered care led to reinstatement of his mental health services. And today, this patient is significantly healthier, drug free, treating his medical and mental illness, and is one less person sitting in the emergency room.

Another NP describes the impact one can have when going the extra step for a patient:

> While at a precollege arts experience, a teen came to the clinic to ask for help with a sore throat. While assessing her I began discussing her comfort with being away from home for the first time. She mentioned that she was really surprised that having three meals a day made her feel so comfortable. (Students eat in the college cafeteria during the program.) Further questioning revealed that she rarely ate except at school as she qualified for free lunch because, "There is an empty refrigerator in my house." When asked if her school had a breakfast program, she said that they did but her mom, "was too busy to apply—says it is too complicated." Her strep culture was positive, so I prescribed antibiotics and had the resident assistant pick them up from the pharmacy. Meanwhile, I asked the young lady if she would like to speak to the nurse practitioner at her school to contact social services for assistance with not only the breakfast program but also what else the assessment would allow. At that point I learned that her mom was in rehab and unable to be reached—that this student had been assigned a foster care person—whom I contacted regarding care and treatment for the strep throat and confirmed the rest of the story. Activation of social services through contact with the NP at the school-based health center started the process in motion. Additional contact with her throughout the 5 weeks proved to positively impact this child's life.

The NPs in this study expressed how much they love being nurse practitioners. They believe in the added value and unique contributions of the NP to health care and get a lot of gratification from putting in extra time and effort. This is supported by a similar study that showed NPs feel that their lives are enhanced and cite internal rewards and gratification from their interactions with patients:

> I think the most gratifying thing is when I sit down with them and explain their disease and really spend the time with them that they need. I feel like they really understand the necessity for the treatment plan that I recommend, and I really feel like if I spend the time with them that they are so grateful because they feel like you've really invested in them. . . . I think that most nurse practitioners will probably say something to this effect, but when they sit down with their patients, they try to treat them like they would want one of their family members treated. And so when people really see that that you're really doing that for them, and distinguish it from the way that they feel like they've been treated by other providers in the past or when they really recognize the amount of energy and the amount of giving—when they really see that—there's nothing more gratifying than that. (Kleinman, 2004)

The preceding studies validate similar components uncovered by Kleinman (2004) regarding nurse practitioners and their relationships with patients. Essential meanings in her phenomenological study included "openness, connection, concern, respect, reciprocity, competence, time, and professional identity" (p. 264).

Based on research and formal and informal interviews, a concept map depicting nurse practitionering was developed (**FIGURE 1-1**). From that, the Stewart Model of Nurse Practitionering was developed to depict this model of nurse practitioner practice (**FIGURE 1-2**). This model has as its core the nursing model—the foundation of NP practice. As the NP student evolves through the educational program, scientific knowledge and attributes of the medical model are incorporated in order to provide

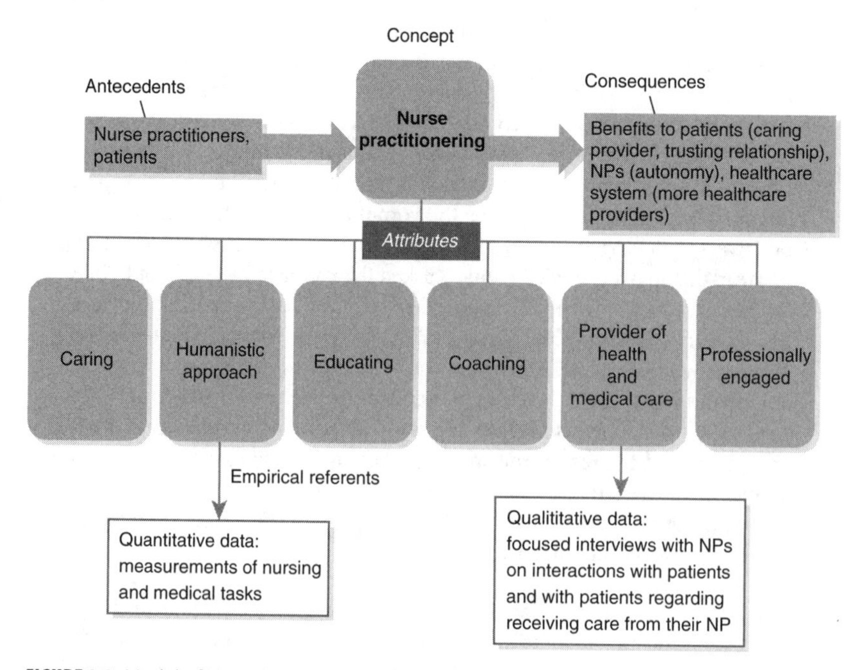

FIGURE 1-1 Model of Nurse Practitioner Practice

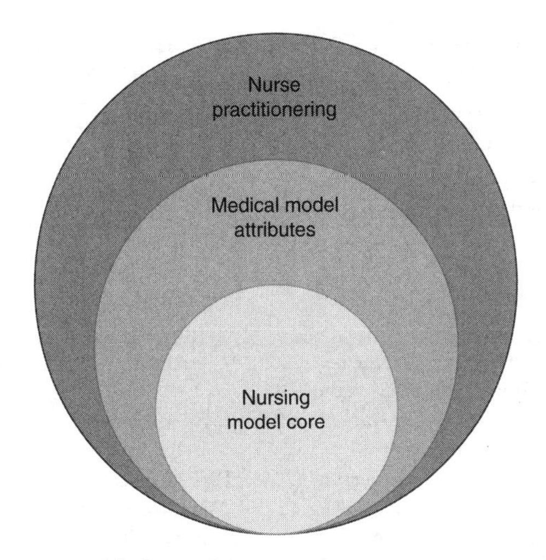

FIGURE 1-2 The Stewart Model of Nurse Practitionering

accurate assessment, medical diagnoses, and appropriate evidence-based treatment modalities to patients needing health care. The circles within the larger circle represent unity and wholeness.

It is evident that in order to function successfully within this model, the NP must retain the crucial interpersonal skills required to provide education surrounding health promotion and disease management. Brykczynski (2012), in an article discussing qualitative research that looked at how NP faculty keep the nurse in the NP student, suggests that holistically focused healthcare providers consider thinking of "patient diagnoses" instead of either medical versus nursing diagnoses (p. 558). Nurse practitioner students and novice NPs need to beware of minimizing the importance of nursing as the core foundation from which excellence in practice develops. Rather, all NPs should emphasize the art and science of nursing philosophies and theories as the building blocks for providing health care to patients. It is these very qualities that make NPs unique—what it is that instills trust and confidence, as well as positive patient–NP relationships—which is the circle labeled in Figure 1-2 as "nurse practitionering." In an opinion article in the *New York Times* (Rosenberg, 2012), it is clearly noted that nurse practitioners approach patient care differently than physicians do and that research has proven that it is as effective and "might be particularly useful for treating chronic disease, where so much depends on the patients' behavioral choices" (para. 5). Sullivan-Marx et al. (2010) posit that the NP encompasses both the holistic nursing caring model and more than the physician's curing model—that NPs have a paradigm flexible enough to be able to move between the two. Who better than NP/DNPs to tackle the inequities in health that have been tied to variations in socioeconomic status, racial and ethnic discrimination, and stressors, as well as policies relating to social and economical justice?

Seminar Discussion Questions

1. What was the purpose for the initial role of the nurse practitioner, and does it differ from the role of the nurse practitioner in today's healthcare system?
2. Who are advanced practice registered nurses (APRNs)?

3. What are the master's and DNP essentials, and what are they used for?
4. Describe the NP core competencies as identified by NONPF, and discuss how students can attain basic mastery of those competencies.
5. What are elements of role transition from RN to NP, and what are you currently experiencing in this process?
6. The concept of "nurse practitionering" has been introduced in this chapter. Comment on your responses to this idea.

References

American Association of Colleges for Nursing. (2006). *The essentials of doctoral education for advanced nursing practice.* Washington, DC: Author.

American Association of Colleges of Nursing. (2011). *The essentials of master's education in nursing.* Washington, DC: Author.

American Association of Colleges of Nursing. (2013). *DNP fact sheet.* Washington, DC: Author.

American Association of Colleges of Nursing. (2015). White Paper: *The doctor of nursing practice: Current issues and clarifying recommendations.* Washington, DC: Author.

American Association of Colleges of Nursing. (2017). *DNP fact sheet.* Washington, DC: Author. Retrieved from http://www.aacnnursing.org/Portals/42/News/Factsheets/DNP-Factsheet-2017.pdf

American Academy of Nurse Practitioners. (2010a). *Quality of nurse practitioner practice.* Austin, TX: Author.

American Academy of Nurse Practitioners. (2010b). *Nurse practitioner cost-effectiveness.* Austin, TX: Author.American Association of Nurse Practitioners. (2017). *Press release: More than 234,000 licensed nurse practitioners in the United States.* Retrieved from Https://www.aanp.org/press-room/press-releases/173-press-room/2017-press-releases/2098-more-than-234-000-licensed-nurse-practitioners-in-the-united-states

American Association of Nurse Practitioners. (June, 2017). *Fact sheet.* Retrieved from https://www.aanp.org/all-about-nps/np-fact-sheet

APRN Consensus Work Group and the National Council of State Boards of Nursing APRN Advisory Committee. (2008). *Consensus model for APRN regulation: Licensure, accreditation, certification & education.* APRN Joint Dialogue Group Report, July 7, 2008.

Auerbach, D. I. (2012). Will the NP workforce grow in the future? New forecasts and implications for healthcare delivery. *Medical Care, 50*(7), 606–610.

Baillie, L. (1996). A phenomenological study of the nature of empathy. *Journal of Advanced Nursing, 24*(6), 1300–1308.

Bauer, J. (2010). Nurse practitioners as an underutilized resource for health reform: Evidence-based demonstrations of cost-effectiveness. *Journal of the American Academy of Nurse Practitioners, 22,* 228–231.

Brown, S. J. (2005). Direct clinical practice. In A. B. Hamric, J. A. Spross, & C. M. Hanson (Eds.), *Advanced practice nursing: An integrative approach* (3rd ed., pp. 143–185). Philadelphia, PA: Elsevier Saunders.

Bruner, K. (2005, May). *Nurse practitioners' program to celebrate 40th anniversary.* Retrieved from http://www.uchsc.edu/news/bridge/2005/may/NP_anniversary.html

Brunton, B., & Beaman, M. (2000). Nurse practitioners' perceptions of their caring behaviors. *Journal of the American Academy of Nurse Practitioners, 12,* 451–456.

Bryant, L. (2009). The art of active listening. *Practice Nurse, 37*(6), 49.

Brykczynski, K. (2012). Clarifying, affirming, and preserving the nurse in nurse practitioner education and practice. *Journal of the American Academy of Nurse Practitioners, 24,* 554–564.

Budzi, D., Lurie, S., Singh, K., & Hooker, R. (2010). Veterans' perceptions of care by nurse practitioners, physician assistants and physicians: A comparison from satisfaction surveys. *Journal of the American Academy of Nurse Practitioners, 22*(3), 170–176. doi:10.1111/j.1745-7599.2010.00489.x

Buerhaus, P. (2010). Have nurse practitioners reached a tipping point? Interview of a panel of NP thought leaders. *Nursing Economics, 28*(5), 346–349.

Carryer, J., Gardner, G., Dunn, S., & Gardner, A. (2007). The core role of the nurse practitioner: Practice, professionalism and clinical leadership. *Journal of Clinical Nursing, 16*(10), 1818–1825. doi: 10.1111/j.1365-2702.2006.01823.x

Charlton, C. R., Dearing, K. S., Berry, J. A., & Johnson, M. J. (2008). Nurse practitioners' communication styles and their impact on patient outcomes: An integrated literature review. *Journal of the American Academy of Nurse Practitioners, 20*, 382–388. doi:10.1111/j.1745-7599.2008.00336.x

Chinn, P. L., & Kramer, M. K. (1999). *Theory and nursing: Integrated knowledge development* (5th ed.). St. Louis, MO: Mosby.

Chitty, K., & Black, B. (2007). *Professional nursing: Concepts and challenges*. St. Louis, MO: Saunders.

Cody, W. (Ed.). (2013). *Philosophical and theoretical perspectives for advanced practice nursing* (5th ed.). Burlington, MA: Jones & Bartlett Learning.

Conrad, D., Hanson, P., Hasenau, S., & Stocker-Schneider, J. (2012). Identifying the barriers to use of standardized nursing language in the electronic health record by the ambulatory care nurse practitioner. *Journal of the American Academy of Nurse Practitioners, 24*(7), 443–451.

Creech, C., Filter, M., & Bowman, S. (2011). *Comparing patient satisfaction with nurse practitioner and physician delivered care*. Poster presented at the 26th Annual American Academy of Nurse Practitioners Conference, Las Vegas, Nevada.

Department of Health & Human Services. (2011). *Over $100 million in new affordable care act grants help fight health insurance premium hikes*. Retrieved from http://www.hhs.gov/news/press/2011pres/09/20110920a.html

Gallop Politics. (2016, December 19). *Ratings of honesty and ethics*. Retrieved from http://www.gallup.com/poll/200057/americans-rate-healthcare-providers-high-honesty-ethics.aspx?g_source=Social%20Issues&g_medium=newsfeed&g_campaign=tiles

Gladwell, M. (2000). *The tipping point: How little things can make a big difference*. New York, NY: Little, Brown & Company.

Green, A. (2004). Caring behaviors as perceived by nurse practitioners. *Journal of the American Academy of Nurse Practitioners, 16*, 283–290.

Hagedorn, M. (2004). Caring practices in the 21st century: The emerging role of nurse practitioners. *Topics in Advanced Practice Nursing eJournal*, 4. Retrieved June 11, 2006, from http://www.medscape.com/viewarticle/496372

Hamric, A., Spross, J., & Hanson, C. (2009). *Advanced practice nursing* (4th ed.). Philadelphia, PA: W. B. Saunders.

Haugsdal, C., & Scherb, C. (2003). Using the nursing interventions classification to describe the work of the nurse practitioner. *Journal of the American Academy of Nurse Practitioners, 15*, 87–94.

Health Resources and Services Administration (HRSA), Bureau of Health Professions. (2004). *A comparison of changes in the professional practice of nurse practitioners, physician assistants, and certified midwives: 1992 and 2000*. Retrieved from http://bhpr.hrsa.gov/healthworkforce/reports/comparechange19922000.pdf

Indiana University. (2009, January 22). The total package: A skillful, compassionate doctor. *Indiana University News Room*. Retrieved from http://newsinfo.iu.edu/web/page/normal/9704.html

Jenning, C. (2002, October 29). *Testimony: American Academy of Nurse Practitioners before the National Committee on Vital and Health Statistics*. Retrieved from http://www.ncvhs.hhs.gov/021029p3.html

King, I. (1981). *A theory for nursing: Systems, concepts, process*. New York, NY: Wiley.

Kleinman, S. (2004). What is the nature of nurse practitioners' lived experiences interacting with patients? *Journal of the American Academy of Nurse Practitioners, 16*(6), 263–269.

Kurtz, S., Silverman, J., & Draper, J. (1998). *Teaching and learning communication skills in medicine*. Oxford: Radcliffe Medical Press.

Laurant, M., Reeves, D., Hermens, R., Braspenning, J., Grol, R., & Sibbald, B. (2005). Substitution of doctors by nurses in primary care. *Cochrane Database of Systematic Reviews, 2*, CD001271.

Leininger, M. (1995). Culture care theory, research and practice. *Nursing Science Quarterly, 9*, 71–78.

Mundinger, M. O., Kane, R. L., Lenz, E. R., Totten, A. M., Tsai, W. Y., Cleary, P. D., . . . Shelanski, M. L. (2000). Primary care outcomes in patients treated by nurse practitioners or physicians: A randomized trial. *Journal of the American Medical Association, 283*(1), 59–68.

Nicoteri, J. A., & Andrews, C. (2003). The discovery of unique nurse practitioner theory in the literature: Seeking evidence using an integrative review approach. *Journal of the American Academy of Nurse Practitioners, 15*, 494–500.

Nightingale, F. (2009). *Florence Nightingale: Notes on nursing*. New York, NY: Fall River Press.

National Organization of Nurse Practitioner Faculties. (2006). *National Organization of Nurse Practitioner Faculties domains and core competencies of nurse practitioner practice.* Retrieved from http://www.nonpf.org/associations/10789/files/DomainsandCoreComps2006.r157pdf

National Organization of Nurse Practitioner Faculties. (2017). *Nurse practitioner core competencies with suggested curriculum content.* Washington, DC: Author.

Ortiz, J., Wan, T. T., Meemon, N., Paek, S. C., & Agiro, A. (2010). Contextual correlates of rural health clinics' efficiency: Analysis of nurse practitioners' contributions. *Nursing Economics, 28*(4), 237–244.

Peplau, H. (1952). *Interpersonal relations in nursing.* New York, NY: Putnam.

Pulcini, J. (2013). Advanced practice nursing: Moving beyond the basics. In S. DeNisco & A. M. Barker, *Advanced practice nursing: Evolving roles for the transformation of the profession* (2nd ed., pp. 19–26). Burlington, MA: Jones & Bartlett Learning.

Roberts, S. J., Tabloski, P., & Bova, C. (1997). Epigenesis of the nurse practitioner role revisited. *Journal of Nursing Education, 36,* 67–73.

Rosenberg, T. (2012, October 24). The nurse as family doctor. *New York Times.* Retrieved from http://opinionator.blogs.nytimes.com/2012/10/24/the-family-doctor-minus-the-m-d

Sullivan-Marx, E., McGivern, D., Fairman, S., & Greenberg, S. (Eds.) (2010). *Nurse practitioners: The evolution and future of advanced practice* (5th ed.). New York, NY: Springer.

U.S. News and World Report (2017, January). *U.S. News & World Report* announces the 2017 best jobs. Retrieved from https://www.usnews.com/info/blogs/press-room/articles/2017-01-11/us-news-announces-the-2017-best-jobs

Van Leuven, K. (2012). Population aging: Implications for nurse practitioners. *Journal for Nurse Practitioners, 8*(7), 554–559.

Visintainer, M. (1986). The nature of knowledge and theory in nursing. *Image: Journal of Nursing Scholarship, 18,* 32–38.

Weiland, S. (2008). Reflections on independence in nurse practitioner practice. *Journal of the American Academy of Nurse Practitioners, 20*(7), 345–352. doi: 10.111/j.1745-7599.2008.00330.x

Whitlock, E., Orleans, T., Pender, N., & Allan, J. (2002). Evaluating primary care behavioral counseling interventions: An evidence-based approach. *American Journal of Preventative Medicine, 22*(4), 267–284.

Wilson, I. B., Landon, B. E., Hirschhorn, L. R., McInnes, K., Ding, L., Marsden, P. V., & Cleary, P. D. (2005). Quality of HIV care provided by nurse practitioners, physician assistants, and physicians. *Annals of Internal Medicine, 143*(10), 729–736.

Zaccagnini, M., & White, K. (2011). *The doctor of nursing practice essentials: A new model for advanced nursing practice.* Sudbury, MA: Jones and Bartlett.

PART 2

The Nurse Practitioner–Patient Relationship

CHAPTER 2

Family-Focused Clinical Practice: Considerations for the Nurse Practitioner

Susan M. DeNisco

As nurse practitioners we interface with the patient at the point of care and often neglect to consider the individual in the context of a family unit. It is our moral and ethical obligation to consider the health of families throughout their life cycle. Despite changing demographics, most patients live with family members, and these relationships can strongly influence the health and illness of its members (Bray & Campbell, 2007). It is imperative that we consider family background, structure, and level of function when caring for the individual patient. The information that we glean from the patient will have a significant effect on the health and well-being of the patient, and it has the potential to improve the health of the family unit when the nurse practitioner collaborates with and involves the family in the framework of the treatment plan.

Family Theory

Family health has been studied by a variety of disciplines, including but not limited to psychology, sociology, medicine, anthropology, and economics. Most family theories important to advanced practice nursing have been developed by other disciplines but have been used effectively by nurse practitioners. We do not often think that we are using "theory" when taking a family history or conducting a review of systems in the examination room, but if we study the components of theory, we are better able to understand its practical application in the clinical area. The usefulness of a theory is based on its ability to systematically describe the wide range of relationships between variables in order to generalize the findings (Loveland-Cherry, 2004).

As nurse practitioners we are continually striving to explain the relationships between symptoms in patients to develop a differential diagnosis. In a simple example we consider the relationship between chest pain on exertion, back pain, palpitations, and dizziness to help us draw conclusions about coronary heart disease in an individual patient. Similarly, we can use family theory to help expand this differential diagnosis by asking about family risk factors and hereditary causes to assist us in completing the framework of what appears to be coronary heart disease. During the past several decades, the nursing literature has emphasized the importance of "family" in nursing practice. Catch phrases such as "family health promotion," "family healthcare nursing," "family interviewing," and "family systems nursing" helped to define family-centered nursing care as an important part of practice (Wright & Leahey, 2009).

According to Denham (2003), a family theory that is meaningful and useful for nurse practitioners must:

- Describe and explain family structure, dynamics, process, and change.
- Describe interpersonal structures and emotional dynamics within the family and the transmission of distress to individuals.
- View the family as the liaison between the individual and culture.
- Describe the process of healthy individuation and differentiation of family members.
- Predict health and pathology within the family.
- Prescribe therapeutic strategies for dealing with family dysfunction, grief, and illness.
- Account for stability and change when viewed within the family's developmental life cycle.

Most of these propositions have been developed out of family social science theories and can be useful for practice.

Application of Macrosystem Family Theory to Clinical Practice

The macrosystem can be described as the larger world in which the family lives and interacts. This can influence the family's overall development and well-being across the family lifespan. The macrosystem includes social expectations, legal and moral perspectives, and cultural traditions that affect the ways individuals treat and are treated by others. Race, ethnicity, religion, gender, social class, and age may alter the ways individuals and families view themselves and others. The macrosystem serves as a social framework that has unintentional influences on values, attitudes, and behaviors through time. On the other hand, the family's microsystem consists of extended family members as well as those in the nuclear family and the roles and expectations that the family holds for its membership.

Structural Approach

All theories, whether at the macrosystem level or microsystem level, have applicability to practice. When the nurse practitioner uses the structural approach to assessing the family unit, he or she is considering the position or status of the family in society. Each position has associated social norms or expectations for society. For example, in most societies a woman in the kinship position of "mother" is expected to act in a nurturing manner toward her child. A social role implies the cluster of expectations or norms for any status position (White & Klein, 2008). An individual may occupy several positions or roles at the same time across the life span. The mother may also be a sister, teacher, wife, volunteer, and daughter simultaneously, which can lead to role strain and conflict.

Interactional Approach

The interactional approach views the family as being constructed by culture and societal norms. Individuals establish their roles and communicate them within the family and to the external environment. It is the way individuals in a family unit frame their behavior. For example, transition to parenthood can be conceptualized when parents form their beliefs about their contributions to parenthood. In a study, new fathers were found to have a greater number of social accounts to justify noninvolvement with childcare activities than the mothers had (White & Klein, 2008).

Developmental Approach

The developmental approach considers normal family changes and experiences over the members' lifetime; this framework assesses both individuals and families as a whole unit. The developmental framework has three major theoretical components: (1) individual life span theory, (2) family development theory, and (3) life course theory. All of these components influence each other and must be considered together. Individual life span theory focuses on the genetic development of the individual and factors that affect that development. The family development theory focuses on the systematic and patterned changes experienced by families as experience stages and events of the family life course. Life course theory examines the event history of an individual and how earlier events, such as marriage, influence later outcomes, such as birth or adoption of a child (White & Klein, 2008). The developmental approach emphasizes dimensions of time and change in the membership structure of the family including the change in content of social roles in the family. These events and roles do not necessarily proceed in a given sequence, but rather constitute the sum total of the individual's actual experience.

Application of Microsystem Family Theory to Clinical Practice

Family Systems Approach

Health professionals have applied general systems theory, introduced in 1936 by von Bertalanffy, to the understanding of families for a number of years (Wright & Leahey 2009). The general belief of systems theory is that all parts of a system are interconnected. Any change in one family member will affect all family members, and understanding the family is only possible by viewing the whole. The nurse practitioner (NP) that is skilled in collecting and analyzing family data within this framework will consider boundaries within the family and external environment, rules of transformation within the family, positive and negative communication patterns, equilibrium in the family unit, and what the relationships are like within the subsystems of the unit, such as sibling to sibling or parent to child (White & Klein, 2008).

Family Stress Theory

Family stress and individual stress must be assessed by focusing on both the individual and family resources and coping skills. The study of stress has emphasized significant events or a pileup of stressors in the individual and family history. Certain normative events such as buying a house, becoming a parent, and changing jobs may occur at the same time as unexpected events such as the death of a parent, infidelity, or divorce. The normative event may be stressful enough; when the compression of unexpected events occurs at the same time, the family unit can become compromised. The NP must consider the general family stressors, specific stressors, and family strengths as identified by the family.

Change Theory

It is well-known that systems of family relationships undergo progressive change. However, a French proverb states, "The more something changes, the more it remains the same." This paradoxical relationship highlights the dilemma frequently faced by families in need of both stability and change (Wright & Leahey, 2009). Changes in family behavior are dependent on the perception of the problem and may or may not be accompanied by insight. The NP must understand that facilitating change is necessary to help stabilize the family unit in the face of major life events such as death, disability, divorce, natural disasters, and addictions.

Family Resilience and Capacity Models

Resilience is the process of "bouncing back" from life's adversities and difficult experiences. It does not mean that individuals and families do not suffer or experience grief when faced with hardship, but it is a quality that can be learned and developed. In the past decade, Americans have witnessed terrorist attacks and random acts of violence on communities. Out of these disasters we have seen individual and community efforts to build capacity in order to heal.

Resilience

Resilience is defined as an individual's or family's abilities to function well and achieve life's goals despite overbearing stressors or challenges that might easily impair the person or family unit (Mullin, 2008). Felten and Hall (2001) define resilience as "the ability to achieve, retain, or regain a level of physical or emotional health after devastating illness or loss" (p. 46). Wagnild and Young's (1993) theoretical model of resilience describes resilience as an enduring personality characteristic that persists through the human life cycle and moderates the negative effects of stress and promotes adaptation. This model describes five themes that constitute resilience: equanimity, self-reliance, existential aloneness, perseverance, and meaningfulness (Wagnild & Young, 1990). Resilience has also been studied from developmental and environmental perspectives. Environmental factors that influence resilience include social support, which can be described as interactions between the individual, family, and environment (Tusaie & Dyer, 2004). Most researchers agree on the basic nature of resilience but use different terms to define it. The most accepted terms connected to the concept of resilience are *adversity*, *stressors*, *adaptation*, *coping*, *risk factor*, and *protective factor* (Mullin, 2008). Resilience is sometimes conceptualized as the ability to withstand a crisis that is brief in nature, but most often it is associated with the ways that an individual or family faces a pervasive social condition such as poverty or a devastating illness or injury.

Resilient individuals preserve hope and construct a meaningful account of their situations (Druss & Douglas, 1988). Resilience is the process of identifying or developing resources and strengths to manage stressors flexibly and gain a positive outcome (Haase, 2004). When they need assistance, resilient individuals reach out to others including their family, their community, their society, and health professionals (Rabkin, Remien, Katoff, & Williams, 1993). In addition, researchers have identified contributing factors to resilience (Dyer & McGuinness, 1996; Rabkin et al., 1993). Patients with AIDS, for example, have identified social support, excellent medical care, personal resources (e.g., intelligence, education), and access to supplementary services (e.g., visiting nurses, home health aides) as contributing factors to resilience (Rabkin et al., 1993).

In a descriptive correlational study of 71 African-American females with type 2 diabetes, the researcher found that high levels of resilience were significantly correlated with low glycosylated hemoglobin levels, suggesting that resilience may play a role in positive health outcomes (DeNisco, 2011). NPs have an opportunity to consider resilience in the care of minority populations with a chronic illness such as type 2 diabetes. Clinical implications based on the findings of this study include preventing complications of poorly controlled diabetes by recognizing holistic approaches to care that integrate not only the physiological aspects of care but also the psychological aspects of the person, including interventions to help build individual resilience (DeNisco, 2011). **FIGURE 2-1** depicts a theoretical model of resilience showing the effect of resilience on physiological stressors.

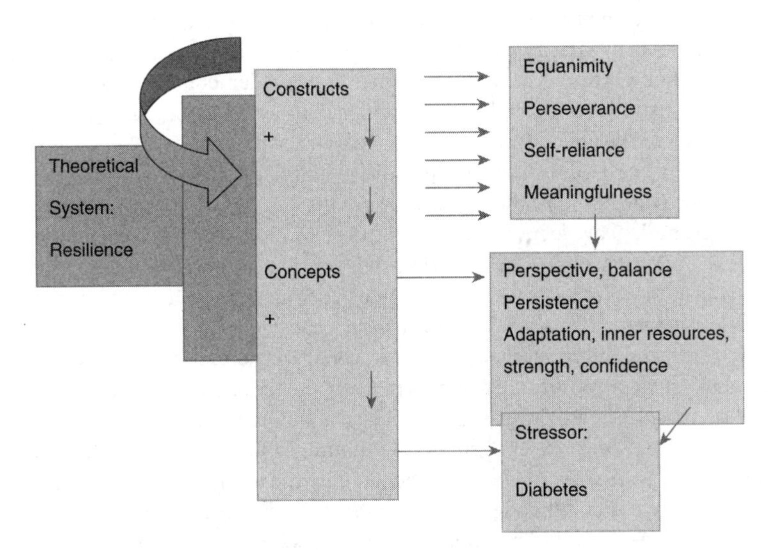

FIGURE 2-1 Theoretical Model of Resilience

Modified from Wagnild, G. M., & Young, H. M. (1993). Development and psychometric evaluation of the resilience scale. *Journal of Nursing Measurement, 1*(2), 165–178. *Journal of Nursing Measurement* by Springer Publishing Company. Reproduced with permission of Springer Publishing Company.

Family Resilience

The system-based resilience model of family stress, adjustment, and adaptation based on the work of McCubbin and McCubbin (1993) is concerned with family development and the family's ability to negotiate change and adapt to stressful life events over time, particularly to stressors such as illness (Kaakinen, Hanson, & Denham, 2010). An approach like this is useful in clinical practice as it analyzes interactions between family members, the family system, and the community or environment to shape the course of family resilience and adaptation. Germain and Bloom (1999) wrote that families are more resilient when there is a "fit" between the family and the environment. They note that specific protective factors or positive characteristics of an individual or family help moderate risk factors or negative characteristics that easily become problematic (Germain & Bloom, 1999).

Resilience was identified recently by the Committee on Future Direction for Behavioral and Social Sciences as a research priority for the National Institutes of Health (Singer & Ryff, 2001). The committee addressed the significance of behavioral and psychosocial processes in disease etiology, well-being, and health promotion. Singer and Ryff (2001) point out the need for the increased study of correlates of resilience including protective factors such as optimism, meaning, purpose, as well as social and emotional support.

Since the 1970s, research on resilience has shifted its focus from the study of personal qualities that predicate positive outcomes to studying the process of resilience, to foster this in all individuals and to develop interventions to promote health (Peterson & Bredow, 2004). The helping professions have been seeking ways to understand the reasons that one individual or family faces insurmountable problems and continues to function well, while others do not. The search to identify the factors of resilience was begun by researchers who focused specifically on children, adolescents, and the elderly (Garmezy, 1993; Gilligan, 2004). Resilient children were seen as having positive temperaments and being easily lovable, autonomous, and intelligent. They were generally seen to have benefited from close relationships with supportive adults or extended family members and others in the community (Garmezy, 1993; Gilligan, 2004).

In a meta-analysis of 24 studies examining the sense of self in children with cancer and in childhood cancer survivors, Woodgate and McClement (1997) found similar themes. Most studies evaluated the psychological functioning of children including self-esteem and the effect on family functioning and adjustment. It was found that the majority of children with cancer do not have significantly lower self-esteem scores than healthy children (Woodgate & McClement, 1997).

Other studies have focused on resilience in children with asthma (Svavarsdottir & Rayens, 2005; Vinson, 2002). In a descriptive correlational survey study of 235 children with asthma, Vinson (2002) found positive correlations between family environment and child characteristics, as well as between the dependent variables of appraisal, coping, quality of life, and illness indices. The researcher also reported that cohesiveness and adaptability were positively correlated with competence and optimism.

Researchers have also investigated resilience in children with cancer. Hockenberry-Eaton, Kemp, and Dilorio (1994) studied 44 children with cancer receiving outpatient chemotherapy. In this descriptive correlational study, the relationship between the independent variables of childhood cancer stressors (protective factors) and the dependent variables of physiologic and psychological responses to stressors experienced during cancer treatment were examined. Findings revealed that family environment, global self-worth, and social support are protective factors that may influence resilience.

The concept of resilience has also been studied in adolescent populations. In a descriptive correlational study, Rew, Taylor-Seehafer, Thomas, and Yockey (2001) explored relationships among resilience and selected protective factors and which factors were the best predictors of resilience in a convenience sample of 59 homeless adolescents. In another descriptive correlational study, the relationship between adaptive and maladaptive coping correlates to health and illness outcomes in 404 female adolescent athletes who have experienced high levels of stress recently (Yi, Smith, & Vitaliano, 2005).

Resilience has been studied in elderly populations to describe characteristics of resilience. In a qualitative study of elderly women over 85 years of age, nine emerging themes were identified as characteristics of resilience: frailty, determination, hardship, access to care, culture, family support, self-care activities, care of others, and efficiency (Felten & Hall, 2001). The researchers concluded that resilience has implications for healthcare providers to facilitate these traits in order to prevent frailty and disability.

Three other studies were conducted to measure resilience in elderly populations (Adams, Sanders, & Auth, 2004; Becker & Newsome, 2005; Hardy, Concato, & Gill, 2004). In a descriptive qualitative study of 38 African-American participants between the ages of 65 and 91 years, it was found that values such as independence, spirituality, and survival were important factors that shaped responses to chronic illness. Thus, resilience may be a culturally important tool as ethnic minority people age (Becker & Newsome, 2005).

A descriptive cross-sectional study of resilience in 546 community-dwelling older adults found that higher stress levels were negatively correlated ($r = -0.48, P < .001$) with lower resilience scores (Hardy et al., 2004). Resilience scores were negatively correlated with depressive symptoms. The authors concluded that more research was needed on the relationship between resilience and future health and functional status as a predication of recovery (Hardy et al., 2004). According to Adams et al. (2004), in a study of 234 elderly participants living in a retirement community, loneliness was seen as a risk factor for depression and associated with a smaller social network.

The following case study represents a model case study of resilience.

ELLEN'S STORY

Ellen Collins is a 63-year-old Jamaican female who has a history of chronic physical problems including type 2 diabetes mellitus, hypertension, asthma, and hyperlipidemia for which she is on numerous medications. Ms. Collins also has a history of depression, but she has maintained well on an antidepressant for a number of years. She visits her primary care provider regularly for the above problems. Ms. Collins cares for her 87-year-old aunt who has a polymorphic adenoma of the salivary glands. Ms. Collins was also awarded custody of her 13-year-old grandson because her son and daughter-in-law are drug addicts and unable to care for their child. Ms. Collins's youngest son is dually diagnosed with bipolar disorder and alcohol abuse, has had legal problems related to domestic violence, and is currently hospitalized for decompensation of his mental illness.

Despite the myriad of adversities, Ms. Collins has a good outlook on life, and she seeks out the support of her healthcare provider and community services. Her chronic health problems are well controlled. She continues to care for her aunt, son, and grandson with a positive attitude and sees hope for the future. She owns her own home, and continues to work with the Department of Children and Families providing foster care for troubled adolescents. She enjoys gardening, raises money for HIV research, and is looking forward to taking her grandson to Niagara Falls this summer.

Family resilience or relational resilience has been defined by Walsh (2006) as having three domains: beliefs systems, family organizational patterns, and communication processes. Walsh redefined resilience as having "reparative" potential on family functioning. The following individual, family, and social factors contribute to family resilience:

- An internal locus of control or the belief that the individual or family is empowered to influence the environment
- Spirituality that fosters personal meaning and a sense of purpose in life
- Downward social comparison
- Positive social supports including emotional support, informational support, social companionship, and instrumental support

When a nurse practitioner encounters an individual in the healthcare system, the following theoretical assumptions should be kept in mind:

- Some individuals recover or "bounce back" better than expected when faced with an adverse condition (Dyer & McGinness, 1996).
- Positive health outcomes (both physiological and psychological) include the absence of disease or low levels of symptoms or impairments (Heinzer, 1995; Hockenberry-Eaton et al., 1994).
- Resilient individuals have inherent personality characteristics that are protective factors in the face of illness or adversity (Haase, Heiney, Ruccione, & Stutzer, 1999; Jacelon, 1997; Polk, 1997; Woodgate & McClement, 1997).
- Nurse practitioners can be helpful in fostering resilience within individuals, families, and communities (Drummond, Kysela, McDonald, & Query, 2002; Hockenberry-Eaton et al., 1994).

Family Capacity

One of the greatest challenges for many healthcare providers is to address the need for family capacity; if a family has not realized their "capacity" or capabilities, they can face significant obstacles in their day-to-day living. Family capacity-building involves increasing the families' competence in implementing strategies to enhance their development and build their problem-solving skills while increasing their confidence that they are able to do so.

Family capacity can be defined as the extent to which the family needs, goals, strengths, capabilities, and aspirations can meet the family's ability to function to its fullest potential (Dunst & Trivette, 2009). It is the nurse practitioner's responsibility to assess the family's capacity to support the family's health and wellness, as well as prevent illness risks, treat medical conditions, and manage tertiary care needs. Similar to resilience, family capacity can be viewed as the family's ability to adapt and change.

The family capacity model is presented in **FIGURE 2-2**.

Traditionally, the literature considered children and families as having deficits and weaknesses that needed treatment by healthcare professionals to correct problems, whereas the capacity-building literature believes that families have varied strengths and assets, and the focus of interventions is on supporting and promoting competence and other positive aspects of family member functioning (Dunst & Trivette, 2009). To understand family capacity, the nurse practitioner needs to understand family structure, function, and roles.

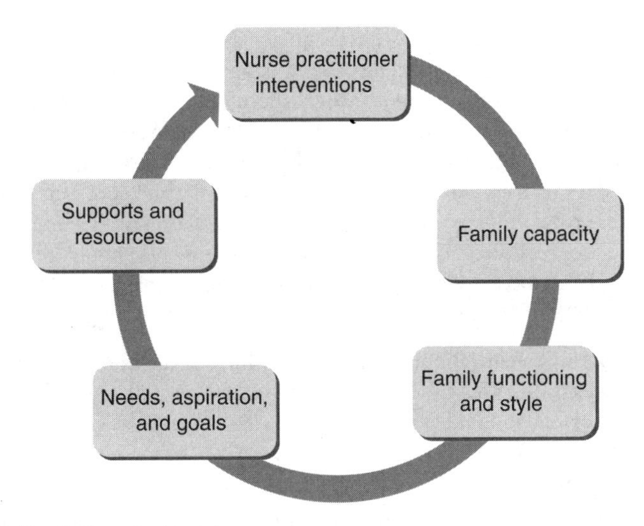

FIGURE 2-2 Family Capacity Model

Modified from Dunst, C. J., & Trivette, C. M. (2009). Capacity building family systems intervention practices. *Journal of Family Social Work, 12,* 119–143. Reprinted by permission of the publisher, Taylor and Francis Ltd., http://wwwtandf.co.uk/journals and the author.

▶ Family Structure, Function, and Roles

There are many clinical family assessment models that the nurse practitioner can use to assess family structure, function, and roles. Some of the popular models are:

1. The Calgary Family Assessment (CFAM) (Wright & Leahey, 2009)
2. The Family Assessment and Intervention Model (Kaakinen et al., 2010)
3. The Friedman Family Assessment Model (Friedman, 1998)

All three models may have different approaches in their theoretical underpinnings, scope, data collection methods (quantitative or qualitative), and unit of analysis, but they have many similarities. Broadly, these assessment tools are available to expand the clinician's understanding and management of family-wide threats to both physiologic and psychologic health.

There are five key goals of family life:

1. Pass on culture (religion, ethnicity).
2. Socialize young people for the next generation (to be good citizens, to be able to cope in society through going to school).
3. Exist for sexual satisfaction and procreation.
4. Serve as a protective mechanism for family members against outside forces.
5. Provide closer human contact and relations.

Family Structure

The nurse practitioner may use a genogram or "family tree" to gather much of the information regarding family structure. A detailed discussion of the genogram will take place later in this chapter. Family structure can be defined as the organizational framework that determines family membership and the way in which a family is organized according to roles, rules, power, and hierarchies. There is no typical family form in the 21st century. Nurse practitioners need to expand their definitions of the traditional nuclear family (or biological family of procreation) to include alternate forms of family life: the single- or sole-parent family, blended families including stepchildren, grandparents raising grandchildren, communal families, and the lesbian, gay, bisexual, queer, intersexed, transgendered, or twinspirited (LGBT) couple or family (Wright & Leahey, 2009).

Whether or not you are using a pictorial representation of the family structure such as the genogram or ecomap, the following components should be included in the interview data collection regarding family structure (Bomar, 2004; McGoldrick & Carter, 1999, 2003).

1. Family constellation: Knowledge of who is in the immediate family, who lives in the house, how the individuals are related, and the relationship to extended family and boundaries
2. Family constellation changes: Permanent (birth or death), temporary (illness, hospitalizations, co-parenting in divorced families, homelessness)
3. Individual family members: Age, gender, sexual orientation, ethnicity, race, health problems, occupation, educational level, and cultural/religious beliefs
4. Environmental: Housing or living situation
5. Social support: Stress management, financial support, entitlements such as Medicaid, WIC, food stamps

Family Function

According to Wright and Leahey (2009), family functioning can be defined as the processes by which the family operates as a whole, including communication patterns and manipulation of the environment for problem solving. Each family possesses a distinctive operating system, and it can influence healthcare outcomes. Some specific areas to assess include:

- Activities of daily living: Eating, sleeping, common tasks including family participation in leisure activities and family rituals
- Nutrition: Food insecurity
- Communication patterns: How family members communicate (Is there one spokesperson when articulating healthcare issues?)
- Family perceptions: How illness affects each family member, concerns for other family members, care-seeking behaviors
- Family members' mental health history: Includes substance, tobacco, and alcohol use
- Problem-solving abilities
- Influence and power: Knowledge of who is dominate, subordinate, controlling, abusive, guilt-inducing, the scape-goat, etc.

Family Development

The nurse practitioner must also consider the developmental life cycle for each family that he or she encounters in the clinical setting. Families are shaped by people who share a past and future history together. As contemporary families move through time, there is a normative sequence by which families develop and change. McGoldrick and Carter (2003) have done extensive work on the family life cycle by describing the underlying factors that influence family development as the family expands and contracts by variables such as birth, death, marriage, divorce, adoption, poverty, and catastrophic illness. These events typically cause realignment of the family system to support the entry, exit, and developmental changes of family members through time. Major life-cycle transitions are marked by fundamental changes in the family system itself (second-order changes) rather than rearrangements within the system (first-order changes). McGoldrick and Carter (1999) have designed a classification system of normative stages that typical middle-class American families go through across the life cycle. When reviewing these "normative" stages of the family life cycle, the nurse practitioner must take into consideration societal influences and sweeping changes in the way the family functions. In this day and age, it is hard to conceptualize what is considered a typical family when there are gay and lesbian couples, sole-parent adoptions, dual-career families, grandparents raising grandchildren, cohabiting couples, military families, and foster families.

In the Calgary Family Assessment Model, Wright and Leahey (2009) propose that family developmental assessment includes an overview of the stages, tasks, and attachments that are important to each stage. The nurse practitioner must also keep in mind common health issues that may accompany each stage.

Divorced Families

According to the U.S. Census Bureau, in 2008 there were over 10.5 million single-parent families in the United States, accounting for 29.5% of all households with children under the age of 16 (U.S. Census Bureau, 2012). This is higher than the reported rates in Canada, Denmark, France, and Japan. Children living with a parent who divorced in 2009 were more likely to live in a household headed by their mother (75%) than in a household headed by their father (25%). Additionally, children living with a parent who divorced in 2009 were more likely to be in a household below the poverty level (28%) compared with other children (19%), and they were more likely to live in a rented home (53%) compared with other children (36%) (U.S. Census Bureau, 2012). While the divorce rate fluctuates given geographic location, population, income, and educational status, single-parent and divorced families are common in our society and have unique challenges.

The term *divorce* invokes a series of images of bitter custody battles, financial hardship, broken families, vulnerable children, hostility, resentment, and failure to live up to commitments. While these images may be true of some divorces, research shows that most families will experience short-term, moderate effects postdivorce (Bowen, 2012; Demo, 2010). However, it is true that families experiencing divorce are under significant emotional pressure during the transition and must fulfill the same developmental tasks as the two-parent nuclear family but without all the means. Shortages in time, money, and energy can cause single parents to experience self-doubt and often feel guilty for not meeting societal expectations of living in a two-parent family (Wright & Leahey, 2009).

Nontraditional Families

If we consider society a generation ago, the average American family might be defined as a married man and woman with two biological children. Divorce rates were lower, optional single parenthood was rare, and surrogacy and in vitro fertilization by sperm or egg donation were not available. The gay and lesbian community had little hope of raising their own children. Grandparents and extended family members played a supportive role during holidays, special events, and illness, but did not have major responsibility to the nuclear family. Adoption was closed if available (Lantz, 2012). While societal perceptions of the "traditional family" may still be a certainty for some, this is clearly dependent on age, gender, education, religious beliefs, socioeconomic status, and geographic location. The reality is that less than 25% of U.S. households are considered "traditional."

Single-Parent Families

Single-parent families are recognized as the most common nontraditional family; in 2006, the number of single-parent households increased to 10 million, accounting for 26% of families with children in the United States. Father-only families are on the rise, accounting for 2 million families, or 5% of all family structures (Kaakinen et al., 2010). Single-parent families by divorce or death are under significant pressure for time, space, adequate finances, social control, and tension management. Single parents typically have the ultimate responsibility for paying the bills, disciplining, and caring for the children's physical and emotional needs. This can be especially challenging for the parent who does not have the financial resources, support of the biological parent, or extended family support. Single-parent mothers and fathers also experience societal pressure to live in a "normal family" and feel like failures in meeting expectations of friends, neighbors, and their extended families (Wright & Leahey, 2013). In working with single-parent families, it is important for the NP to help the parent explore his or her feelings, develop coping mechanisms, and find community and financial resources to support the parent through issues of custody, visitation, social networks, and effective parenting.

Same-Sex Couple Families

Until recently gay and lesbian families have been "invisible" in our culture. With changes in the laws recognizing the legal union of same-sex couples, more attention is being focused on these relationships, their structures, challenges, strengths, and issues. In 2010, the American Community Survey (ACS) results showed that 19.4% of households were headed by same-sex couples with children. By conservative estimates, there are at least 400,000 to 500,000 gay or lesbian parents living with children in the United States. Of these families (Lofquist, 2011):

- 72.8% reported having biological children from previous heterosexual relationships or artificial insemination.
- 21.2% reported as having stepchildren or adopted children.
- 6% reported having a combination of biological, stepchildren, and adopted children.

While research studies on children raised by gay and lesbian parents are still relatively new, to date the majority of evidence suggests that children who grow up in families headed by same-sex parents fare as well as children who grow up in families headed by opposite-sex parents. In addition, children who have gay, lesbian, bisexual, or transgender parents do not appear to differ from children who have heterosexual parents in terms of psychological health, social relationships, or cognitive or emotional functioning (Burkholder & Burbank, 2012). State laws and rights of same-sex parents and children vary widely. It is important for the nurse practitioner to understand these differences in order to assist the family to navigate a complicated legal system that may not support the family, or one that may place legal limitations on the family. Child custody issues, adoption rights, and a variety of other rights and benefits offered to married couples, such as insurance coverage and spousal benefits, are not available to same-sex couples. The NP must gain expertise in assessments and interventions that address the unique needs of these families in order to help parents and children to deal with social stress from being perceived as different by other children, or as problematic and threatening by other parents.

Foster Families

Other types of nontraditional families include foster parenting and grandparents raising grandchildren. In the United States, 30%–60% of children residing in urban school districts live with caretakers that are not their biological parents (Lantz, 2012). The nurse practitioner must be cognizant of the intensity of the health and emotional issues that a child residing in foster care may present with; many children have been victims of emotional and physical abuse and have special medical and physiological needs (Lenora, 2009).

In a descriptive study of physical examination findings of 5,181 children taken into protective custody, the researchers found that nearly half (44%) had an identified health problem, including acute infections (otitis media, sexually transmitted diseases), anemia, and lead poisoning. In addition, approximately 5% of the children evaluated for physical abuse were found to have occult fractures not suspected by their caseworkers (Chernoff, Coombs-Orme, Risley-Curtiss, & Heisler, 1994). In another large study of 2,419 children assessed shortly after placement in foster care almost all (92%) had at least one abnormality on physical examination, including disorders of the upper respiratory tract (66%), skin (61%), genitals (10%), eyes (8%), abdomen (8%), lungs (7%), and extremities (6%). Nearly one-quarter (23%) of younger children failed a developmental screening, and 22% of older children were already receiving special education services before placement. As a result of these evaluations, 53% of the children were referred for further medical services (Flaherty & Weiss, 1990).

Because of the high rate of physical, mental, and developmental problems in foster children, they often require more frequent healthcare visits than most children. Many states require that children newly placed in foster care have a comprehensive health assessment within 30 to 60 days of placement (Simms, 2000). The clinician needs to negotiate a management plan with the foster parents and their children to ensure timely routine health maintenance visits including close developmental screening and mental health interventions as appropriate. This plan needs to be updated with each patient care encounter, and communicated to the caseworker and the foster family. NPs play a significant role in coordinating services for foster children and ensuring they receive care in a timely manner.

Grandparents Raising Grandchildren

Recent U.S. census reports show that there are more than 4.5 million children being raised in grandparent-headed households (Conway, 2011). The phenomenon of grandparent caregiving is prevalent among African-American and Latino grandparents: African-Americans and Latino grandparents have a 38% and 13% chance, respectively, of becoming caregivers for their grandchildren (Conway, 2011).

The increase in the numbers of grandparents in caregiving roles parallels the increase in the growing number of older adults. According to the federal Administration on Aging (AOA, 2011), it is estimated that the number of adults age 65 and older will make up 20% of the population in the year 2030 as compared to 12% in the year 2000. The grandparenting role is a stressful one; typically, the caregiver attains responsibility for the child secondary to a family crisis where the biological parents cannot effectively care for their child. Factors that may contribute to the shift in parenting include substance abuse, mental health issues, lack of money, incarceration, death, and abuse or neglect of the children. These unexpected life events can cause significant emotional and financial strain on the grandparents as they assume new parenting responsibilities for children.

Grandparents who are primary caregivers usually face a number of challenges, including higher rates of depression, health problems, and fatigue, as compared to noncaregivers or to others their age (Kaakinen et al., 2010). Grandparents often are dealing with their own chronic health issues, may be raising their own adolescent children, and are often providing care for their aging parents. Grandparents report having less time for themselves, experiencing social isolation, and feeling increased financial pressures, especially if they need to reduce their hours at work or draw on their savings in their efforts to provide a home for their grandchildren. Grandchildren are affected, too; research shows that these children have higher rates of asthma, decreased immunity, poor eating and sleep patterns, physical disabilities, and hyperactivity compared to children in parental households (Kaakinen et al., 2010). The nurse practitioner plays a key role in assisting the grandparents to seek out and use existing community resources and social supports to prevent social isolation, ease financial burdens, and promote the health and well-being of the family unit.

Structural Assessment and Family Interviews

Structural assessment tools are helpful to discern the internal and external functioning of the family. Family interviews can be gathered by drawing a genogram, ecomap, or family pedigree. The genogram is essentially a diagram of the family constellation, while the ecomap displays the important contacts that are external to the immediate family. The family pedigree is a risk assessment tool for conditions that have familial genetic predisposition.

The relationship between family history and health risks has long been recognized. Indeed, family history is a risk factor for many pediatric and adult onset diseases and disorders. It represents genetic susceptibility, shared environment, common behaviors, and the interactions between and among the family members. The genogram and ecomap are tools that can assist the nurse practitioner in assisting a family as a whole system, as well as assisting the individuals within the family system. The therapeutic relationship between the nurse practitioner and patient can begin in the waiting room, the examination room, or at the hospital beside. When using a genogram or an ecomap, it is impossible to differentiate between its value to the nurse practitioner–patient relationship, or on the quality and quantity of information acquired and its effect on that family or individual. At the most superficial level, either of these tools gives family members a new framework with which to understand themselves as individuals and as an active part of a system (Denham, 2003).

The family pedigree is another interview tool that includes a three-generational assessment of medical conditions in each relative, including specific genetic disorders, birth defects, Down syndrome, and questions about certain behaviors (e.g., alcohol, substance abuse, and tobacco use), as well as questions about consanguinity and ethnicity (Yoon, 2003).

Genograms

A genogram is an assessment tool or clinical method of taking, storing, and processing family information for the benefit of the patient and the family. It is displayed as a graphic representation of family members and their relations over three generations (McGoldrick, 2008). The three-generation family genogram was developed primarily out of the family systems theory and is a popular tool among social workers, psychologists, physicians, and nurses. According to Bowen (2012), people are organized into family systems by age, generation, sex, or other similar features. Where the person fits into the family structure influences the person's functioning, relational patterns, and type of family he or she forms in the next generation. It is also believed that sex and birth order shape sibling relationships and individual characteristics (Rakel & Rakel, 2015). Families repeat themselves over generations in the phenomenon called the transmission of family patterns; what happens in one generation repeats itself in the next, so that the same issues are played out from generation to generation (Bowen, 2012).

The information collected for the genogram may include genetic, medical, social, behavioral, and cultural aspects of the family.

Because the process of creating a genogram involves extensive interviewing, it is a way for the nurse practitioner to establish a therapeutic relationship with the family. Families tend to become engaged in the process of developing the genogram and often gain insight into their potential health issues and missing support systems (Schilsin, 1993). Despite the clear advantages the genogram offers, many primary care clinicians often neglect to use it as it can take up extra time in an already overburdened office schedule (Schilsin, 1993). The genogram does not have to be completed in one sitting but can be started on the initial visit and completed on subsequent visits. While some primary care clinicians may not feel skilled at delving into psychosocial issues and sensitive family matters, nurse practitioners by virtue of their education and experience are poised to assist families to identify strengths as individuals and in a family unit to promote their mutual support and growth. Some key indications for the nurse practitioner to develop a family genogram are represented in **BOX 2-1**.

Process of Developing the Genogram

The manner in which a genogram is taken is perhaps more important than what is elicited and the technique of recording. The nurse practitioner needs to be sincere,

BOX 2-1 Key Indicators to Develop a Family Genogram

Depression
Somatic problems (e.g., headache, abdominal pain, chest pain)
Frequent office visits
Poor school or work attendance
Behavioral problems
Problems between family members
Stepfamilies with problems
Obesity, smoking, alcohol, substance abuse
Nonadherence to treatment regimen

open-minded, interested, and nonjudgmental, and even occasionally prepared to share anecdotes of his or her own family to put the patient at ease. It is a mutual scientific inquiry with members of a family and they often get enthusiastic about drawing their "family tree" and want it be accurate, complete, and relevant. You may use a flip chart, or in a hurried practice setting a pad of paper or progress note. The diagramming of a family genogram must comply with the use of specific symbols to ensure that the family and the nurse practitioner have the same understanding and interpretations of the genogram. Authors may vary on symbols used for different nodal events, but all genograms are similar in terms of gathering information on family membership, structure, interaction patterns, and other important information. The genogram does not have to be completed in one session; in general, nurse practitioners working in a primary care setting will see patients and their families over time, and data can be collected and added as a continuous process.

See **BOXES 2-2**, **2-3**, and **2-4** for the three types of family genogram interview data: factual events, expanded events, and relationships.

Understanding and Interpreting the Genogram

Discussion of the completed genogram can offer alternatives to the family for their current behaviors, and it offers a chance to escape from repetitive family patterns if the family views this as helpful. Furthermore, a genogram will help the family make sense of unexplained fears and anxieties about family patterns and illness.

BOX 2-2 Family Genogram Interview Data: Factual Events

Family composition: Who is the immediate family? Who has the identified health problem?
Who lives with the immediate family, and how are they related?
Dates of births, miscarriages, abortions, and stillbirths
Dates of any adoptions
Dates and causes of deaths
Major illnesses and dates
Dates of marriages, separations, divorces, remarriages, retirements, and relocations

BOX 2-3 Family Genogram Interview Data: Expanded Events

Religion, ethnic factors, occupations, social class, education, military service
Additional births, abortions, miscarriages, adoptions, and infertility
Congenital abnormalities, mental disabilities, learning problems
Illnesses similar to presenting illness
Cancer, heart disease, hypertension, asthma, hyperlipidemia, diabetes, depression, alcoholism, substance abuse
Common causes of death in that family
Family secrets
Troubles with the law, incest

BOX 2-4 Family Genogram Interview Data: Relationships

Who is close to whom? Is there too much closeness? Are there "favorites" or "isolates"?

Relationships and alliances between:

- Marriage partners
- Siblings
- Children and parents
- Children and grandparents

Boundaries between family members:

- Permeable
- Loose
- Rigid

Power and patterns of avoidance
Patterns of friendships and relationships with work colleagues
Matters that cannot be talked about in the family

One of the challenges for nurse practitioners is to take the vast amount of information collected during the interview process and consolidate the data into categories that can be analyzed for repetitive relationship patterns between generations. Categorizing the data groups can assist in the identification of the most pertinent family problem that needs immediate attention. In a family where emotions can be neither recognized nor displayed, distress may present as somatic symptoms resulting in frequents office visits. **BOX 2-5** lists themes in a family genogram that should raise a red flag and help you identify problems and patterns that may affect family functioning and individual family members' well-being.

Family Pedigree

Similar to a genogram, a family pedigree is a graphic representation of a person's medical and biological history and is often referred to as the "family tree." Like the genogram, the pedigree is a family history assessment tool developed in an interview with a patient; it includes three generations and involves the use of standardized

BOX 2-5 Family Genogram Red-Flag Themes

Repetitive patterns between generations, such as alcoholism, drug addiction, divorce, or mental illness
Chronological coincidences, such as births, marriages, and deaths
Similarity of names, possible personality resemblances, or identity in upbringing, such as family favorites, family scapegoat
Cultural, educational, ethnic, and religious backgrounds—differences and similarities
Family patterns from husband's and wife's relations—similarities and differences
Family secrets, such as abortions, adoptions, or secret affairs
Significance of nicknames
Too much closeness between generations (absence of boundaries)
Poor or loose contact between the generations, as in cut off
Inappropriate alliances
Fighting and domestic abuse

symbols, which clearly mark individuals affected with a specific diagnosis to allow for easy identification (Yoon, 2003). Advances in genetics and genomics have brought pedigree analysis from the traditional prerogative of genetic specialists into mainstream primary care practice. When appropriately used, a pedigree generated from a family history can be one of the nurse practitioner's most powerful clinical tools for health risk identification, diagnosis, and intervention, yet it provides little insight into family dynamics or the complex context of the patient and family in the community.

Nurse practitioners need a comprehensive, three-generation pedigree that records a patient's medical, social, and environmental history, thereby communicating an expansive scenario for holistic primary care practice. Such a tool can guide the identification of risk factors to inform the patient and family clinical decisions regarding care management strategies, psychosocial support, and education for reproductive decisions, risk reduction, and the prevention, screening, diagnosis, referral, and long-term management of disease. The family pedigree should indicate the age of individuals; if deceased, the age and cause of death; and any relevant health history, illnesses, and age of onset. If any genetic testing has been performed on family members, the results should be indicated on the pedigree. The ethnic background of each grandparent should be listed as well as any known consanguinity. A general inquiry about the more distant relatives should be made in case there is a possible X-linked disorder or autosomal dominant disorder with reduced penetrance (National Genetics Education and Development Centre, 2012).

While the genogram focuses on the family relationships and communication patterns, the pedigree is a collection of the family health history and an assessment of disease risk factors. It is used to develop a differential diagnosis for identified familial traits. Family history plays a critical role in assessing the risk of inherited medical conditions and single gene disorders. Certain types of cancer, such as breast cancer and colon cancer, appear more frequently in some families, as do some adverse birth outcomes. Coronary artery disease, type 2 diabetes, depression, and thrombophilias also have familial tendencies (Yoon, 2003). The U.S. Surgeon General's Family History Initiative was launched in 2004. The goal of this initiative is to educate both healthcare providers and patients about the value of collecting a family history as a screening tool and to increase its use and effectiveness in clinical care by simplifying the collection process and analysis of the family history (Office of the Surgeon General, 2012).

Over the past 20 years, the Human Genome Project has afforded us a better understanding of the effect of genetic variation on health and disease. This has furthered research in identifying genotype–phenotype correlations and enhanced the ability to predict those at risk of developing inherited medical conditions (National Genetics Education and Development Centre, 2012). With increased awareness of the importance of using the family history as a screening tool and of the value of preventive measures and increased surveillance, there is hope for improved outcomes.

Although it may be best to take a systematic approach to enquiring about each branch of a family, sometimes this may not be possible in a busy primary care practice. There are some useful general questions, however, that can help the NP to gain a quick overview of the medical conditions in a family. Answers to these questions may trigger a need for drawing out how the people with the condition are related to each other. This would inform a preliminary assessment of whether there is an increased genetic risk that warrants further investigation, a detailed family pedigree, or specialist referral. **BOX 2-6** provides some key questions to ask individuals about their family history.

FIGURES 2-3 and **2-4** show the process of drawing a family tree and the symbols used.

More samples of pedigree diagrams for healthcare professionals can be found by visiting http://www.geneticseducation.nhs.uk. A PowerPoint presentation showing the process of creating a pedigree as well as exercises to practice making family histories and pedigrees can also be found on this website.

Family Risk Assessment Tools

The screening tool selected should be tailored to the practice setting and patient population, taking into consideration patient education level and cultural background. Whether a pedigree diagram or questionnaire is used, it is important to review and update the family history periodically for new diagnoses within the family as appropriate. A family history screening tool will allow the healthcare provider to stratify levels of risk (Centers for Disease Control and Prevention, 2012). Moreover, the use of

BOX 2-6 Key Questions for a Family History Warranting a Detailed Pedigree

Do you have any concerns about diseases or conditions that seem to run in either your or your partner's side of the family?
Does anyone have a major medical, physical, or mental problem?
Has anyone ever needed treatment in a hospital?
Has anyone ever had any serious illnesses or operations?
How old was this person at diagnosis?
(Avoid just asking "Is everyone well?" as past medical history may not be offered!)
Have any adults, children, or babies died?
How old were they, and what was the cause of death?
Have there been any miscarriages or babies who were stillborn?

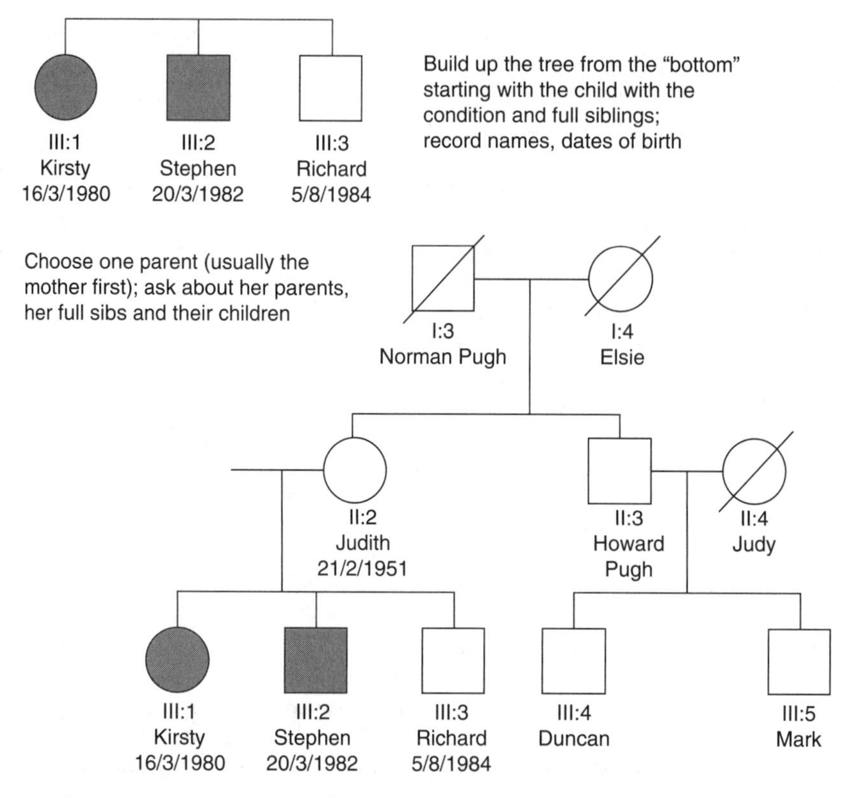

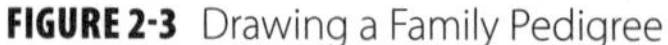

FIGURE 2-3 Drawing a Family Pedigree

Genetic family history pedigree images reproduced with permission from the NHS National Genetics Education and Development Centre.

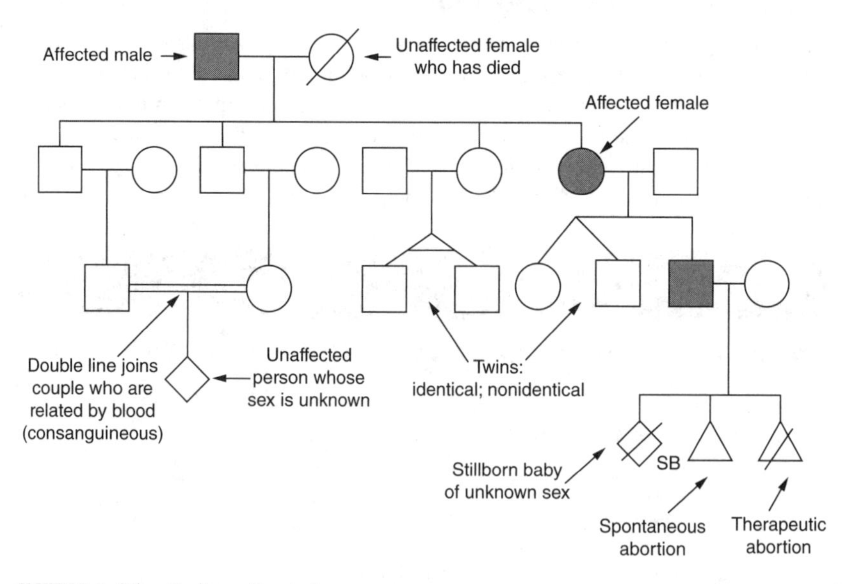

FIGURE 2-4 Other Pedigree Symbols

Genetic family history pedigree images reproduced with permission from the NHS National Genetics Education and Development Centre.

BOX 2-7 Red Flags for Genetic Conditions

Family history of a known or suspected genetic condition
Ethnic predisposition to certain genetic disorders
Close biological relationship between parents (consanguinity = blood relationship of parents)
Multiple affected family members with the same or related disorders
Earlier than expected age of onset of disease
Diagnosis in less-often-affected sex
Multifocal or bilateral occurrence of disease (often cancer) in paired organs
Disease in the absence of risk factors or after application of preventive measures
One or more major malformations
Developmental delays or mental retardation
Abnormalities in growth (growth restriction, asymmetric growth, or excessive growth)
Recurrent pregnancy losses (>2)

Reproduced from The National Coalition for Health Professional Education in Genetics (NCHPEG). Available online at http://www.NCHPEG.org

a family history screening tool (pedigree or questionnaire) has been shown to increase by 20% the likelihood of detecting a patient at high risk of developing an inherited medical condition compared with medical record review alone (Yoon, 2003). **BOX 2-7** lists red flags for genetic conditions that may warrant referral to a genetic specialist (National Coalition for Health Professional Education in Genetics, 2012).

Ecomap

Similar to the genogram, the ecomap is a pictorial representation of a family's contact with larger systems. These systems can include school, work environment, place of worship, healthcare agencies, social support agencies, courts, recreation, housing, and friends. The ecomap is used to clarify reciprocal relationships between family members and the broader community. It provides a way of assessing resources and strengths of family relationships with significant others, organizations, and institutions (Bomar, 2004; Reed, 1994). The ecomap allows the nurse practitioner to view both the nurturing aspects of a family's world and the family's stress-producing connections. Often the ecomap shows deprivation of resources, which can assist the nurse practitioner in developing an adequate plan of care for the family (Wright & Leahey, 2009).

Typically a simplified version of the genogram is developed first and can be placed in the center of the ecomap circle. Outer circles represent significant people, agencies, or institutions in the family's context. Lines are drawn between the circles and the family members to depict the nature and quality of the relationships and to show what kinds of resources are moving in and out of the family. Straight lines denote strong or close relationships. Wider or thicker lines show stronger relationships. Straight lines with slashes show stressful or strained relationships. Broken or dotted lines show tenuous, weak, or distant relationships. Arrows are drawn to indicate the flow of energy and resources between people and the environment. The ecomap provides the nurse practitioner with a more integrated perception of the family situation and can be helpful in assisting the family to define goals and increase its use of community resources (Kaakinen et al., 2010).

Family Problem List

Following careful assessment of the individual in the context of the family unit, the nurse practitioner must develop a comprehensive prioritized problem list. The problem oriented medical record (POMR) and the "problem list" date back to the 1960s; they were developed by Dr. Lawrence Weed as a simple way to document and manage important health problems facing a patient (Holmes, 2011). Today the problem list still exists as an acceptable model of documentation in both paper and electronic medical records. The contents of the problem list may vary from one healthcare organization to the next and may vary depending on the healthcare provider's preference. In general, nurse practitioners and other primary care providers agree that the problem list should contain the following general information:

- A list of chronic diseases or illnesses
- An ongoing or active problem that you are working on with the patient
- A summarization of the most important things about a patient

There is some debate about what diagnosed illnesses are worthy of the problem list. Currently the decision of which problems are included or excluded remains largely up to the judgment of the practitioner. Some practitioners will exclude certain information as it may "clutter up" the record with extraneous information (e.g., lab results or "sensitive issues" such as sexually transmitted infections or mental health issues). Primary care nurse practitioners provide integrated, accessible healthcare services and are accountable for addressing a large majority of personal healthcare needs, developing a sustained partnership with patients, and practicing in the context of family and community (DeNisco & Barker, 2015). In caring for the individual patient in the context of the family unit, it is important for the nurse practitioner to maintain clear documentation of the family's healthcare needs. At minimum, the problem list should include the following elements: acute self-limiting problems, routine health maintenance issues, allergies, family planning, social problems, and chronic health problems.

Acute self-limiting problems are problems that may be acute or short term. For example, streptococcal pharyngitis is an example of an acute self-limiting problem. Nocturnal leg cramps, upper respiratory infection, and contact dermatitis are other problems that fall into this category. Routine health maintenance refers to health promotion and screening activities that are needed by the patient per age and risk factor analysis. This includes but is not limited to mammograms, annual physical examinations, pap smears, immunizations, and well-child care. Allergies would include allergies to medications, food, dust, and mold. Family planning would address contraceptive needs of the family including infertility issues. Social problems take into account the toxic history of the patient or family members (e.g., tobacco use, substance abuse, alcohol use). Chronic health problems include long-standing diagnoses the healthcare provider is following (e.g., hypertension, type 2 diabetes, hyperlipidemia, asthma, migraine headaches).

The other category is a net to catch all other problems that may be important to remember as you care for the patient. This may include family problems (death of family member, mental health issues, school truancy), financial problems (unemployment, entitlements such as food stamps), sexual preferences, and so on.

There are many issues complicating the maintenance of a patient problem list. If the list is messy, unorganized, or partially completed because the healthcare provider did not have time to add problems, the list will not be used effectively. The usefulness of problem lists in the care of the individual patient and family is based on the ability of the nurse practitioner to articulate patient problems (when identified) and follow consistent guidelines that ensure the lists are current and useful.

The family problem list includes these categories:

- Acute self-limiting problems
- Routine health maintenance
- Allergies
- Family planning
- Social
- Chronic problems and other

Family Problem List/Case Study Exercises

Read the following cases and develop a comprehensive problem list for each case. If you do not have enough information to develop a list for each problem category as described in this chapter, propose what questions you would need to ask the patient and family to gather the information you need.

CASE STUDY ONE

Ms. Belcher is a 48-year-old married white female and has two children and three grandchildren. Ms. Belcher has a long history of schizoaffective disorder and also has chronic medical problems including type 2 diabetes mellitus, hypertension, and coronary artery disease. She is on a laundry list of medications and visits her primary care provider and psychiatrist regularly. She also attends a day psychiatric program three times a week for socialization and vocational skills. Ms. Belcher has resided at the same low-income housing project for many years. Her husband, who is African-American, also suffers from schizoaffective disorder and has a multitude of chronic health problems and has been hospitalized recently for renal insufficiency. Ms. Belcher's daughters, age 19 and 15, reside at home and are very important in Ms. Belcher's life. The youngest daughter was hospitalized last year for a new diagnosis of bipolar disorder, and Ms. Belcher was very concerned about this. She was worried that Department of Children and Families would take her daughter out of the home.

Despite these adversities, Ms. Belcher has an optimistic view regarding her family life and does her best to care for her husband and daughters. She does have moments when she becomes very somatic and visits her healthcare provider frequently for reassurance. Ms. Belcher reaches out to her psychiatric visiting nurse and her primary care provider for support when the going gets tough.

CASE STUDY TWO

Ms. Dora Roman is a 50-year-old Hispanic female who resides in her car on the streets of Bridgeport. She relocated to Connecticut 1 year ago after she left an abusive relationship with her husband while residing in Florida. Ms. Roman is educated as an LPN and has worked in long-term care settings in the past. She has a history of sarcoid and other chronic medical problems. She seeks medical care at the local community

(continues)

CASE STUDY TWO *(continued)*

health center since relocating to Connecticut and had her medical records sent to Connecticut so she can have continuity of care. Ms. Roman has a sister in Connecticut and uses her house occasionally in the bitterest cold nights, but mostly sleeps in her car and uses the public beach bath house for hygiene purposes. Since relocating to Connecticut, she has worked seasonally at a Halloween store in the local mall.

Ms. Roman has filled out applications for subsidized housing and Medicaid entitlements for health care, but for unknown reasons she has not been successful in obtaining them. Ms. Roman does not speak to her daughter who lives in Connecticut and feels that she is alone in the world. She has many somatic complaints and seeks narcotics to help her back pain and to "get to sleep in my car."

CASE STUDY THREE

Ms. Tamika Jenkins is a 30-year-old African-American single mother of three children and resides in an economically disadvantaged housing project in the inner city. She frequently visits the health center with a multitude of complaints typically focused around injury. In the past 6 months, Ms. Jenkins has been seen for a miscarriage, a fractured wrist related to a fall while rollerblading, and a head injury related to an altercation with another woman for unknown reasons. Ms. Jenkins states that her husband is incarcerated and she has no family support; her mother died of HIV when she was a teenager, and she doesn't speak to her father. When she presents to the health center she is anxious and despondent and seeks pain medication. She seems to have little insight into her problems. She is currently being investigated by the Department of Children and Families for child neglect.

Seminar Discussion Questions

1. Describe the characteristics that constitute a healthy family.
2. Develop a three-generation family genogram on a partner and build a comprehensive problem list for one family constellation.
3. Draw your family ecomap, and outline the various family relationships to institutions, leisure activities, and agencies. Define which relationships are stress producing and which foster support. Discuss how the individuals in the family are linked to significant people and how they engage in social support.
4. Consider the family capacity model when reading the case of Dora Roman, and outline family strengths, function, needs, goals, and supports needed to maximize the family potential.

References

Adams, K. B., Sanders, S., & Auth, E. A. (2004). Loneliness and depression in independent living retirement communities: Risk and resilience factors. *Aging and Mental Health, 8*(6), 475–485.

Administration on Aging. (2011). *Aging statistics*. Retrieved from http://www.aoa.gov/AoARoot/Aging_Statistics/index.aspx

Becker, G., & Newsome, E. (2005). Resilience in the face of serious illness among chronically ill African Americans in later life. *Journal of Gerontology, 60*(4), S214–S223.

Bomar, P. (2004). *Promoting health in families: Applying family research and theory to practice* (3rd ed.). Philadelphia, PA: Saunders.

Bowen, M. (2012, October 12). *Bowen theory.* The Bowen Center. Retrieved from http://www.thebowencenter.org/pages/theory.html

Bray, J. H., & Campbell, T. L. (2007). The family's influence on health. In R. Rakel, *Textbook of family medicine* (7th ed., pp. 25–34). Philadelphia, PA: Elsevier.

Burkholder, G., & Burbank, P. (2012). Caring for lesbian, gay, bisexual and transsexual parents and their children. *International Journal of Child Birth Education, 27*(4), 12–18.

Centers for Disease Control and Prevention. (2012, October 13). *Chronic disease prevention and health promotion.* Retrieved from http://www.cdc.gov/chronicdisease/resources/guidelines.htm

Chernoff, R., Coombs-Orme, T., Risley-Curtiss, C., & Heisler, A. (1994). Assessing the health status of children entering foster care. *Pediatrics, 93*, 594–601.

Conway, F. J. (2011). Emotional strain in caregiving among African American grand-mothers raising their grandchildren. *Journal of Women and Aging, 23*(2), 113–128.

Demo, D. F. (2010). *Beyond the average divorce.* Thousand Oaks, CA: Sage.

Denham, S. F. (2003). *Family health: A framework for nursing.* Philadelphia, PA: F. A. Davis.

DeNisco, S. (2011). Exploring the relationship between resilience and diabetes outcomes in African Americans. *American Journal of Nurse Practitioners, 23*(11), 602–610. doi:10.1111/j.1745-7599.2011.00648.x

DeNisco, S., & Barker, A. (2015). *Advanced practice nursing: Evolving roles for the transformation of the profession* (3rd ed.). Burlington, MA: Jones & Bartlett Learning.

Drummond, J., Kysela, G. M., McDonald, L., & Query, B. (2002). The family adaptation model: Examination of dimensions and relations. *Canadian Journal of Nursing Research, 34*(1), 29–46.

Druss, R. G., & Douglas, C. J. (1988). Adaptive responses to illness and disability. *General Hospital Psychiatry, 10*, 163–168.

Dunst, C. J., & Trivette, C. M. (2009). Capacity building family systems intervention practices. *Journal of Family Social Work, 12*, 119–143.

Dyer, J. G., & McGuinness, T. M. (1996). Resilience: Analysis of the concept. *Archives of Psychiatry Nursing, 10*(5), 276–282.

Felten, B. S., & Hall, J. M. (2001). Conceptualizing resilience in women older than 85: Overcoming adversity from illness or loss. *Journal of Gerontological Nursing, 27*(11), 46–53.

Flaherty, E. G., & Weiss, H. (1990). Medical evaluation of abused and neglected children. *American Journal of Diseases of Children, 144*, 330–334.

Friedman, M. (1998). *Family nursing* (4th ed.). Stamford, CT: Appleton & Lange.

Garmezy, N. (1993). Children in poverty: Resilience despite risk. *Psychiatry, 56*, 127–136.

Germain, C., & Bloom, M. (1999). *Human behavior in the social environment: An ecological view.* New York, NY: Columbia University Press.

Gilligan, R. (2004). Promoting resilience in child and family social work: Issues for social work and policy. *Social Work Education, 23*, 93–104.

Haase, J. E. (2004). The adolescent resilience model as a guide to interventions. *Journal of Pediatric Oncology Nursing, 21*(5), 289–299.

Haase, J. E., Heiney, S. P., Ruccione, K. S., & Stutzer, C. (1999). Research triangulation to derive meaning based quality of life theory: Adolescent resilience model and instrument development. *International Journal of Cancer Supplement, 12*, 125–131.

Hardy, S. E., Concato, J., & Gill, T. M. (2004). Resilience of community dwelling older persons. *Journal of the American Geriatrics Society, 52*(2), 257–262.

Heinzer, M. M. (1995). Loss of a parent in childhood: Attachment and coping in a model of adolescent resilience. *Holistic Nursing Practice, 9*(3), 27–37.

Hockenberry-Eaton, M., Kemp, V., & Dilorio, C. (1994). Cancer stressors and positive factors: Predictors of stress experienced during treatment for childhood cancer. *Research in Nursing and Health, 17*, 351–361.

Holmes, C. (2011). The problem list beyond meaningful use: The problem with problem list. *Journal of AHIMA* (February), 30–33.

Jacelon, C. S. (1997). The trait and process of resilience. *Journal of Advanced Nursing, 25*, 123–129.

Kaakinen, J. R., Hanson, S. M. H., & Denham, S. A. (2010). *Family health nursing: Theory, practice and research* (4th ed.). Philadelphia, PA: Davis.
Lantz, N. (2012). Nontraditional family: Who do we live as a family today? *International Journal of Child Birth Education, 27*(4), 8–9.
Lenora, M. (2009). Supporting resilience in foster families: A model for program design that supports recruitment, retention, and satisfaction of foster families who care for infants with prenatal substance exposure. *Child Welfare, 89*(1), 7–29.
Lofquist, D. (2011). *Same-sex couple households: American Community Survey Briefs*. Retrieved from http://www.census.gov/prod/2011pubs/acsbr10-03.pdf
Loveland-Cherry, C. (2004). Family health promotion and health protection. In P. Bomar (Ed.), *Promoting health in families* (pp. 61–89). Philadelphia, PA: Saunders.
McCubbin, M. A., & McCubbin, H. I. (1993). Family stress theory and the development of nursing knowledge about family adaptation. In S. Feetham, S. Meister, J. Bell, & C. Gillis (Eds.), *The nursing of families* (pp. 46–58). Newbury Park, CA: Sage.
McGoldrick, M. S. (2008). *Genograms: Assessment and intervention*. New York, NY: W. W. Norton & Company.
McGoldrick, M., & Carter, B. (1999). *The expanded family life cycle: Individual, family, and social perspectives*. Boston, MA: Allyn & Bacon.
McGoldrick, M., & Carter, B. (2003). The family life cycle. In F. Walsh (Ed.), *Normal family processes*. New York, NY: Guilford Press.
Mullin, W. A. (2008). Resilience of families living in poverty. *Journal of Family Social Work, 11*(4).
National Coalition for Health Professional Education in Genetics. (2012, October 13). *Red flags*. Retrieved from http://www.nchpeg.org
National Genetics Education and Development Centre. (2012, October 12). *Genetics education: Supporting education in genetics and genomics for health*. Retrieved from http://www.geneticseducation.nhs.uk/teaching-genetics/medical-practitioners/resources.aspx#concepts
Office of the Surgeon General. (2012, October 12). *Surgeon General's Family Health History Initiative*. Retrieved from http://www.hhs.gov/familyhistory
Peterson, S. J., & Bredow, T. S. (2004). *Middle range theories*. Philadelphia, PA: Lippincott Williams Wilkins.
Polk, L. V. (1997). Toward a middle range theory of resilience. *Advanced Nursing Science, 19*(3), 1–13.
Rabkin, J. G., Remien, R., Katoff, L., & Williams, J. B. (1993). Resilience in adversity among long-term survivors of AIDS. *Hospital and Community Psychiatry, 44*(2), 162–167.
Rakel, R. (2007). *Textbook of family medicine* (7th ed.). Philadelphia, PA: Elsevier.
Rakel, R., & Rakel, D. (2015). *Textbook of family medicine* (9th ed.). Philadelphia, PA: Elsevier.
Reed, M. (1994). Digging up family plots: Analysis of axes of variation in genograms. *Teaching Sociology, 22*, 255–259.
Rew, L., Taylor-Seehafer, M., Thomas, N. Y., & Yockey, R. D. (2001). Correlates of resilience in homeless adolescents. *Journal of Nursing Scholarship, 33*(1), 33–40.
Schilsin, E. B. (1993). Use of genograms in family medicine: A family physician/family therapist collaboration. *Family Systems Medicine, 11*, 201–208.
Simms, M. D. (2000). Health care needs of children in the foster care system. *Pediatrics, 106*(909), 909–918.
Singer, B. H., & Ryff, C. (2001). *New horizons in health: An integrative approach*. Washington, DC: National Academy Press.
Svavarsdottir, E. K., & Rayens, M. K. (2005). Hardiness in families of young children with asthma. *Journal of Advanced Nursing, 50*(4), 381–390.
Tusaie, K., & Dyer, J. (2004). Resilience: A historical review of the construct. *Holistic Nursing Practice, 1*, 3–9.
U.S. Census Bureau. (2012, September 27). *Population, households*. Retrieved from http://www.census.gov/compendia/statab/2012/tables/12s1337.pdf
Vinson, J. A. (2002). Children with asthma: Initial development of the child resilience model. *Pediatric Nurse, 28*(2), 149–158.
Wagnild, G., & Young, H. M. (1990). Resilience among older women. *Image: Journal of Nursing Scholarship, 22*(4), 252–255.

Wagnild, G. M., & Young, H. M. (1993). Development and psychometric evaluation of the resilience scale. *Journal of Nursing Measurement, 1*(2), 165–178.
Walsh, F. (2006). *Strengthening family resilience* (2nd ed.). New York, NY: Gilford.
White, J. M., & Klein, D. M. (2008). *Family theories* (3rd ed.). Los Angeles, CA: Sage.
Woodgate, R., & McClement, S. (1997). Sense of self in children with cancer and in childhood cancer survivors: A critical review. *Journal of Pediatric Oncology Nursing, 14*(3), 137–155.
Wright, L. M., & Leahey, M. (2009). *Nurses and families: A guide to family assessment and intervention* (5th ed.). Philadelphia, PA: F. A. Davis.
Wright, L. M., & Leahey, M. (2013). *Nurses and families: A guide to family assessment and intervention* (6th ed.). Philadelphia, PA: F. A. Davis.
Yi, J. P., Smith, R. E., & Vitaliano, P. P. (2005). Stress-resilience, illness, and coping: A person-focused investigation of young women athletes. *Journal of Behavioral Medicine, 28*(3), 257–265.
Yoon, P. S. (2003). Research priorities for evaluating family history in the prevention of common chronic diseases. *American Journal of Preventative Medicine, 24*(2), 128–135.

Additional Resources

Belcher, J. P. (2011). Family capital: Implications for interventions with families. *Journal of Family Social Work, 14*, 68–85.
McKenry, P. (2000). *Families and change: Coping with stressful events and transitions* (2nd ed.). Thousand Oaks, CA: Sage.
Walsh, F. (2002). A family resilience framework: Innovative practice approaches. *Family Relations, 5*(2), 130–137.

CHAPTER 3

Vulnerable Populations

Susan M. DeNisco and Julie G. Stewart

Section One: Overview of Vulnerabilities and Disparities

Healthcare disparities generally refers to differences in the quality of health care across individuals or groups in regard to access, treatment options, and preventative services. Vulnerability as a concept originated from a variety of disciplines including economics, sociology, anthropology, and environmental science. Segments of the global population experience social inequalities and are at risk for poor health outcomes. Nurse practitioners (NPs) are keenly aware that any individual can become vulnerable at any point in their life; however, it is well documented in the literature that health outcomes and vulnerability fall along a social gradient and that poorer people experience poorer health (Grabovschi, Loignon, & Fortin, 2013; Marmot, 2005). This global phenomenon is seen in low-, middle-, and high-income countries. The World Health Organization (WHO) has been bringing to the forefront a sense of urgency for healthcare leaders to address health inequities across the globe. Health inequities or disparities refers to systematic gaps in health outcomes between different groups of people that are judged to be avoidable and therefore are considered unfair and unjust. It is the inherent human right to primary, secondary, and tertiary medical care, food, housing, and other resources. Primary care nurse practitioners with a strong educational base have a longstanding commitment to cultural competence and social justice. As integral members of the healthcare delivery team, NPs are well positioned for leadership roles in addressing the gaps in health prevention and treatment the rehighlight certain groups as vulnerable populations and attempt to build an understanding of the needs within the various groups.

Social Determinants of Health

The social determinants of health (SDH) are the conditions in which people are born, grow, work, live, and age (Healthy People, 2020). There are four well-established factors that influence individual and aggregate health outcomes including but not limited to (1) lifestyle and behaviors, (2) genetic factors, (3) social and environmental forces, and (4) medical care. For a brief representation see **TABLE 3-1**. Primary care clinicians must be astute at assessing all of these factors whether seeing a patient at point of care or assessing community needs and developing responsive programs for the particular population in which they serve.

Despite significant medical advances in this country, poor and nonwhite ethnic minorities are ranked lower in health status on numerous measures. According to the Centers for Disease Control and Prevention (CDC), morbidity and mortality rates remain higher for African-Americans who continue to die disproportionally more than whites from chronic disease (CDC, 2017). Reasons for the lower health status ranking may include genetic and gender differences, stereotyping, perceived discrimination, and mistrust of healthcare providers. Language barriers, ineffective use of translators, and lack of cultural humility can influence the nurse practitioner's ability to properly diagnosis and treat patients.

Literacy and Advocacy

Health literacy is a concept grounded in the literature on health promotion and education. Health literacy can be defined as the degree to which individuals have the cognitive and social capacity to access, process, and utilize basic health information and services to maintain good health, make appropriate health decisions, and meet their goals. According to the National Assessment of Adult Literacy, only 12% of adults have proficient health literacy and 14% have below basic health literacy, with 42% reporting health is poor (Kutner, Greenberg, Jin, & Paulsen, 2006). Low literacy has been linked with being underinsured and having poor health outcomes, higher rates of hospitalization, and less frequent use of preventive services. Populations most likely to experience low health literacy are older adults, racial and ethnic minority

TABLE 3-1 Social Determinants of Health

Life Style	Social/ Environmental	Genetic	Medical Care
■ Diet ■ Food ■ Exercise ■ Tobacco use ■ Illicit drug use ■ Unsafe sex ■ Irresponsible motor vehicle use	■ Education ■ Employment ■ Socioeconomic status ■ Food insecurity ■ Social cohesion ■ Quality of housing ■ Crime and violence ■ Discrimination ■ Environmental conditions	■ Predisposed to certain diseases ■ Inherited diseases	■ Access to preventative measures ■ Access to curative measures ■ Health literacy ■ New technology ■ Clinical trials

groups, individuals with low educational levels, those living below the poverty level, and non-native speakers of English (U.S. Department of Health and Human Services [USDHHS], 2017). Individuals with low literacy will find it difficult to navigate the healthcare system, provide accurate health histories, fill out complex forms, and engage in self-care and chronic disease management. According to research studies, persons with limited health literacy skills are less likely to receive preventive measures such as mammograms, Pap smears, colonoscopies, and vaccines when compared to those with adequate health literacy skills. Studies have shown that patients with limited health literacy skills enter the healthcare system when they are sicker, which impacts healthcare utilization and cost (USDHHS, 2017).

Advocacy

With advanced education and extensive experience caring for patients and their families, nurse practitioners are equipped to serve as advocates by providing a voice for patients, communities, and the healthcare profession at large. An advocate is defined as an individual or group that pleads, defends, or supports a cause or interest of another. Much of the literature on advocacy comes from nonprofit and special-interest groups that prepare potential advocates to influence public policy. Advocates are often thought of as individuals who lead change through influence and help decision makers work through solutions to problems. At the macrosystem level, advocacy often requires working through formal decision-making bodies to achieve desired goals and outcomes. This process could include working through the "chain of command" within a healthcare organization, state legislature, or other groups at the healthcare system's policy level (Basch, 2014). Ensuring that every individual has access to the health care they need is of paramount importance. Advocacy for social justice and human rights protection for populations who are powerless and dependent on others to address their complex vulnerabilities is a challenge at best. Patients and families often find themselves overwhelmed and lacking the essential information they need to make informed choices. Such vulnerability is cited as a key reason for advocacy at the point of care. At the microsystem level, nurse practitioners must become motivated to act on another's behalf, gain insight into one's self and others, develop cultural skills, and actively engage with diverse groups to promote effectiveness of care (Pacquiao, 2008).

Poverty, Vulnerability, and Resilience

The single, most important determinant of social injustices is poverty and the social and environmental factors that coexist with it. Poverty is a widely recognized global issue and a major determinant of poor health; and this association has been extensively studied and verified. It is a growing problem in the United States and in other developed nations as well as a continuing and devastating problem in the least developed countries (Conway, 2016). The cycle of poverty is more than a socioeconomic issue. It impacts health, well-being, and quality of life for generations to come. Factors that coexist with poverty include poor housing; inadequate nutrition; lack of clean water; increased exposure to violence; fragmented health care; and a higher prevalence of physical illness, mental health issues, and disabilities (Basch, 2014). Despite these well-established linkages, little work has been done to determine what family nurse practitioners can do to address poverty status at point of care and be stewards of sustainable change. For purposes of this chapter, we will consider poverty in the United

States given the steady influx of immigrants and the projected tipping point at 2040, where minorities will become the numerical majority.

Definition of Poverty

The U.S. Census Bureau uses a set of monetary income thresholds that vary by family size and composition to determine who is in poverty. If a family's total income is less than the family's threshold, then that family and every individual in it is considered as living in poverty. As defined by the federal government, those who make less than the official poverty threshold earn less than $24,000 annually for a family of four. In 2015, 43.1 million people lived in poverty in the United States at a rate of 13.5%. Poverty impacts certain groups disproportionately; single-parent families, women, children, seniors, and the disabled experience greater rates of poverty (Proctor, Semegaand, & Kollar, 2015).

Ethnic Groups and Poverty

Certain ethnic and population groups also face greater challenges than the general population in terms of economic advantage. According to 2015 U.S. census data, the highest poverty prevalence by race is among African-Americans (24.1%), with Hispanics (of any race) having the second-highest poverty rate (21.4%). Whites had a poverty rate of 9%, and Asians 11.4% (Proctor et al., 2015).

Women and Children Living in Poverty

Poverty does not strike all demographics equally. For example, in 2015, 12.2% of men lived in poverty, and 14.8% of women lived in poverty. Along the same lines, the poverty rate for married couples in 2014 was only 5.4%, but the poverty rate for single-parent families with no wife present was up to 14.9%, and for single-parent families with no husband present 28.2% (Proctor et al., 2015).

According to the National Center for Children in Poverty (NCCP) approximately 15 million children in the United States, or 21% of all children, live in families with incomes below the federal poverty threshold, a measurement that has been shown to underestimate the needs of families (NCCP, 2016). On average, families need an income of about twice that level to cover basic expenses. Using this standard, 43% of children live in low-income families. Children living in poverty are more likely to experience hunger, which has secondary effects of lower reading and math scores, more physical and mental health problems, more emotional and behavioral problems, and a greater chance of obesity (Yang, Granja, & Koball, 2017).

Elderly and Poverty

While poverty was once far more prevalent among the elderly than among other age groups, today's elderly have a poverty rate similar to that of working-age adults and much lower than that of children. For people aged 65 and older, the 2015 poverty rate declined to 8.8% from 10% in 2014, while the number in poverty declined to 4.2 million, down from 4.6 million (Proctor et al., 2015). Social security income is often mentioned as a likely contributor to the decline in elderly poverty; however, increases in the life expectancy of the elderly over time mean that financial resources have to last longer. At the same time, healthcare and housing costs are on the rise and employer benefit pension plans have decreased. This means seniors face significant insecurity about whether or not their resources are sufficient to cover the duration of their lives after retirement (Borrowman, 2012). In addition, it is well-known that poverty rates among Hispanics and African-Americans ages 65 and older are below the threshold when compared to white adults in this age group (Cubanski, Casillas, & Damico, 2015).

Vulnerability and Resilience

Resilience may be an approach to understanding the vulnerability of families and the community in which the nurse practitioner serves. Resilient communities promote or encourage diversity, flexibility, inclusion, and participation among its members. At a systems level, recognition of social values, accepting uncertainty and change, and fostering an educational environment are approaches that facilitate the building of social capacity (deChesney & Anderson, 2016). Understanding the social capacity of a community will help the nurse practitioner identify important differences within communities in terms of access to resources and entitlements for the poor. Individuals with few financial assets may be less resilient, meaning less adaptive to withstanding adversities in terms of poor housing and lack of adequate food, clothing, education, and medical care. Families with low incomes are generally viewed as households with substantial problems putting themselves at risk for homelessness, exposure to violence, school failure, and social deprivation. Helping families assess their strengths in terms of economic resources, problem-solving capabilities, family cohesion, communication, and social support will make them less risk adverse (Orthner, 2004). As individuals and families living in poverty build their resilience and adaptive capacities, positive consequences may be realized in terms of maintaining school attendance, avoidance of violence and crimes, engagement in developmentally appropriate activities, and maintaining stable housing.

Section Two: Overview of Select Special Populations, Direct Care, and Access

Adverse Childhood Events

A large epidemiological research study founded by collaborative researchers from the Centers for Disease Control (CDC) and Kaiser Permanente examined the relationship between adverse childhood experiences (ACEs) and adult health issues in over 17,000 patient members (CDC, 2016). Childhood experiences that have been examined include emotional abuse, physical abuse, sexual abuse, violence against the respondent's mother, living with substance abusing household members, living with mentally ill or suicidal household members, and living with household members who have been imprisoned (CDC, 2016). Results have demonstrated that exposure to one ACE is likely to increase exposure to other ACEs as well as positively correlate to a large variety of adult illnesses. Adult disease associated with

ACEs include cancer, autoimmune conditions, heart disease, chronic obstructive pulmonary disease, alcoholism, depression, and high-risk behaviors (CDC, 2016). Researchers suggest that high-risk behaviors may well be coping strategies used to manage stress associated with surviving ACEs. In the mental health chapter of this book there is a discussion on the effect of ACEs on the neurocognitive development of children. The ACEs Pyramid, in **FIGURE 3-1**, can be used as a tool for NPs to use in understanding risk factors that may lead to increased morbidity and mortality later in life.

Nurse practitioners have a unique approach to patients and families and stress both care and cure. Nurse practitioners are in an ideal position to increase the practice of assessing and screening for patients who are survivors of ACEs, and encouraging those who are appropriate for therapy to mental health services. **BOX 3-1** provides a sample questionnaire that covers topics from the original ACEs; however, research has uncovered that bullying and witnessing violence in the community are just as or perhaps more stressful. Therefore, the NP may prefer to ask the patient about general issues as they relate to the patient's childhood, such as:

- How well do you remember your childhood?
- Are there things that happened to you when you were a child that shouldn't have happened to you or anyone?
- Would you like your children to grow up as you did?
- Sometimes we feel guilty about things that happened to us in the past. Are you feeling any sense of guilt or shame? (Clarke, Schulman, McCollum, & Felitti, 2015)

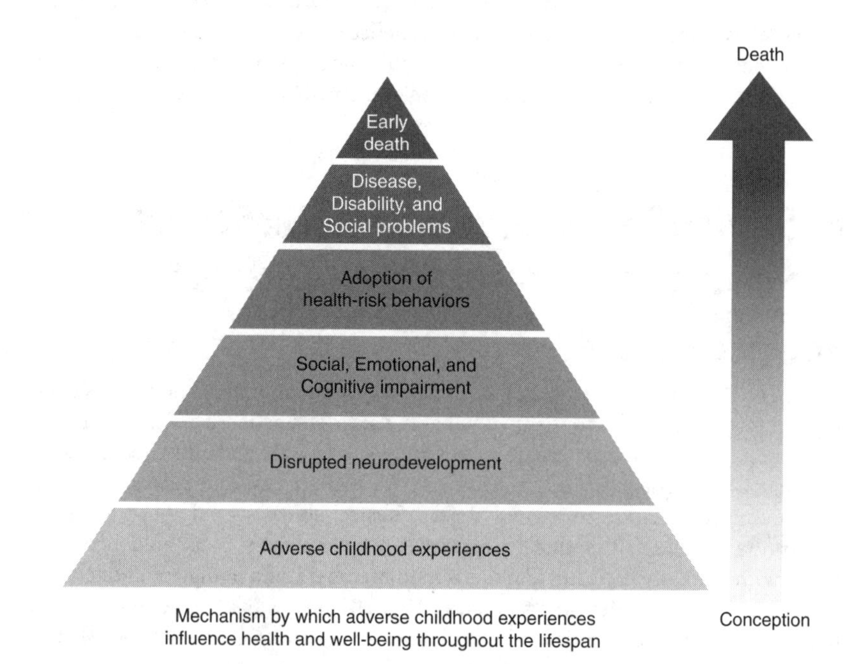

FIGURE 3-1 ACEs Pyramid

Reproduced from CDC. (2016). About the CDC-Kaiser ACE study. Retrieved from https://www.cdc.gov/violenceprevention/acestudy/about.html

BOX 3-1 BRFSS Adverse Childhood Experience (ACE) Module Prologue: (CDC, 2016)

I'd like to ask you some questions about events that happened during your childhood. This information will allow us to better understand problems that may occur early in life, and may help others in the future. This is a sensitive topic and some people may feel uncomfortable with these questions. At the end of this section, I will give you a phone number for an organization that can provide information and referral for these issues. Please keep in mind that you can ask me to skip any question you do not want to answer. All questions refer to the time period before you were 18 years of age. Now, looking back before you were 18 years of age:

1. Did you live with anyone who was depressed, mentally ill, or suicidal?
2. Did you live with anyone who was a problem drinker or alcoholic?
3. Did you live with anyone who used illegal street drugs or who abused prescription medications?
4. Did you live with anyone who served time or was sentenced to serve time in a prison, jail, or other correctional facility?
5. Were your parents separated or divorced?
6. How often did your parents or adults in your home ever slap, hit, kick, punch, or beat each other up?
7. Before age 18, how often did a parent or adult in your home ever hit, beat, kick, or physically hurt you in any way? Do not include spanking. Would you say?
8. How often did a parent or adult in your home ever swear at you, insult you, or put you down?
9. How often did anyone at least 5 years older than you or an adult, ever touch you sexually?
10. How often did anyone at least 5 years older than you or an adult, try to make you touch them sexually?
11. How often did anyone at least 5 years older than you or an adult, force you to have sex?

RESPONSE OPTIONS:

Questions 1–4:	1=Yes	2=No	7=DK/NS	9=Refused
Question 5:	1=Yes 9=Refused	2=No	8=Parents not married	7=DK/NS
Questions 6–11:	1=Never 9=Refused	2=Once	3=More than once	7=DK/NS

Free access to review and use survey questionnaires about health and family history are available on the CDC website at https://www.cdc.gov/violenceprevention/acestudy/about.html.

Reproduced from CDC. (n.d.). BRFSS Adverse Childhood Experience (ACE) Module. Retrieved from https://www.cdc.gov/violenceprevention/acestudy/pdf/brfss_adverse_module.pdf

Transgenerational Trauma

Transgenerational or intergenerational trauma is a wounding from a traumatic event that has effects upon generations after the initial trauma. This type of trauma can occur in individual families, or groups who have experienced genocide, terrorism, natural disasters, etc., as collective trauma. In either case, there can be long-lasting harmful effects on physiological processes in the body, which can cause chronic disease.

An example of this can be found in the Native American population, which suffers from some of the highest health disparities in the United States. The median age of death in South Dakota Native Americans is 58 compared to whites, where 81 years of age is the median (Warne & Lajimodiere, 2015). Native Americans have experienced centuries of inequities adding to the root causes for these poor health disparities. From the 15th to the 19th century, millions of Native Americans died from warfare and infectious diseases, including smallpox which was intentionally spread to the indigenous people by giving them blankets that had been used by smallpox patients (Warne & Lajimodiere, 2015). In the late 1890s up to the 1930s, there were multitudes of off-reservation boarding schools developed to destroy the Native American culture by teaching the children reading, writing, and arithmetic and keeping them away from their parents and tribal culture and customs. Children from ages 4 and up were taken and sent away to boarding schools—their parents often having no choice. These children were exposed to all forms of abuse, homesickness, infectious diseases, lack of love and parenting, and loss of tradition and culture identity, resulting in the deaths of many of these children. Those who survived lack the skills and knowledge to parent, have not been able to heal, and therefore suffer from alcoholism, substance abuse, poverty, depression, and the like. Homicides, suicides, and interpersonal violence injuries beset this population. The trauma has been passed down to the next generation.

Homeless Health Care

According to the National Alliance to End Homelessness, the annual Housing and Urban Development (HUD) point-in-time count identified 564,708 people experiencing homelessness in 2015. Though the vast majority of the homeless population lived in some form of shelter or in transitional housing at the time of the point-in-time count, approximately one-third lived in a place not meant for human habitation, such as the street or an abandoned building. Subpopulations experiencing homelessness are individuals, which accounts for more than half of the homeless; families are the second largest subgroup. Other subgroups are those individuals who were chronically homeless, chronically homeless families, veterans, and unaccompanied youth and children. Although most homeless persons live in urban areas, a surprising 16.1% live in rural areas where they sleep in the woods, campgrounds, cars, and abandoned farm buildings.

Defining Homelessness

According to the National Health Care for the Homeless Council (NHCHC, 2017) there is more than one "official" definition of homelessness. Health centers funded by the USDHHS use the following definition:

> A homeless individual is defined in section 330(h)(5)(A) as "an individual who lacks housing (without regard to whether the individual is a member of a family), including an individual whose primary residence during the night is a supervised public or private facility (e.g., shelters) that provides temporary living accommodations, and an individual who is a resident in transitional housing." (NHCHC, 2017)

The Federal Bureau of Primary Health Care expands the definition of homelessness to include the following: an individual may be considered to be homeless if that person is "doubled up," a term that refers to a situation where individuals are unable to maintain their housing situation and are forced to stay with a series of friends and/or extended

BOX 3-2 Assessing for Homelessness at Point of Care

- Patient self-defines as homeless.
- Patient lives place to place.
- Patient lives with family or friends because there is no other option.
- Patient is staying in a place that restricts number of nights (including pays rent by hours, days, or weeks).
- Patient lives in overcrowded situation.
- Patient lives in housing that is based on illegal/unwanted acts (e.g., prostitution).
- Patient is separated from family members because of limited housing choice.

family members (see **BOX 3-2**). In addition, previously homeless individuals who are to be released from a prison or a hospital may be considered homeless if they do not have a stable housing situation to which they can return. A recognition of the instability of an individual's living arrangements is critical to the definition of homelessness (HRSA, 1999; NHCHC, 2017).

Programs funded by the U.S. Department of Housing and Urban Development (HUD) use a different, more limited definition of homelessness that is restricted to individuals living on the streets or in shelters. Advocates of homeless states that HUD needs to expand its definition to allow communities flexibility in providing cost-effective housing and support services to this currently underserved group.

Clinical Practice Guidelines

With the start of the new millennium a group of clinicians from the National Health Care for the Homeless Council in collaboration with the Agency for Health Care Quality and Research (AHCQR) began to adapt clinical practice guidelines for patients who are considered homeless. In 2004, the National Guidelines Clearinghouse placed NHCHC-published guidelines for specific disease processes and general care of the homeless (NHCHC, 2017). There are now nine specific clinical guidelines as well as a standard clinical practice guideline to address the special challenges faced by homeless patients that may limit their ability to adhere to a plan of care (see **BOX 3-3** and **TABLE 3-2**). In addition, the NHCHC website provides information on diseases and

BOX 3-3 National Health Care for the Homeless Council Adapted Clinical Guidelines: 10 Areas of Focus

Asthma
Cardiovascular Diseases: Hypertension, Hyperlipidemia, and Heart Failure
Chlamydial or Gonococcal Infections
Chronic Pain
Diabetes Mellitus
General Recommendations for the Care of Homeless Patients
HIV/AIDS
Opioid Use Disorder
Otitis Media
Reproductive Health Care

Reproduced from NHCHC. (2017). Adapted Clinical Guidelines. Retrieved from https://www.nhchc.org/resources/clinical/adapted-clinical-guidelines/

TABLE 3-2 Health Care for Homeless Patients: Summary of Recommendations

History	Physical examination
■ Living situation ■ Prior homelessness ■ Acute/chronic illness history ■ Medications ■ Mental illness/cognitive deficit ■ Developmental/behavioral problems ■ Alcohol/nicotine/other drug use ■ Health insurance and other assistance ■ Sexual history—gender identity, sexual orientation, behaviors, partners, pregnancies, hepatitis/HIV/other STIs ■ History and current risk of ■ Legal problems/violence ■ Work history—longest time held a job, veteran status, occupational injuries/toxic exposures ■ Education level ■ Nutrition/hydration—diet, food resources, preparation skills, liquid intake ■ Cultural heritage/affiliations/supports ■ Strengths—coping skills, resourcefulness, abilities, interests	■ Comprehensive exam—at first encounter if possible ■ Serial, focused exams—for patients uncomfortable with full-body, unclothed exam at first visit ■ Special populations—victims of abuse, sexual minorities ■ Dental assessment—age-appropriate teeth, obvious caries, dental/referred pain, diabetes patients
Education, self-management	**Diagnostic tests and screening**
■ Protection from communicable diseases, risk of delayed/interrupted treatment ■ Behavioral change—individual/small group/community interventions, motivational interviewing ■ Education of shelter/clinical staff—regarding special problems/needs of homeless people	■ Baseline labs, including EKG, lipid panel, potassium and creatinine levels, HbA1c, LFTs ■ Asthma—spirometry or peak flow monitoring ■ TB screening for patients living in shelters and others at risk for tuberculosis ■ STI screening—for chlamydia, gonorrhea, syphilis, HIV, HBV, HCV, and trichomonas ■ Mental health—Patient Health Questionnaire (PHQ-9, PHQ-2), MHS-III, MDQ ■ Substance abuse—SSI-AOD ■ Cognitive assessment—Mini-Mental Status Examination (MMSE) ■ Developmental assessment ■ Interpersonal violence—Posttraumatic Diagnostic Scale ■ Forensic evaluation—if strong evidence of child abuse ■ Healthcare maintenance—cancer screening for adults, EPSDT for children

TABLE 3-2 Health Care for Homeless Patients: Summary of Recommendations *(continued)*

Medications	**Follow-up/Outreach and Engagement**
■ Simple regimen—low pill count, once-daily dosing where possible ■ Storage/access—in clinic/shelters; if no access to refrigeration, don't prescribe meds that require it. ■ Patient assistance—entitlement assistance, free/low-cost drugs if readily available for continued use ■ Aids to adherence—harm reduction, outreach/case management, directly observed therapy	■ Contact information—phone, email for patient/friend/family/case manager ■ Medical home—to coordinate/promote continuity of health care ■ Frequent follow-up, incentives, nonjudgmental care regardless of adherence ■ Drop-in system—Anticipate/accommodate unscheduled clinic visits ■ Transportation assistance—provide car fare, tokens, help with transportation services ■ Outreach, case management ■ Referrals—linkage with specialists, providers sensitive to underserved populations
Associated Problems and Complications	**Model of Care**
■ No place to heal—efficacy of medical respite/recuperative care, supportive housing ■ Fragmented care—multiple providers ■ Masked symptoms/misdiagnosis ■ Developmental discrepancies ■ Functional impairments—assist with SSI/SSDI applications ■ Dual diagnoses—integrated treatment for concurrent mental illness/substance use disorders ■ Loss of child custody - support for parent of child abused by others, and for abused parent	■ Integrated, interdisciplinary—coordinated medical, dental, and psychosocial services ■ Therapeutic ■ Multiple points of service ■ Flexible service system—walk-ins permitted, help with resolving systems barriers ■ Outreach sites—streets, soup kitchens, shelters, other homeless service sites ■ Clinical standard guidelines ■ Consumer and peer involvement ■ Access to supportive housing

Modified from Bonin, E., Brehove, T., Carlson, C., Downing, M., Hoeft, J. Kalinowski, A., . . . Post, P. (2010). Adapting your practice: General recommendations for the care of homeless patients. Nashville: Health Care for the Homeless Clinicians' Network, National Health Care for the Homeless Council, Inc. Retrieved from http://www.nhchc.org/wp-content/uploads/2011/09/GenRecsHomeless2010.pdf

conditions including but not limited to cognitive impairments, cold- and heat-related injuries, mental health, oral health, trauma, infectious disease, and end-of-life care.

Barriers to Health Care for the Homeless

Homeless populations face many barriers to healthcare services. Financial barriers and ability to get health insurance are obvious. Transportation to medical appointments is problematic; and competing needs for food, shelter, and money take priority.

Homeless individuals suffering from mental illness may be paranoid, disorganized, have nontraditional health beliefs, lack social support, and fear authority figures. Conditions living on the street make adherence to medical care problematic in terms of medication storage, inadequate sanitation, and poor nutrition (Montauk, 2006). To help homeless individuals overcome some of these barriers, nurse practitioners must work with a team of healthcare professionals poised to meet this population's unique circumstances. Federal efforts to provide care to homeless populations include bringing services to where homeless populations gather such as shelters, parks, soup kitchens, transportation centers, and places of worship. Outreach teams such as the aforementioned most often are based in healthcare centers where patients can be referred for additional care. Providing bus tokens for transportation, free medication, and a walk-in appointment system are other examples of strategies that can help remove obstacles to care.

Building trust is paramount and can be established by emphasizing patient strengths and capacity. Acknowledging that patients kept their appointment or took medication prescribed are examples of basic patient assets that should be recognized. The NHCHC guidelines point out that just meeting survival needs while homeless takes resourcefulness, patience, and tenacity.

Substance Use Disorders and Addiction

Substance use is a major public health problem in the United States. According to the Substance Abuse and Mental Health Services Administration (SAMHSA), 10.1% of people age 12 years or older used illicit drugs in the past month, and 7.8% had a substance use disorder (SUD) in the past year (SAMHSA, 2015). Substance use disorders can mimic or coexist with other medical and mental health disorders; and nurse practitioners are in a unique position to provide screening for, urgent care to, and continuity of care for individuals and families who are at risk. Recurrent use of alcohol, tobacco, cannabis, stimulants, hallucinogens, and opioids can have devastating consequences causing clinically significant impairment, including health problems, disability, and failure to meet major responsibilities at work, school, or home. Reducing SUDs and related problems among adults is critical for mental and physical health, safety, and quality of life. Alcohol use in the United States remains the most widely abused, with marijuana and illicit drug use (including nonmedical use of prescription painkillers) most prevalent (see **FIGURE 3-2**).

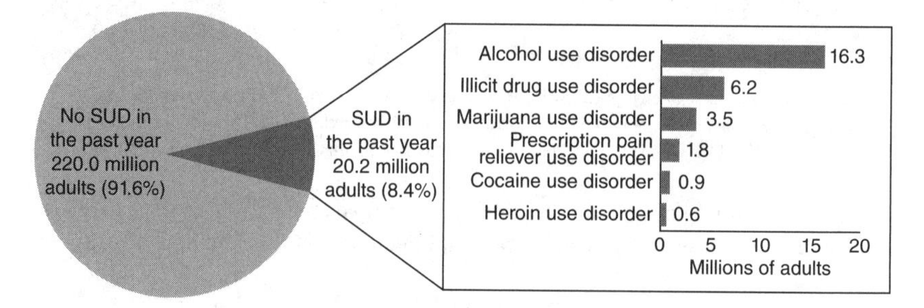

FIGURE 3-2 Trends in Substance Use Disorders

Reproduced from SAMHSA. (2017, June 29). Trends in substance use disorders among adults aged 18 or older. The CBHSQ Report. Retrieved from https://www.samhsa.gov/data/sites/default/files/report_2790/ShortReport-2790.html. Data from SAMHSA, Center for Behavioral Health Statistics and Quality, National Survey on Drug Use and Health (NSDUH), 2014.

Impact on Patients

Patients with SUD and addiction have health, emotional, family, social, legal, and spiritual issues that can be troublesome to the patient, the family, and the healthcare provider. Major vulnerabilities include overdose, withdrawal symptoms, unintentional injuries, unintended pregnancy, neonatal complications, long-term health sequela, and disruption to the family unit. SUD is a constellation of cognitive, behavioral, and physiological symptoms that an individual displays but continues to use a harmful substance despite the associated negative consequences. The *Diagnostic and Statistical Manual of Mental Disorders, Fifth Edition* (*DSM-5*), no longer uses the terms *substance abuse* and *substance dependence*; rather, it refers to substance use disorders, which are defined as mild, moderate, or severe to indicate the level of severity, which is determined by the number of diagnostic criteria met by an individual (SAMHSA, 2015).

Addiction

According to the American Society of Addiction Medicine (ASAM, 2017), addiction is a primary, chronic disease of brain reward, motivation, memory, and related circuitry. Dysfunction in these circuits leads to an individual pathologically pursuing reward and/or relief by substance use and other behaviors. Addiction is characterized by the inability to consistently abstain from and control behavior and cravings. It is characterized with diminished recognition of significant problems with one's behaviors and interpersonal relationships, and a dysfunctional emotional response (see **FIGURE 3-3**). Like other chronic diseases, addiction often involves cycles of relapse and remission. Without treatment or engagement in recovery activities, addiction is progressive and can result in disability or premature death. The term *dependence* implies both psychological craving and physiological symptoms of tolerance and withdrawal.

Vulnerable Populations and SUDs

In addition, the nurse practitioner must be aware of the special populations that are susceptible to substance use disorders. Adolescents are a high-risk population for marijuana, alcohol, and prescription pain medication obtained from the family medicine cabinet. Drugs used by gay men and men who have sex with men (MSM) at circuit parties can

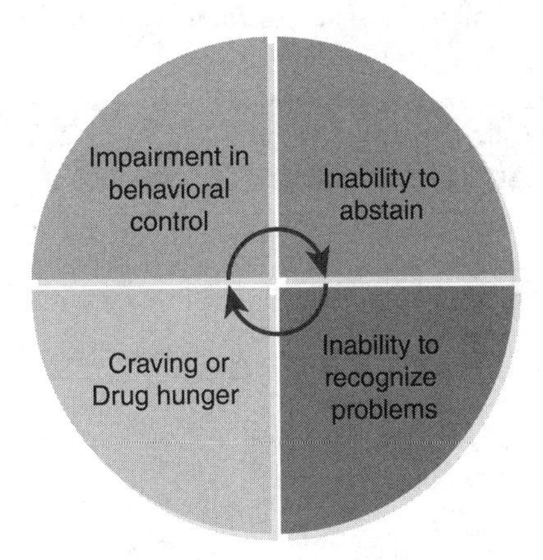

FIGURE 3-3 Characteristics of Addiction

impair judgment and result in risky sexual behavior. Adults that use illicit drugs may have a mental illness they are self-medicating for. As with any population, nurse practitioners working with the LGBT population must practice with competence and sensitivity. It is also important to recognize that chronic pain sufferers who are appropriately prescribed opioids are not substance users or necessarily considered "dependent."

Evaluation

Identifying and treating addiction or SUDs requires proactive assessment, awareness of signs and symptoms associated with abuse, the ability to develop an individual treatment plan, and the willingness to promote community-level policy change as appropriate. Important factors in deciding when and how to treat addiction include the patient's willingness to undergo treatment, social support network, health insurance coverage, financial resources, programs available in the community, and provider's skill level in treating addiction. When taking a patient history, the nurse practitioner must be cognizant of the red flags, which can provide clues to areas that will prompt further screening (see **BOX 3-4**).

Screening

The U.S. Preventative Services Task Force (USPSTF, 2014) concludes that the current evidence is insufficient to assess the balance of benefits and harms of screening adolescents, adults, and pregnant women for illicit drug use. There are, however, many self-report screening tools to assess alcohol misuse and some are validated for detecting substance abuse. The CAGE questionnaire is thought to be 60–90% sensitive when two or more responses are positive and 40–60% specific for excluding alcohol abuse. The CAGE-AID has been modified for drug use. The CRAFFT test has been validated for screening adolescents for substance-related disorders (Conners & Volk, 2004). It should be noted the screening test is less important than the actual act of the clinician asking the patient about substance use.

Management and Treatment of SUDs

Patients who are addicts continue to use substances despite negative consequences. They may be frequently reluctant to stop using even when their plight gets desperate. The nurse practitioner will be most successful in improving their patients' chances

BOX 3-4 Red Flags for Substance Abuse Disorders

- Family history of alcohol or substance abuse
- Partner who is a substance abuser
- Frequent encounters with the police
- Arrests for driving under the influence (DUIs)
- Behavior changes reported by family members
- Sudden loss of job, financial problems
- Absence from school and work
- Depression or anxiety
- Sleep problems
- Complaints of sexual dysfunction

for change by understanding their desire to stop or reduce use. The NP can use a wide variety of therapeutic options including but not limited to brief motivational interventions, cognitive behavioral therapy, and targeted pharmacological treatment. Assuring medical and psychological stability is of paramount importance. Decisions regarding outpatient versus inpatient interventions must be considered carefully and long-term monitoring and follow-up care in the community should be part of the treatment plan. Obviously family members and friends are almost always impacted by the addicted patient's tobacco, alcohol, and/or drug use so that the nurse practitioner is in a key position to influence family dynamics and refer patients and families to support programs such as Al-Anon, Nar-Anon, or Alateen.

Refugee and Immigrant Health

The United Nations High Commission for Refugees (UNHCR, 2017) reports an unprecedented 65.6 million people around the world have been forced from home. Among them are nearly 22.5 million refugees, over half of whom are under the age of 18. Refugees, by definition, are fleeing their countries due to a well-founded fear of being persecuted "for reasons of race, religion, nationality, membership in a particular social group, or political opinion" (CDC, 2013).

By definition, asylum seekers have submitted a claim for refugee status and are waiting for this claim to be accepted or rejected. Refugees and asylees comprise the majority of displaced persons resettled to the United States (CDC, 2013). In the new millennium, nurse practitioners can contribute to improving the quality of life for displaced families, refugees, and immigrants by understanding the needs of new immigrants.

Top Countries of Origin

In 2016, the Syrian Arab Republic was the most common country of origin with some 824,400 newly recognized refugees fleeing the conflict there. Crises in sub-Saharan Africa led to new displacements with almost 737,400 from South Sudan. The next largest numbers of new refugees were from Burundi, Iraq, Nigeria, and Eritrea (UNHCR, 2016).

Major Host Countries

According to UNHCR, for the third consecutive year, Turkey hosted the largest number of refugees worldwide, with 2.9 million people (2016). It was followed by Pakistan (1.4 million), Lebanon (1 million), the Islamic Republic of Iran (979,400), Uganda (940,800), and Ethiopia (791,600) (see **FIGURE 3-4**). In 2016, UNHCR referred 162,600 refugees to states for resettlement. According to government statistics, 37 countries admitted 189,300 refugees for resettlement during the year, including those resettled with UNHCR's assistance. The United States admitted the highest number (96,900) with the top states for resettlement being Nebraska, North Dakota, Idaho, Vermont, and Arizona (Lopez & Bialik, 2017).

Resettlement Issues

When refugees arrive in the United States, not only are they leaving what they know, but they are also being introduced to an entirely new culture, language, food, and

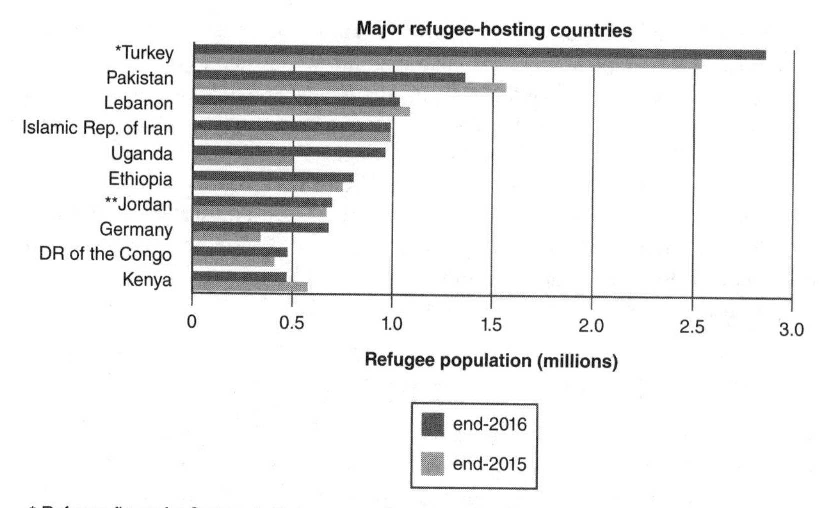

* Refugee figure for Syrians in Turkey was a Government estimate.

** Includes 33,100 Iraqi refugees registered with UNHCR in Jordan. The Government estimated the number of Iraqis at 400,000 individuals at the end of March 2015. This include refugees and other categories of Iraqis.

FIGURE 3-4 Major Host Countries

Reproduced from UNHCR. (2017). Global trends: Forced displacement in 2016. Geneva, Switzerland: Author. Retrieved from http://www.unhcr.org/globaltrends2016/

climate. To support the immediate transition, the U.S. Department of State (USDS, 2017) has cooperative agreements with national resettlement agencies to provide "Reception and Placement" services. Local affiliates of national refugee resettlement agencies arrange food, housing, clothing, employment, counseling, medical care, and other immediate needs for refugees during the first 90 days after arrival. Longer-term transitional support is also available for refugees by the Department of State's Bureau of Population, Refugees, and Migration.

Common Health Care Issues and Torture

Providing health care for resettled refugees is challenging. It requires knowledge of the healthcare and social conditions of the country of origin, attention to subtle expressions of acute and chronic illnesses, and a culturally sensitive approach to the individual and family. Historical estimates of the percentage of refugees who endure the trauma of torture have ranged between 5% and 35%. Studies of more recent waves of refugees from Somalia and Ethiopia have indicated torture prevalence rates as high as 69% (Miles & Garcia-Peltoniemi, 2012). Of immigrants from countries where torture is practiced, 6–12% say they have been tortured, but often refugees remain silent about the trauma they experienced (Miles & Garcia-Peltoniemi, 2012). Torture rates are highest in people seeking political asylum and persecution. Of asylum-seeking refugees from Somalia, Ethiopia, Eritrea, Senegal, Sierra Leone, Tibet, and Bhutan, 20–40% report being tortured (Miles & Garcia-Peltoniemi, 2012). The aftermath of witnessing and surviving cruelty and the violence of war leaves many refugees with significant symptoms of psychological distress including post-traumatic stress disorder (PTSD), depression, and anxiety (Shannon, O' Dougherty, & Mehta, 2012). Chronic pain, post-concussion syndromes, sleep disturbance, and musculoskeletal symptoms can complicate the detection of other infectious and/or chronic conditions. The NP must become astute at identifying victims of torture. Asking direct questions has high sensitivity and specificity. **TABLE 3-3** represents possible physical and psychological morbidities that individuals may have endured in their home country or refugee camp. Eliciting this information is valuable for legal medical documentation for evidence should the refugee go to court to rule on asylum status as well as to be able to properly treat and refer the individual to reduce disability, pain, and distress.

Other concurrent health problems to consider include oral health problems, tuberculosis, hepatitis B, malaria, lead poisoning, anemia, and malnutrition. Infections such as sexually transmitted diseases (STDs) or intestinal parasites are also common. The NP must evaluate risk factors and potential exposures in the countries of origin. Catchup vaccinations and cancer screenings, both routine and as indicated by various risk factors, are important parts of complete health care for refugees (CDC, 2016).

Refugee Health Profiles

Health information and refugee health profiles can be an invaluable reference which provides key health and cultural information about specific refugee groups resettling in the United States.

The refugee health profiles information is a collaborative effort between the World Health Organization, the International Organization for Migration (IOM), the United Nations High Commissioner for Refugees, the U.S. Department of State, scientific research, and other sources (CDC, 2017).

The information gleaned from the profiles is provided to assist healthcare providers, public health and resettlement agencies to facilitate medical screening, and determine appropriate interventions and services for individuals of a specific refugee group. This comprehensive resource describes the demographic, cultural, and health characteristics of the specific population. It is the responsibility of the NP to gain an understanding of where refugees come from, the circumstances of their displacement, living conditions during asylum, and health conditions for which they may be at increased risk (see **TABLE 3-4**).

TABLE 3-3 Physical and Psychological Morbidities in Refugees

Physical Morbidity	Psychological Morbidity
■ Concussive trauma ■ Suspension, hyperflexion ■ Ligatures, binding, and compression ■ Sexual torture and genital mutilation ■ Burns, electrical shock, and cutting ■ Injurious environmental factors	■ Humiliation and degradation ■ Extreme fear witnessing torture ■ Isolation ■ Sleep deprivation ■ PTSD sequela from physical torture

TABLE 3-4 Refugee Health Profiles

Refugee Topic Information	Refugee Groups Currently Represented
Priority Health Conditions Background Population Movements Healthcare and Conditions Pre-arrival Medical Screening of U.S.-bound Refugees Post-arrival Medical Screening Health Information	Bhutanese Refugees Burmese Refugees Central American (Guatemalan, Honduran, Salvadoran) Refugees Minor Refugees Congolese Refugees Iraqi Refugees Syrian Refugees

Prison Health

The United States is home to 5% of the world's population, but houses 25% of its prisoners. According to statistics from the U.S. Department of Justice (USDJ), approximately 6,899,000 Americans are under correctional supervision; 4,751,400 people were under the supervision of probation and parole, and 2,220,300 individuals were incarcerated in prisons and jails (Kaeble, Glaze, Tsoutis, & Minton, 2016). During their lifetime, 1 in 9 American men and 1 in 56 American women are likely to spend time in prison (Center for Prisoner Health and Human Rights, 2017). When factoring in racial disparities the picture becomes bleak. The statistics on race and incarceration in the United States present an alarming view of a criminal justice system in which people of color are vastly overrepresented and face harsher penalties than their white peers. With an overwhelming number of African-Americans and Latinos in the criminal justice system who already come from impoverished backgrounds, the consequences on their incarceration have a grave impact on their ability to find adequate housing, employment, and health care in the post-incarceration period. Disruption to the family unit is high, with 1.7 million children under the age of 18 having an incarcerated parent (Center for Prisoner Health and Human Rights, 2017).

Healthcare Needs of Prisoners

The healthcare needs of prisoners are diverse and cover the range of conditions found in the general population; however, there tends to be an increased ratio of incarcerated individuals who enter with health problems confounded by alcohol and substance use and a history of general poor health and self-neglect prior to their sentence. Nurse practitioners are in a unique position to intervene at three distinct periods in the incarceration timeline including identifying risk factors prior to the incarceration, providing direct care during incarceration, and lastly providing interventions following release from prison and transition into society (see **TABLE 3-5**) (Daniels, 2016).

Clinical Practice Guidelines for Prison Health

The Federal Bureau of Prisons (BOP, 2017) makes clinical practice guidelines available for the public for information purposes and transparency. There are more than 30

TABLE 3-5 Incarceration Timeline Risk Factors

Pre-Incarceration Risk Factors	Incarceration Care	Post-Incarceration Stressors
African-American Poverty Urban-centered crime Mental illness Substance abuse Homelessness Parent who was incarcerated Failure to complete high school Childhood neglect and abuse	Screening and treatment of infectious disease Health education Preventative health Management of mental health disorders Oral health Managing issues of aging prisoners Encouraging family communication Referring prisoners for internal and external services	Lack of safety net, routine and boundaries Transition issued to halfway house living Lack of housing Lack of social network Stigma of being a felon Legal barriers Lack of rehabilitation while incarcerated (i.e., acquiring job training, GED) Lack of healthcare and community services

healthcare management guidelines including but not limited to the most common health problems prison populations encounter. Infectious disease guidelines include treatment for hepatitis, HIV, MRSA, tuberculosis, and sexually transmitted infections. Mental health guidelines include treatment for depression, bipolar disorder, schizophrenia, and chemical detoxification. Guidelines for management of chronic health problems such as diabetes, asthma, hypertension, and osteoarthritis are also available. The BOP also utilizes a medication formulary, which is a list of medications that are considered to be high-quality, cost-effective drug therapy for the population served. The primary goals of formulary management are to optimize therapeutic outcomes, maintain cost-effective care, and ensure drug usage is conducive within the correctional environment.

Interventions for Reintegration Post Incarceration

Developing a community transition plan is essential for reducing vulnerabilities the prisoner may encounter post-incarceration. As patient advocates, nurse practitioners must assist individuals to achieve their highest level of health and well-being post-incarceration. When working with these populations, understanding the prison discharge process and community resources in your catchment area is essential. Often ex-offenders find themselves obtaining care through federally qualified health centers (FQHCs) in medically underserved communities. Becoming familiar with all the services a FQHC can provide under one umbrella (e.g., internal medicine, dental, mental health, women's health, pharmacy assistance) will make for increased access to services with healthcare providers skilled at working with underserved populations. Working in a team with social and outreach services the NP can assist the client to identify new social networks and resources to meet basic needs including but not limited to church groups, legal aid, and vocational services. See **BOX 3-5** for an abbreviated community transition checklist for post-incarceration.

BOX 3-5 Transitioning to Life in the Community

Community Transition Checklist for Reentry

- Housing
- Basic Living Needs
- Income Sources
- Medical Care
- Prescriptions
- Mental Health
- Substance Abuse, After Care and Maintenance
- Disability Benefits and Compensation
- Legal Aid
- Social/Community Supports
- U.S. Veteran Services
- Dental Care
- Vocational Services
- HIV/AIDS Services
- Domestic Violence
- Senior Services
- Offenders: Sex, Female, and Ex-offenders

Data from Federal Bureau of Prisons. (2002). Clinical guidelines for social work professionals: Discharge assistance. Retrieved from https://www.bop.gov/resources/pdfs/discharge.pdf

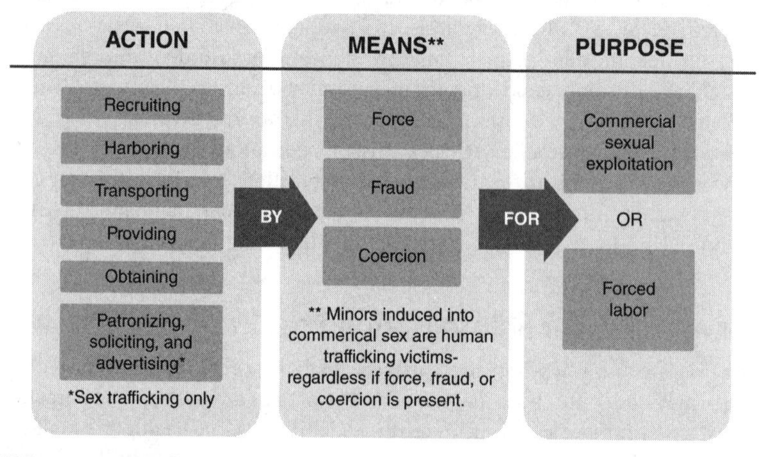

FIGURE 3-5 Human Trafficking

Reproduced from U.S. Department of Health & Human Services, Office on Trafficking in Persons. (2017). What is human trafficking? Retrieved from https://www.acf.hhs.gov/otip/about/what-is-human-trafficking

Human Trafficking

There are millions of persons across the globe who are victims of human trafficking (Morris & Vega, 2016). Human trafficking encompasses labor trafficking as well as sex trafficking and includes children, women, and men. The Office of Administration of Children and Families has within it an office that focuses on human trafficking, which likens human trafficking to modern slavery. Action, meaning, and purpose are three facets of criminal activities and exploitation, as depicted in **FIGURE 3-5**.

All of the vulnerable persons discussed in this chapter are at risk of being targeted for trafficking. Globally, there are approximately 1.2 million children being exploited for sex (Ernewein & Nieves, 2015). Human trafficking for sexual exploitation is one of the most lucrative criminal activities in our time period. Those that are brought here from other countries typically arrive in New York, Miami, or Los Angeles. However, looking within the United States we might think there are more foreign persons being exploited, but that is a false assumption. There are more U.S. citizens of all ages being trafficked within our own country (Ernewein & Nieves, 2015).

Gorenstein (2016) reported almost 88% of victims of sex trafficking visit an emergency department at some point. Nurse practitioners are therefore in a prime position to assess patients who may be victims of human trafficking. As mandatory reporters, NPs must recognize and report abuse. Providing confidentiality, safety, and a nonjudgmental manner is crucial to reduce barriers to communication.

Potential indicators of persons being trafficked include having someone with them who appears to be controlling them and the scenario, fear, sadness, bruises and other traumatic injuries, lack of documentation, poor health, discrepancy of behavior and reported age, and generally poor health (Ernewein & Nieves, 2015; Morris & Vega, 2016). Polaris Project (2016) suggests asking patients privately after assuring safety and confidentiality where they live and if they are free to come and go as they please, if they have been threatened or harmed, and if they have been forced to have sex or perform sex acts. Useful laboratory testing includes complete blood count, STD testing (including HIV), ova and parasites, hepatitis B and C, as well as tuberculosis. Nurse practitioners need to be astute at identifying the short- and long-term effects of human trafficking on individuals in order to develop a sound treatment (see **TABLE 3-6**).

Working with social services and law enforcement as a team can assist the NP to help get the victim to safety and into services to assist transitioning to safe housing with long-term treatment for psychological and medical issues. It is imperative that NPs be educated on identifying victims of human trafficking, developing culturally appropriate caring patient/provider relationships, becoming knowledgeable on reporting laws, and assisting colleagues to better identify and refer potential victims. **BOX 3-6** has a list of useful telephone numbers for victims and healthcare providers.

TABLE 3-6 Impact of Sex Trafficking on Victims

Short-Term Effects	Long-Term Effects
■ Higher risk behaviors (i.e., drug and alcohol abuse) ■ Impaired judgment ■ Emotional exhaustion ■ Depersonalization ■ Fear, anxiety, and nervousness ■ Muscle tension	■ Post-traumatic stress disorder ■ Trauma bonding ■ Severe depression ■ Suicidal ideation ■ Spiritual questions ■ Feelings of being mentally broken ■ Sexual dysfunction ■ Difficulty establishing/maintaining relationships

BOX 3-6 Telephone Numbers for Victims and Health Care Providers

- The Childhelp National Child Abuse Hotline: (800)-4ACHILD
- National Runaway Safeline: (800)-RUNAWAY
- National Human Trafficking Resource Center: (888)-373-7888

Gender Identity, Expression, and Sexual Preference

Recently a baby was born in Canada that was not given a genital inspection at the birth, which was outside the medical system, and was given a health card by the government with a "U" (unidentified/unknown) for gender/sex (Rahim, 2017). The parent, who identifies as nonbinary, transgender, wants the child to choose a gender identity when ready to. This is likely the first known documentation of an infant to not have a gender/sex assigned upon birth by the choice of the parent(s). Approximately 1.4 million people in the United States identify as transgender (Flores, Herman, Gates, & Brown, 2016). Facebook has over 60 options for choosing gender. Unfortunately, in 2016 there were at least 28 known transgender women reported killed, and the vast majority were of color (Schmider, 2016). Harassment, bullying, assault, homelessness, and health disparities are issues that lesbian, gay, bisexual, transgender, queer, questioning, and intersex (LGBTQ/QI) face daily. Nurse practitioners need to be aware of the issues surrounding children and adults whose gender identity, gender expression, and/or sexual preference(s) are different from the binary, cultural norm that the NP may be comfortable with.

Gender dysphoria is a term that defines a person who has distress with clinical symptomatology because their gender identity is not consistent with the gender assigned at birth. Terminology is critical to be familiar with, to maintain open communication with patients, potential patients, and their significant others. For some, gender may be fluid, as well as sexual partner(s) preference, meaning that one may identify more with female one day and more with male on another day, or may be more attracted to male, female, both, or none at varying times (see **TABLES 3-7** and **3-8**).

TABLE 3-7 Commonly Used Gender Identity Terminology (not all-inclusive)

Agender	Does not identify with a gender
Androgynous	Identifies as mixed or neutral gender
Bigender	Identifies as a combination of male and female gender
Cisgender	Identifies with the gender assigned at birth
Gender fluid	Gender is not static, but shifts
Genderqueer	Does not identify with a gender, falls in between or beyond gender
Pangender	Identifies as all genders

TABLE 3-8 Commonly Used Sexual Preference or Affectional Orientation Terminology (not all-inclusive)

Asexual	Not attracted to any gender
Bisexual	Attracted to male and female genders, but does not have to be at the same time or with the same intensity
Gay	A male attracted to males
Heterosexual	Attracted to a gender/sex that is not one's own
Homosexual	Attracted to the same gender/sex as one's own
Lesbian	A female attracted to females
Pansexual	Attracted to people regardless of gender, gender identity, or gender expression

Health-related disparities are significant in these populations, and sadly many do not seek health care because of fears of being judged or marginalized by healthcare providers and those working in the health system. In addition to the routine health maintenance needs for all children and adults, providers must be aware of health issues that are significantly associated with LGBTQ/QI. These issues include depression, which could be associated with gender dysphoria but may be related to other causes, anxiety, prevention, and/or treatment from being victims of bullying and violence, substance abuse, and suicide attempts. In addition, the provider must be aware of where to refer patients to appropriate mental health specialists, substance abuse counselors, HIV testing and treatment, and specialists for hormone therapy, as well as surgical options for those who are seeking these interventions. As noted earlier, transgender women of color are at high risk of being victims of violence, including homicide, so that providing education regarding safety is a priority if the patient is agreeable to discussing options.

Children and adolescents who are gender nonconforming require support and acceptance of parents/caregivers and healthcare providers (Alegria, 2011). While transient role-play of opposite gender occurs in young children, some may continue to express themselves in nonconforming genders, and a subset may continue to identify as other gender. The NP should be aware of experienced counselors and providers to refer families to so that they can have accurate information and support services if needed. This is very important if there are decisions to be made for an adolescent to transition (Alegria, 2011). It is imperative for NPs to be aware of the distress and dysphoria experienced by many as they move into puberty as this is a time when severe depression and suicidal attempts may occur (Alegria, 2011). Approximately 50% of gender nonconforming youth do not have the support of their family, and the risk of abuse, homelessness, substance abuse, and sex work increases (Grossman & D'Augelli, 2007). NPs must be aware of these potential issues and provide compassionate, sincere support in these instances.

Offering an environment in the clinic/office that is safe, inclusive, and nonjudgmental is also paramount. All healthcare providers must be able to put any biases aside. Reflecting on how one views and feels about these issues in advance can help to avoid uncomfortable interactions. If one cannot put biases aside, then it is imperative to know where to refer people to for care. The clinic/office can hang a rainbow flag to show visible support. Another important item is to not assume that anyone (whether adult or child) has a partner or parent(s) who are male, female, or has one or more mothers or fathers. When approaching patients who identify or express themselves as non-cisgender, asking how they would prefer to be addressed is acceptable if done in a considerate manner. Some people may prefer "he" or "she," or perhaps "they" or "ze." Providing care to persons of all backgrounds and beliefs requires NPs to keep up to date with issues facing patients and to continue to reach out to offer assistance with compassion and honesty in a confidential and safe environment.

HIV/AIDS

Human immunodeficiency virus (HIV) and acquired immunodeficiency syndrome (AIDS) have been around for almost 100 years that we are aware of (CDC, 2017). The virus is believed to have been spread to humans from chimpanzees during the 1920s in the Republic of Congo. Yet the stigma and discrimination associated with HIV infection remains a huge concern as well as cause for many who either do not get tested and/or do not seek health care. Those most at risk for acquiring HIV globally include women, children, men who have sex with men, transgenders, injection drug users, sex workers, and prisoners. These populations are often marginalized and suffer discrimination in many parts of the world. Educating our communities and patients about HIV/AIDS can help to get more people into care early, which can increase their life span, reduce the community viral load, and decrease the stigma associated with HIV/AIDS.

In 1981, there were initial reports of five gay men who were infected with *Pneumocystis carinii* pneumonia (Gottlieb, 2001); and in 1982, there were reports of women being infected as well as reports of infections from transfusions and vertical transmission (Sepkowitz, 2001). One of the most famous cases of AIDS discrimination occurred in the 1980s. Ryan White, age 13, was infected by a blood transfusion containing HIV. His school prevented him from attending classes, due to unfounded fears of him infecting other students. The case gained much attention, which helped to educate many about HIV. Unfortunately, White died before the Ryan White Comprehensive AIDS Resources Emergency (CARE) Act was passed by Congress (HRSA, 2016), which would have protected him from discrimination.

Globally, in 2015, there were over 36.7 million people living with HIV (World Health Organization [WHO], 2016). Twenty-seven percent of newly infected people in 2015 were between the ages of 15 and 24 (Kaiser Family Foundation, 2017). In the 1990s the addition of protease inhibitors for the treatment of HIV significantly decreased morbidity and mortality of those infected with HIV. Over the past 35 years, treatment options have improved so much that there are many who view HIV infection as a chronic disease if patients adhere to medication regimens and medical monitoring and visits. However, stigma and discrimination around HIV/AIDS continues across the world and are the leading barriers to prevention and early treatment (UNAIDS, 2014).

According to the United Nations Programme on HIV/AIDS, "HIV-related stigma refers to the negative beliefs, feelings and attitudes towards people living with HIV, groups associated with people living with HIV (e.g. the families of people living with HIV) and other key populations at higher risk of HIV infection. HIV-related discrimination refers to the unfair and unjust treatment (act or omission) of an individual based on his or her real or perceived HIV status" (UNAIDS, 2014, p. 2). They have been measuring stigma faced by HIV-infected persons internationally for years. The program also guides nations and communities on best practices for reducing the stigma and discrimination facing persons living with or at risk of HIV infection. Strategies promote developing strategies Emphasis is placed on developing strategies to care for HIV-infected persons and their families, paying close attention to discrimination against women, girls, sex workers, transgenders, and drug users. Programs are targeted to specific groups represented in the community, including families, the workplace organizations, and healthcare facilities. Strengthening the legal system to protect the human rights of those infected or at risk of infection with HIV is paramount. Nurse practitioners need to educate their office/clinic staff, colleagues, and communities about the myths and facts of HIV transmission and infection. Maintaining a level of knowledge to best serve patients is the best approach, to play a part in reducing the stigma and discrimination fears surrounding HIV/AIDS.

More information on HIV/AIDS is covered in chapter eightthe Population Health chapter in this book.

Section Three: Developing Population-Based Programs for the Vulnerable

Needs Assessment for a Vulnerable Population

A *needs assessment* is the process of *identifying* and *measuring* areas for improvement in a target population, and determining the methods to achieve improvement. It is different than a list of needs. All of the populations discussed in this chapter, as well as many others not specifically addressed in this book, require initial and periodic assessments of the needs of the population within a certain community. That community may be a local, state, national, or virtual community. For example, it may be within a prison system or a school system. There are different approaches to conducting community needs assessments. All needs assessments begin with target population identification and development of an action plan.

Needs Assessment Framework and Plan

Once you have identified the population of interest, it is necessary to write out the plan, starting with bullet points to develop the framework for the needs assessment. Tasks that need to be considered include the following:

- Formulate a clear description of the population that will be the focus of the needs assessment.
- Create a rationale for why this assessment is being done: What is the purpose and what are the objectives and goals?

- Establish the current problems and the strengths of existing conditions and resources.
- Survey other agencies/organizations in the community to avoid unnecessary overlap in program activities and to identify emerging issues and new resources.
- Interview key informants and community members who have knowledge of or experience with the problem.
- Identify the stakeholders (community members, families, friends, businesses, hospitals, sports organizations, etc.).
- Determine if this needs assessment fits in with a local or state organization's mission and strategic plan. If so, will you be working with someone from that organization in developing and/or implanting the needs assessment?
- Identify who you might collaborate with for best outcomes, if appropriate. For instance, this might require an interprofessional team/committee.
- Discover how the assessment relates to local and global healthcare trends, systems, and policies with the focus on future trends, professional standards, clinical practice guidelines, etc.
- Determine barriers and gaps that exist, to address in the needs assessment.
- Recognize any available resources already in place.

Process Measures

Once you have identified the key issues that the needs assessment will address, it is necessary to decide what process measures will be utilized. For instance, is there a valid survey or questionnaire for data collection, and/or will focus groups be a part of the assessment? Interviews, community forums, public meetings, etc. are all excellent ways to collect information from the community of interest, but you must have the right questions for each key issue that the needs assessment is seeking to assess. Develop a sampling plan for a small pilot group which will help identify any problem issues that need to be redesigned or addressed prior to the larger sample needs assessment.

Gap Analysis and Results

Using appropriate statistics and analysis for the results of the needs assessment, include the following gap analysis:

- Findings about met and unmet needs from the assessment data
- Information about existing prevention services, resources, funding, and populations served
- Secondary data about availability, accessibility, and appropriateness of existing services for the target population
- Cross reference of needs with existing assets

Consider potential uses of the results; summarize the gap analysis by target population and proposed service needs. Develop an action plan to address the unmet needs of the target population. The action plan should have objectives with corresponding timelines. Short-term, intermediate, and long-term goals should be identified. Recommendations must include budgetary considerations including a cost-benefit analysis if appropriate. Be specific, including timelines and people responsible for data collection. Share this information with the key stakeholders and community members to obtain needed support for implementation of the action plan.

Chapter Summary

Given the ever-changing demographic population in the United States and demands for globalization, there is a growing body of knowledge regarding vulnerability and health disparities. Whether your interactions with vulnerable populations is a vocation or an avocation, the rewards are worth the effort put forth to improve the health of those in need. Advocacy is a key role that nurse practitioners can play to benefit patients, families, and communities alike. With advanced education, nurse practitioners have the ability to design, implement, and evaluate individual and population-focused models to ensure that the needs of the vulnerable are met.

Seminar Discussion Questions

1. Identify factors which makes a person or population vulnerable?
2. Is there a specific vulnerable population that you want to learn more about and why?
3. How would you begin developing a needs assessment on a particular vulnerable population?
4. Mary comes in to the urgent care clinic with a broken nose. She appears to be a young teen, perhaps 13 or 14, but says she is 21 years old. She is disheveled and very quiet, answering only with a few words and keeps her eyes downcast. There is a couple (man and woman) who appear to be in their 30s accompanying the girl to be treated. They continue to stare at her and refuse to leave her side. Your attending physician colleague is busy transferring a trauma patient. What are your next steps in specific order?
5. Reach out to an NP working in the prison system or with the homeless. Interview this person about how to approach patients. Does the interviewee deal with legal issues on a daily basis that impede providing health care in the manner preferred?

References

Alegria, C. A. (2011). Transgender identity and health care: Implications for psychosocial and physical evaluation. *Journal of the American Academy of Nurse Practitioners, 23*, 175–182. doi:10.1111/j.1745-7599.2010.00595.x

American Society of Addiction Medicine. (2017). *Public policy statement: Definition of addiction/short definition of addiction.* Retrieved from https://www.asam.org/resources/definition-of-addiction

Basch, C. H. (2014). Poverty, health, and social justice: The importance of public health approaches. *International Journal of Health Promotion and Education, 52*(4), 181–187. doi:10.1080/14635240.2014.894669

Borrowman, M. (2012). Understanding elderly poverty in the U.S.: Alternative measures of elderly deprivation. Schwartz Center for Economic Analysis and Department of Economics, The New School for Social Research, Working Papers Series.

Centers for Disease Control. (2013). *Immigrant and refugee health. Refugee health guidelines.* Retrieved from https://www.cdc.gov/immigrantrefugeehealth/guidelines/refugee-guidelines.html

Centers for Disease Control. (2016a). *Adverse childhood experiences.* Retrieved from https://www.cdc.gov/violenceprevention/acestudy/about_ace.html

Centers for Disease Control. (2016b). *Immigrant and refugee health. Evaluating and updating immunizations during the domestic medical examination for newly arrived refugees.* Retrieved from http://refugeehealthta.org/physical-mental-health/health-conditions/

Centers for Disease Control. (2017a). *HIV/AIDS*. Retrieved from https://www.cdc.gov/hiv/basics/whatishiv.html

Centers for Disease Control. (2017b). QuickStats: Age-adjusted death rates, by race/ethnicity—National Vital Statistics System, United States, 2014–2015. *Morbidity and Mortality Weekly Report, 66*, 375. Retrieved from https://www.cdc.gov/mmwr/volumes/66/wr/mm6613a6.htm

Centers for Disease Control. (2017c). *Refugee health profiles*. Retrieved from https://www.cdc.gov/immigrantrefugeehealth/profiles/index.html

Center for Prisoner Health and Human Rights. (2017). *Incarceration in the United States*. Retrieved from http://www.prisonerhealth.org/educational-resources/factsheets-2/incarceration-in-the-united-states/

Clarke, D., Schulman, E., McCollum, D., & Felitti, V. (2015). *Clinical approaches for adult ACE survivors experiencing unexplained physical symptoms and health problems*. Retrieved from http://www.avahealth.org/aces_best_practices/clinical-approaches-for-adults.html

Connors, G. J., & Volk, R. J. (2004). *Self-report screening for alcohol problems among adults*. Retrieved from https://pubs.niaaa.nih.gov/publications/AssessingAlcohol/selfreport.htm

Conway, C. (2016). *UCSF news brief. Poor health: When poverty becomes a disease*. Retrieved from https://www.ucsf.edu/news/2016/01/401251/poor-health

Cubanski, J., Casillas, G., & Damico, A. (2015). Poverty among seniors: An updated analysis of national and state level poverty rates under the official and supplemental poverty measures. *The Henry J. Kaiser Family Foundation*. Retrieved from http://files.kff.org/attachment/issue-brief-poverty-among-seniors-an-updated-analysis-of-national-and-state-level-poverty-rates-under-the-official-and-supplemental-poverty-measures; https://www.healthypeople.gov/2020/data-search/Search-the-Data#topic-area=3499

Daniels, J. (2016). Negotiating the world: Nursing interventions for a vulnerable prison population before and after parole. In M. De Chesnay & B. A. Anderson (Eds.), *Caring for the vulnerable: Perspective in nursing theory, practice, and research* (4th ed., chap. 25, pp. 365–380). Sudbury, MA: Jones and Bartlett Publishers.

de Chesnay, M., & Anderson, B. A. (2016). *Caring for the vulnerable: Perspectives in nursing theory, practice, and research* (4th ed.). Sudbury, MA: Jones and Bartlett Publishers.

Ernewein, C., & Nieves, R. (2015). Human sex trafficking: Recognition, treatment, and referral of pediatric victims. *Journal for Nurse Practitioners, 11*(8), 797–803.

Federal Bureau of Prisons. (2017). *Health management resources. Clinical practice guidelines*. Retrieved from https://www.bop.gov/resources/health_care_mngmt.jsp

Flores, A., Herman, J., Gates, G., & Brown, T. (2016). How many adults identify as transgender in the United States. *The Williams Institute*. Retrieved from https://williamsinstitute.law.ucla.edu/research/how-many-adults-identify-as-transgender-in-the-united-states/

Gorenstein, D. (2016). *Health care takes on the fight against trafficking*. Retrieved from http://www.marketplace.org/2016/03/02/health-care/health-care-takes-fight-against-trafficking

Gottlieb, M. S. (2001). AIDS—Past and future. *New England Journal of Medicine, 344*, 1788–1791.

Grabovschi, C., Loignon, C., & Fortin, M. (2013). Mapping the concept of vulnerability related to health care disparities: A scoping review. *BMC Health Services Research, 13*(1), 1.

Grossman, A. H., & D'Augelli, A. R. (2007). Transgender youth and life-threatening behaviors. *Suicide and Life-Threatening Behavior, 37*, 527–537. doi:10.1521/suli.2007.37.5.527

Healthy People 2020 [Internet]. Washington, DC: U.S. Department of Health and Human Services, Office of Disease Prevention and Health Promotion [cited September 16, 2017]. Retrieved from https://www.healthypeople.gov/2020/topics-objectives/topic/social-determinants-of-health.

Homeless Clinician's Network. (2010). *Adapting your practice: General recommendations for the care of homeless patients*, pp. ix–x. Retrieved from http://www.nhchc.org/wp-content/uploads/2011/09/GenRecsHomeless2010.pdf

HRSA. (2016). *About the Ryan White HIV/AIDS program*. Retrieved from https://hab.hrsa.gov/about-ryan-white-hivaids-program/about-ryan-white-hivaids-program

HRSA/Bureau of Primary Health Care (1999). Program assistance letter 99-12. *Health Care for the Homeless Principles of Practice*. Retrieved from https://bphc.hrsa.gov/policiesregulations/policies/pal199912.pdf

Kaeble, D., Glaze, L., Tsoutis, A., & Minton, T. (2016). *U.S. Department of Justice: Correctional populations in the United States, 2014*. Retrieved from https://www.bjs.gov/content/pub/pdf/cpus14.pdf

Kaiser Family Foundation. (2017). *The global HIV/AIDS epidemic*. Retrieved from http://www.kff.org/global-health-policy/fact-sheet/the-global-hivaids-epidemic/

Kutner, M., Greenberg, E., Jin, Y., & Paulsen, C. (2006). *The health literacy of America's adults: Results from the 2003 National Assessment of Adult Literacy* (NCES 2006–483). U.S. Department of Education. Washington, DC: National Center for Education Statistics.

Lopez, G., & Bialik, K. (2017). *Key findings about U.S. immigrants*. Retrieved from http://www.pewresearch.org/fact-tank/2017/05/0 key-findings-about-u-s-immigrants/

Marmot, M. (2005). Social determinants of health inequalities. *Lancet, 365,* 1099–1104.

Miles, S. H., & Garcia-Peltoniemi, R. E. (2012). Torture survivors: What to ask, how to document. *Journal of Family Practice, 61*(4), E1–E5.

Montauk, S. L. (2006). The homeless in America: Adapting your practice. *American Family Physician, 74*(7), 1132–1142.

Morris, R., & Vega, C. (2016). Detecting human trafficking: Guidelines for clinicians. *Medscape*. Retrieved from http://www.medscape.org/viewarticle/859358

National Alliance to End Homelessness. (2016). *The of state of homelessness America: An examination of trends in homelessness, homeless assistance, and at-risk populations at the national and state levels*. Retrieved from https://endhomelessness.org/homelessness-in-america/homelessness-statistics/state-of-homelessness-report

National Center for Children in Poverty. (2017). *Child poverty*. Retrieved from http://www.nccp.org/topics/childpoverty.html

National Health Care for the Homeless Council. (2017a). *What is the official definition of homelessness?* Retrieved from https://www.nhchc.org/faq/official-definition-homelessness/

National Health Care for the Homeless Council. (2017b). *Adapting your practice: Treatment and recommendations for homeless patients*. Retrieved from https://www.nhchc.org/resources/clinical/adapted-clinical-guidelines/

Orthner, D. (2004). The resilience and strengths of low-income families/Low-income and working-poor families. *Family Relations, 53*(2), S159–S167.

Pacquiao, D. F. (2008). Nursing care of vulnerable populations using a framework of cultural competence, social justice and human rights. *Contemporary Nurse, 28,* 189–197.

Pearson, G. S., Hines-Martin, V. P., Evans, L. K., York, J. A., Kane, C. F., & Yearwood, E. L. (2015). Addressing gaps in mental health needs of diverse, at-risk, underserved, and disenfranchised populations: A call for nursing action. *Archives of Psychiatric Nursing, 29,* 14–18.

Polaris Project. (2016). 2016 Statistics from the National Human Trafficking Hotline and BeFree Textline. Retrieved from http://www.polarisproject.org/ resources/hotline-statistics/human-trafficking-trends-in-the-United States

Proctor, B. D., Semegaand, J. L., & Kollar, M. A. (2015). U.S. Census Bureau, Current Population Reports, P60-256(RV), *Income and poverty in the United States: 2015*. Washington, DC: U.S. Government Printing Office. Retrieved from https://www.census.gov/content/dam/Census/library/publications/2016/demo/p60-256.pdf

Rahim, Z. (2017). Canadian baby given health card without sex designation. *CNN*. Retrieved from http://www.cnn.com/2017/07/04/health/canadian-baby-gender-designation/index.html

Schmider, A. (2016). 2016 was the deadliest year on record for transgender people. *GLADD*. Retrieved from https://www.glaad.org/blog/2016-was-deadliest-year-record-transgender-people

Septowitz, K. (2001). AIDS—The first 20 years. *New England Journal of Medicine, 344,* 1764–1772. doi:10.1056/NEJM200106073442306. Retrieved from http://www.nejm.org/doi/full/10.1056/NEJM200106073442306#t=article

Shannon, P., O' Dougherty, M., & Mehta, E. (2012). Refugees' perspectives on barriers to communication about trauma histories in primary care. *Mental Health in Family Medicine, 9,* 47–55.

Substance Abuse and Mental Health Services Administration (SAMHSA). (2015). *Substance use disorders*. Retrieved from https://www.samhsa.gov/disorders/substance-use

UNAIDS. (2014). *Reduction of HIV-related stigma and discrimination*. Retrieved from http://www.unaids.org/sites/default/files/media_asset/2014unaidsguidancenote_stigma_en.pdf

United Nations High Commissioner for Refugees. (2016). *Global trends: Forced displacement in 2016*. Retrieved http://www.unhcr.org/en-us/statistics/unhcrstats/5943e8a34/global-trends-forced-displacement-2016.html

United Nations High Commissioner for Refugees. (2017). *Statistical year book 2015*. Retrieved from http://www.unhcr.org/en-us/statistics/country/59b294387/unhcr-statistical-yearbook-2015-15th-edition.html

U.S. Department of Health and Human Services. (2017a). *Office of Disease Prevention and Health Promotion quick guide to health literacy*. Retrieved from https://health.gov/communication/literacy/quickguide/Quickguide.pdf

U.S. Department of Health and Human Services, Office on Trafficking in Persons. (2017b). *What is human trafficking?* Retrieved from https://www.acf.hhs.gov/otip/about/what-is-human-trafficking

U.S. Department of State. (2017). *The reception and placement program*. Retrieved from https://www.state.gov/j/prm/ra/receptionplacement/index.htm

U.S. Preventative Services Task Force. (2014). *Final recommendation statement: Drug use, illicit: Screening*. Retrieved from https://www.uspreventiveservicestaskforce.org/Page/Document/RecommendationStatementFinal/drug-use-illicit-screening

Warne, D., & Lajimodiere, D. (2015). *American Indians health disparities: Psychosocial influences*. Hoboken, NJ: John Wiley & Sons, Ltd.

World Health Organization. (2017). *Social determinants of health*. Retrieved from http://www.who.int/social_determinants/en/

Yang, J., Granja, M. R., & Koball, H. (2017). *Basic facts about low-income children. Children under 6 years, 2015*. Retrieved from http://www.nccp.org/topics/childpoverty.html

CHAPTER 4

Mental Health and Primary Care: A Critical Intersection

Brandi Parker Cotton

Nurse practitioners (NPs) routinely provide services to vulnerable populations. The unique needs of individuals suffering from acute and chronic mental illness, substance use disorder, homelessness, and intimate partner violence must be addressed in order to provide comprehensive care. Nurse practitioners across diverse practice settings and geographical locations are well positioned at the forefront of clinical care. Susceptible to a wide range of physical, mental, and psychosocial challenges, patients often present with complex symptomatology and complicated differential diagnoses that are among the most challenging in clinical practice.

Untreated mental health symptoms potentially result in problems securing and maintaining employment and may create financial struggles that lead to housing instability and homelessness. Access to care is a prevailing issue; limited social and financial resources create challenges in navigating complex healthcare systems and pose logistical problems, such as travelling to and from appointments and managing co-pays for provider visits and laboratory testing. Psychiatric symptoms, such as those reported during depressive episodes, affect not only the individual but also significantly the nation's economy (Stewart, Ricci, Chee, Hahn, & Morganstein, 2003). It is widely accepted that depression is a leading cause of absenteeism in the workforce (Stewart et al., 2003). Researchers estimated that approximately $31 billion is lost on reduced productivity when employees struggle with depression (Stewart et al., 2003).

Health Disparities in Mental Health

Health disparities are a critical issue within the context of mental health. For example, access to—and satisfaction with—mental health services vary considerably by race and ethnicity (Carpenter-Song, Whitely, Lawson, Quimby, & Drake, 2011). African-Americans, when compared to other minority groups, are the most unsatisfied with services and receive less mental health treatment than other minority groups. White Americans are 1.5 times more likely to receive mental health or substance abuse services than either African-Americans or Latinos (Carpenter-Song et al., 2011; Wells, Klap, Koike, & Sherbourne, 2001). Additionally, case management services are also underutilized by minority groups (Barrio et al., 2003; Carpenter-Song et al., 2011) and African-Americans are more likely to be involuntarily hospitalized than White Americans with equally severe mental illness. A recent study of justice-involved adolescents serving in long-term residential facilities found considerable racial disparities in diagnoses of conduct disorder and attention-deficit hyperactivity disorder (ADHD) between white and black adolescents; black adolescents were more likely to be diagnosed with conduct disorder (40% for males; 54% for females) and whites were 40% more likely to receive a diagnosis of ADHD when compared to black adolescents. Even more troubling is the fact that black males were 32% less likely to receive psychiatric treatment when compared to white males (Baglivio, Wolff, Piquero, Greenwald, & Epps, 2017).

Especially relevant to NPs, this research suggests that the majority of disparate care is occurring when patients receive mental health services within the primary care setting. The U.S. Department of Health and Human Services (USDHHS) identified four areas of health disparity in mental health treatment, including limited availability and access to care, less likelihood of receiving needed care, poorer quality of care, and the fact that minorities are not adequately represented in research (Carpenter-Song et al., 2011; USDHHS, 2001). The Dartmouth-Howard Collaboration was created to better understand the disparities that exist within the mental health system. The collaborative goals of this multidisciplinary team include the following:

> (1) situating disparity research in the context of social justice; (2) understanding the trends in disparities; (3) promoting a sophisticated understanding of "culture" and its role in disparities; (4) critically assessing strategies that attempt to mitigate disparities; and (5) developing a reflexive research agenda. (Carpenter-Song et al., 2011)

Several suggestions have been proposed to deal with this challenge. Addressing racial disparities within clinical education would promote a greater capacity for culture competency. For example, training medical professionals on diverse help-seeking behaviors and diversity within groups would assist in avoiding stereotypes that create barriers to mental health treatment (Carpenter-Song et al., 2011). Another proposed suggestion is increasing diversity among professionals in the mental health field through academic admissions policies, ameliorating financial barriers to mental health professional trainings, and using accreditation efforts to promote institutional diversity (Carpenter-Song et al., 2011).

▸ Patients with Co-occurring Disorders

Consider the following patient scenario:

> Adrian presents to the NP for refills on his sertraline and bupropion. He is diagnosed with recurrent major depressive disorder and has been

medicated with various antidepressants for the past 3 years. Today he complains that "the medications aren't working." He is reporting depression, irritability, insomnia, fatigue, and thoughts of self-harm. He denies any recent stressors and reports he is adherent to the prescribed medication regimen. Having denied on several occasions any history of substance abuse, the NP requests a urine toxicology screen to rule out a co-occurring substance abuse disorder. The results are positive for cocaine metabolites. The NP discusses the results with Adrian and refers him to a substance-abuse treatment program, explaining that his symptoms will likely not improve while he is actively using cocaine. Adrian refuses to attend the treatment program, asserting that he is a "recreational user" and "clearly not addicted."

Patients with co-occurring diagnoses (at least one mental health diagnosis plus substance abuse) are among the most vulnerable populations. Patients with psychiatric diagnoses are at increased risk for substance abuse problems. The National Alliance on Mental Illness (NAMI) estimates that as many as 50% of all individuals with psychiatric diagnoses also meet criteria for substance use disorders (Substance Abuse and Mental Health Services Administration [SAMHSA], n.d.). Self-medicating with illegal substances while experiencing medically untreated or undertreated mental illness often leads to substance use disorders that exacerbate existing mental health conditions and symptomatology (Santucci, 2012). Predictably, antisocial behaviors are potentially exacerbated with substance use, and can lead to increased criminal activity and involvement with the criminal justice system. Suicide risk is also increased for this population (National Association of Mental Illness, 2003).

General risk factors are often present for both mental illness and substance use; substance use may be secondary to a psychiatric disorder, but a psychiatric disorder may also develop secondary to substance abuse. Commonly, dual-diagnosis is *bidirectional*, meaning each contributes to each other (Santucci, 2012). Practitioners should exercise caution when assessing routine patients for mental illness, carefully distinguishing symptoms present and absent during prolonged periods of sobriety and the possible effect of a substance use disorder on cognitive functioning, behaviors, and mood. Research findings are discovering the benefits of improved collaborative care for dually diagnosed patients, asserting that treatment compliance and patient outcomes improve when care is less fragmented (Santucci, 2012).

Parents with substance use disorders (SUD) are a unique subset of an at-risk cohort. Substance abuse is the most common reason for out-of-home placement for children (Suchman, McMahon, Zhang, Mayes, & Luthar, 2006). Factors most strongly associated with children's out-of-home placement are severity of parental substance use disorder as well as parental psychosocial maladjustment (Suchman et al., 2006). Out-of-home placement is also more prevalent among women with SUD who have experienced childhood adverse events (e.g., exposure to violence, physical or sexual abuse, or other factors such as teen pregnancy and unemployment) (Suchman et al., 2006). These risk factors emphasize the importance of confounding variables that place families at increased risk for further traumatization and destabilization.

In 2001, the Substance Abuse and Mental Health Services Administration created National Outcome Measures (NOM) for individuals with co-occurring disorders. The efforts to improve treatment interventions led to the development of 10 domains that are used to measure the efficacy of services and treatment modalities: reduced morbidity, employment/education, crime and criminal justice, stability in housing, social connectedness, access/capacity, retention, perception of care, cost effectiveness, and use of evidence-based practices (http://www.samhsa.gov/co-occurring/topics/data/nom.aspx). NOM reflect the interconnectedness of substance use and the psychosocial factors influencing addictive behaviors (SAMHSA, n.d.).

The past decade has produced considerable research on both screening and treatment for substance abuse (Carroll, 2005). Several approaches have proven to be effective, including a method of therapy known as contingency management (CM), a theory based on the fundamental principle of psychology that reinforced behaviors are likely to be repeated (Carroll, 2005). Higgins and Silverman conducted a research study exploring the efficacy of CM with statistically significant treatment results after offering rewards in the form of goods and services in exchange for periods of sobriety (Carroll, 2005). The results proved effective in promoting periods of abstinence based on the behavioral principle of positive reinforcements. CM has also proved efficacious when used in other health domains. One study proved that CM was effective in increasing medication adherence to antiretrovirals in HIV-positive persons (Carroll, 2005), indicating that its usage in promoting positive behavioral changes can potentially address a multitude of diverse health problems.

Motivational interviewing (MI) (Miller & Moyers, 2017; Miller, Benefield, & Tonigan, 1993) is another treatment model that has earned its place within evidence-based practice for the treatment of SUD. MI has an added benefit in that it can be implemented in relatively short amounts of time, positioning it well within the primary care practice (Carroll, 2005). Please refer to **EXHIBITS 4-1** and **4-2** for self report screening tools that can facilitate the MI process and treatment goals. Studies have shown encouraging results for promoting sobriety among individuals struggling with opioid, cocaine, and marijuana dependencies (Carroll, 2005). The structural components of motivational interviewing allow it to stretch beyond the limits of substance abuse. Similar to contingency management, MI has also been proven successful when applied to a variety of treatments. For example, MI has successfully increased adherence to antiretroviral medications among HIV-infected persons (Golin et al., 2012), improved glycemic outcomes in type II diabetes mellitus (Chen, Creedy, Lin, & Wollin, 2012), and weight loss among Latino females using culturally sensitive techniques (Corsino et al., 2012). These cross-sectional research findings suggest that such treatment modalities could potentially demonstrate far reaching effects on large-scale public health issues.

Finally, medication-assisted treatment for opioid use disorders is becoming more common in the primary care setting. Medications such as buprenorphine (Suboxone), a partial opioid agonist, is used in both primary and mental health clinics to reduce the use of illicit opioids. Taken daily, buprenorphine prevents opiate withdrawal by administering a long-acting opioid formula which does not produce euphoria but prevents opioid withdrawal. Also used to treat opioid use disorder is long-acting naltrexone (Vivitrol), an opioid antagonist which blocks the opioid receptor. Considering the current rise in opioid use disorders, the prescribing of these medications is likely to become even more common within the primary care setting.

EXHIBIT 4-1 The Alcohol Use Disorders Identification Test: Self-Report Version

PATIENT: Because alcohol use can affect your health and can interfere with certain medications and treatments, it is important that we ask some questions about your use of alcohol. Your answers will remain confidential so please be honest. Place an X in one box that best describes your answer to each question.

Questions	0	1	2	3	4
1. How often do you have a drink containing alcohol?	Never	Monthly or less	2–4 times a month	2–3 times a week	4 or more times a week
2. How many drinks containing alcohol do you have on a typical day when you are drinking?	1 or 2	3 or 4	5 or 6	7 to 9	10 or more
3. How often do you have six or more drinks on one occasion?	Never	Less than monthly	Monthly	Weekly	Daily or almost daily
4. How often during the last year have you found that you were not able to stop drinking once you had started?	Never	Less than monthly	Monthly	Weekly	Daily or almost daily
5. How often during the last year have you failed to do what was normally expected of you because of drinking?	Never	Less than monthly	Monthly	Weekly	Daily or almost daily

(continues)

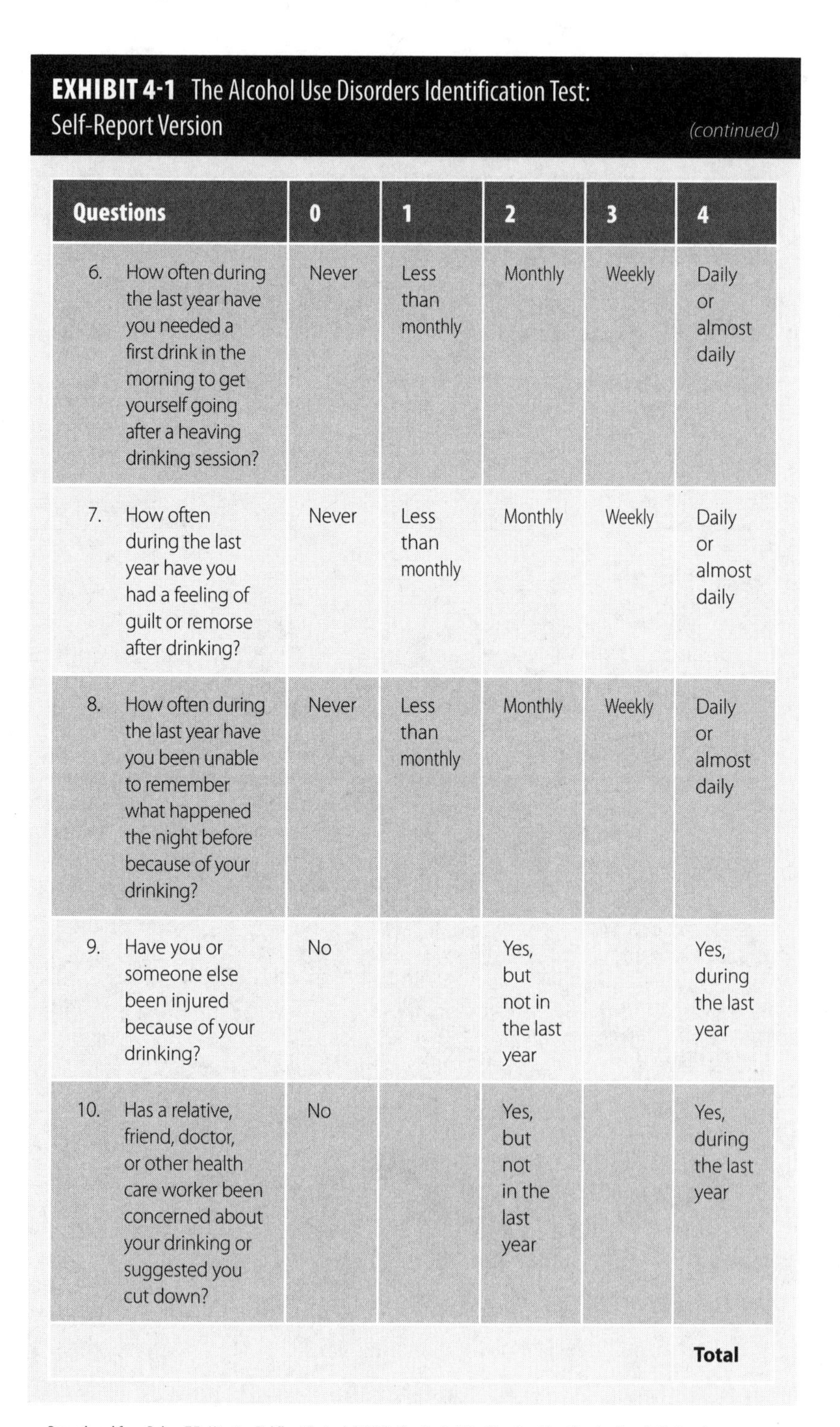

EXHIBIT 4-1 The Alcohol Use Disorders Identification Test: Self-Report Version *(continued)*

Questions	0	1	2	3	4
6. How often during the last year have you needed a first drink in the morning to get yourself going after a heaving drinking session?	Never	Less than monthly	Monthly	Weekly	Daily or almost daily
7. How often during the last year have you had a feeling of guilt or remorse after drinking?	Never	Less than monthly	Monthly	Weekly	Daily or almost daily
8. How often during the last year have you been unable to remember what happened the night before because of your drinking?	Never	Less than monthly	Monthly	Weekly	Daily or almost daily
9. Have you or someone else been injured because of your drinking?	No		Yes, but not in the last year		Yes, during the last year
10. Has a relative, friend, doctor, or other health care worker been concerned about your drinking or suggested you cut down?	No		Yes, but not in the last year		Yes, during the last year
					Total

Reproduced from Babor, T.F., Higgins-Biddle, J.C. et. al. (2001). *The Alcohol Use Disorders Identification Test: Guidelines for use in primary care* (2nd ed.). The Alcohol Use Disorders Identification Test: Self-Report Version (pp. 31, Box 10). © World Health Organization 2001.

EXHIBIT 4-2 Drug Abuse Screening Test (DAST-10)

I'm going to read you a list of questions concerning information about your potential involvement with drugs, excluding alcohol and tobacco, during the past 12 months.

When the words "drug abuse" are used, they mean the use of prescribed or over-the-counter medications/drugs in excess of the directions and any nonmedical use of drugs. The various classes of drugs may include cannabis (e.g., marijuana, hash), solvents, tranquilizers (e.g., Valium), barbiturates, cocaine, stimulants (e.g., speed), hallucinogens (e.g., LSD), and narcotics (e.g., heroin). Remember that the questions *do not include alcohol or tobacco.*

If you have difficulty with a statement, then choose the response that is mostly correct.

You may choose to answer or not answer any of the questions in this section.

These questions refer to the past 12 months:	No	Yes
1. Have you used drugs other than those required for medical reasons?		
2. Do you abuse more than one drug at a time?		
3. Are you always able to stop using drugs when you want to? (If never use drugs, answer "Yes.")		
4. Have you had "blackouts" or "flashbacks" as a result of drug use?		
5. Do you ever feel bad or guilty about your drug use? (If never use drugs, choose "No.")		
6. Does your spouse (or parents) ever complain about your involvement with drugs?		
7. Have you neglected your family because of your use of drugs?		
8. Have you engaged in illegal activities in order to obtain drugs?		
9. Have you ever experienced withdrawal symptoms (felt sick) when you stopped taking drugs?		
10. Have you had medical problems as a result of your drug use (e.g., memory loss, hepatitis, convulsions, bleeding)?		

Children and Mental Health

Assessing and diagnosing psychiatric conditions of childhood requires a comprehensive understanding of cognitive, emotional, and social developmental stages in children. Consider the following clinical case:

> A 13-year-old pubescent male reports he was suspended from school for exposing his genitals to a fellow student. The clinical picture changes considerably if the provider has knowledge that the child's full scale IQ is 62 and a corresponding developmental age of 4 years old. Consider how this scenario changes again if cognitive testing instead reveals a full scale IQ of 110 and during the interview, the child discloses a history of sexual molestation by an older female cousin. The exhibited sexualized behavior would suggest trauma reactivity.

This scenario exemplifies the importance of making a thorough assessment, history-taking, and collecting collaborative information. This is perhaps most important when treating children who may lack the ability to verbalize certain emotions, behaviors, or psychosocial stressors. Collaborative efforts such as communicating with teachers, day care workers, and referrals for neurodevelopmental testing is important for accurate diagnoses as well as treatment planning.

Consider the following clinical case:

> A nurse practitioner evaluates a 12-year-old male with a history of ADHD, currently medicated with extended-release methylphenidate. The child's elementary school has referred the child for assessment after he made repeated threats to another student. This school reports that the student ruminates obsessively over a violent video game, and school staff suspect that he may be susceptible for aggressive acts. When speaking about the video game characters, the child seems to confuse the virtual world with reality. He has repeatedly threatened peers with violent comments, the content of his speech reflecting the grotesque acts observed within the virtual video world. School has forbidden him to return to school until he receives a full psychiatric evaluation by a specialist. The nurse practitioner evaluates the child and confirms that the child exhibits circumscribed interest around the game, specifically a perseverative rigidity and inability to change conversation topics. After a lengthy evaluation, the NP learns that the child has a history of social awkwardness, is unable to read emotions and general social cues, and exhibits multiple sensory issues. The NP administers the Childhood Autism Rating Scale (CARS) and determines that the child meets diagnostic criteria for an autism spectrum disorder (ASD) diagnosis. Additionally, it becomes clear that he can successfully distinguish between virtual characters and reality. This is elucidated once the provider learns that several of the characters in this game are based on human counterparts, with actual names and personalities reflected in the virtual characters. The child successfully identifies which characters have real-life counterparts and which are fictional. He has no history of violence or aggressive behavior and denies any intentions to hurt others. He reports he is easily agitated by peers and often exhibits poor boundaries, impulsively commenting in anger and frustration without ill intent.

The NP recommends that psychotherapy include encouraging him to substitute a nonviolent and age-appropriate interest in place of his current perseveration. After parents restrict access to video games and introduce him to a variety of new activities, the child is eventually able to move past his obsession and become interested in Legos. Family therapy is recommended to provide psychoeducation regarding symptoms of an ASD diagnosis. Parents are cautioned to monitor the child's activities closely and limit his exposure to games and movies with violent content. He returns to school, receives a tailored educational plan to accommodate challenges associated with ASD symptoms, and completes a successful year.

The previous scenario illustrates the importance of a thorough assessment. Collateral information is undeniably important when treating children with psychiatric symptoms. It is also critical to remember that although a clinician may have substantial information from family members and school staff, it is not a substitution for the subjective experience reported by the child. Subjective reports and private interviewing without family members in the room allows the child to reveal clinical information that can be central to the presenting problem.

Children as Victims of Trauma

Children are dependent members of the interconnecting network of family systems, schools, and communities that create their world. Considered one of the most vulnerable populations, children possess little power to alter their environment or life circumstances. Currently, researchers are seeking to understand the implications of childhood trauma and behavioral, emotional, and physical problems that endure far into adulthood. It is widely accepted that early traumatization causes lifelong problems with relationships, learning, and overall level of functioning. The Adverse Childhood Experience study (Felitti et al., 1998) was conducted in 1998 highlighting the relationship between childhood adverse events (abuse and household dysfunction) with adult diseases and health behaviors. The study focused on the public health impact of childhood trauma. Using a standard questionnaire, adults were queried in seven categories:

1. Psychological abuse
2. Physical abuse
3. Sexual abuse
4. Violence against mother
5. Living with household members who were substance abusers
6. Family members who were mentally ill or suicidal
7. Family members with a history of imprisonment

The results of the study revealed the causal relationship between childhood traumatic events and high-risk behaviors exhibited by adults, subsequently making adults more vulnerable to disease and early death (Felitti et al., 1998). This study illustrated that abusive childhood events had a marked effect on overall adult health behaviors, revealing considerable health disparities among adults with histories of childhood trauma. A follow-up study published in 2007 measured the degree of adverse childhood experiences and adult use of psychotropic medication (Anda et al., 2007). Predictably, the study highlighted the connection between childhood trauma and mental illness in adulthood (Anda et al., 2007). Changes in the hypothalamic-pituitary-adrenal (HPA) axis have been noted secondary to traumatic events. Systemic cortisol release is important in human stress reactions and enables the body to respond to stressful stimuli, increasing the processing of glucogenesis (Ouellet-Morin et al., 2011). However, when humans are subject to chronic stress, this process can become maladaptive, with cortisol excretion occurring in excessive amounts—or released in response to nonthreatening stimuli (Ouellet-Morin et al., 2011). Animal studies have concluded that excessive cortisol and increased HPA axis reactivity cause an increased risk of depression. However, cortisol also appears to be important when HPA reactivity is reduced and cortisol response is blunted. Lower HPA reactivity is associated with difficulties in childhood and adulthood, both socially and behaviorally; this biochemical change has been studied with childhood victims of abuse and bullying (Ouellet-Morin et al., 2011). Low cortisol response rate can be detected as early as 12 years of age. Further, children did not need to be direct victims; witnessing adverse events is potentially harmful. For example, low cortisol response rate was observed in children witnessing interpersonal conflict between caregivers (Ouellet-Morin et al., 2011).

Additional studies have identified other brain regions that undergo permanent changes with trauma exposure. A study in 2012 conducted by the Developmental Biopsychiatry Research Program and Brain Imaging Center at McClean Hospital concluded that childhood maltreatment was associated with changes in hippocampal subfield development (Teicher, Anderson, & Polcari, 2012). Additional research has shown that children witnessing violence show reduced fractional anisotropy values when compared to controls; children between the ages of 7 and 13 years are more sensitive to changes in the inferior longitudinal fasciculus, which is part of the visual-limbic pathway (Choi, Jeong, Polcari, Rohan, & Teicher, 2012). Imaging that reflects the physiological changes occurring in the brain during traumatic events offers a new approach to understanding and contextualizing the impact of childhood trauma as a major public health issue.

The implication of childhood trauma and its connection with health disparities in adulthood make assessment and prevention the responsibility of every provider. Nurse practitioners in every practice setting must incorporate trauma screening into routine office visits. Lack of screening and identification of victims of trauma perpetuates the intergenerational cycle of violence. Delayed referral for appropriate therapeutic interventions places children at increased risk for difficulties in the school, home, and community. Post-traumatic stress disorder (PTSD) requires immediate treatment; failure to refer to appropriate therapeutic services can have deleterious effects. **BOX 4-1** offers a brief screening tool that can be used in the primary care setting to help assess for PTSD. This need for thorough assessment cannot be overemphasized. Consider the following clinical example:

> A 6-year-old male presents with inattention, high distractibility, oppositionality, and low frustration tolerance. He is often exhibiting defiant behaviors such as crawling under the desk and refusing to complete work. He frequently appears off-task and has difficulty remaining in his seat. The Connors Rating Scale for ADHD reveals clinically significant ratings of both hyperactivity and inattention. The prescriber offers the parent a prescription for methylphenidate to treat symptoms of ADHD; however, the provider fails to screen for trauma and possible comorbid PTSD. The family leaves with a

BOX 4-1 PC-PTSD Screen

In your life, have you ever had any experience that was so frightening, horrible, or upsetting that in the past month you:
Have had nightmares about it when you did not want to?
YES/NO
Tried hard not to think about it or went out of your way to avoid situations that remind you of it?
YES/NO
Were constantly on guard, watchful, or easily startled?
YES/NO
Felt numb or detached from others, activities, or your surroundings?
YES/NO

Reproduced from Prins, A., Ouimette, P., Kimerling, R., Cameron, R. P., Hugelshofer, D. S., Shaw-Hegwer, J., . . . Sheikh, J. I. (2003). The primary care PTSD screen (PC-PTSD): Development and operating characteristics. *Primary Care Psychiatry, 9*, 9–14. PC-PTSD is in the Public Domain and available at www.ptsd.va.gov.

prescription in hand, despite the fact the provider failed to discover that the mother has been physically abused and verbally degraded by a boyfriend who has been living with the family for over 1 year. The family is financially dependent on the boyfriend's support, and the mother is afraid of losing her home if she asks him to leave. The child is exposed daily to the intimate partner violence between the two. He often intervenes between the couple in order to "protect mom" and is called vulgar names by the boyfriend. The child is unable to sleep at night secondary to distressing nightmares, experiences flashbacks during the day, and exhibits a heightened startle response. These symptoms go unnoticed and untreated.

One year later, the child continues to struggle academically and socially. The school refers the child to a therapist at which point the therapist conducts a full psychiatric evaluation and administers the Childhood Trauma Questionnaire; scores indicate high levels of trauma reactivity.

The previous scenario is common within both the primary care and mental health settings. Lack of a comprehensive assessment can lead to misdiagnoses and lack of appropriate treatment for debilitating conditions. Childhood psychiatric disorders can be difficult to differentiate clinically. For example, ADHD is frequently diagnosed and treated within the primary care setting, yet is often comorbid with other diagnoses. In *Treating ADHD and Comorbid Disorders*, Pliszka (2009) discusses differential diagnosis and offers various treatment algorithms for children who meet criteria for ADHD as well as one additional diagnosis. Anxiety disorders are often comorbid with—as well as mistaken for—ADHD. Determining treatment priorities and symptom management requires thorough clinical assessment and skilled use of medication algorithms (Pliszka, 2009). Symptoms are often reported initially during routine well-child visits; comprehensive history-taking from both child and caregiver is required to determine when a patient can be treated within the primary care setting and when referrals are warranted.

Housing Instability and Homelessness

Homelessness and housing instability are strong predictors of adverse health outcomes. *Housing instability* is a term used to describe individuals and families who are forced to live in overcrowded homes, relocate frequently (for children this means constantly changing schools), and struggle to pay rent and monthly expenses (Rollins et al., 2012). Women are especially vulnerable to housing issues. For example, women who are financially dependent on an abusive partner are less likely to leave a dangerous situation due to lack of housing options (Rollins et al., 2012). The Centers for Disease Control and Prevention (CDC) estimate 2 million injuries and 1,200 deaths annually due to intimate partner violence (Rollins et al., 2012). The SHARE study investigated housing instability and its connection to the level of dangerousness within violent interpersonal relationships (Rollins et al., 2012). Whereas women without financial resources experiencing housing instability will be less likely to leave an abusive partner, it also has a bidirectional influence with intimate partner violence—future housing problems can be predicted by intimate partner violence (Rollins et al., 2012). In fact, a survey conducted in 2005 identified interpersonal violence as the primary cause of homelessness (Rollins et al., 2012). Exposure to intimate partner violence causes comorbid PTSD, which compounds existing mental health issues, creates new symptomatology, and impairs overall functioning. Survivors of interpersonal violence, as well as their children, are at increased risk for both negative physical and social outcomes (Rollins et al., 2012). Surprisingly, housing instability was more strongly associated with negative outcomes than alcohol abuse (Rollins et al., 2012).

Properly assessing patients for housing instability can result in critical clinical information that will considerably alter treatment modalities, barriers, and timetables. The SHARE study developed a method of assessment for the degree of housing instability termed the Housing Instability Index. It is a collection of 10 domains assessing an individual's vulnerability to housing instability and homelessness (Rollins et al., 2012). See **BOX 4-2**.

BOX 4-2 Housing Instability Index (HII)

1. In the past 6 months, how many times have you moved?
2. In the past 6 months, have you lived somewhere you did not want to live? (Yes/No)
3. In the past 6 months, have you had difficulty (or been unable to) pay for your housing? (Yes/No)
4. In the past 6 months, have you had to borrow money or ask friends or family or others for money to pay your rent/mortgage? (Yes/No)
5. Have you had trouble with a landlord in the last 6 months? (Yes/No)
6. In the past 6 months, has your landlord threatened to evict you? (Yes/No)
7. In the past 6 months, have you been served an eviction notice? (Yes/No)
8. Do you expect that you will be able to stay in your current housing for the next 6 months? (Yes/No)
9. Have you had trouble getting housing in the past 6 months? (Yes/No)
10. How likely is it that you will be able to pay for your housing (rent or mortgage) this month? (very likely, somewhat likely, somewhat unlikely, very unlikely)

Note: 1 point is assigned to question 1 if the answer is 3 or more moves. 1 point for each "yes" response to items 2–7 and item 9. 1 point for "no" response on item 8. 1 point for "somewhat likely" or "very unlikely" response on item 10.

Funding was provided to Multnomah County Oregon by Centers for Disease Control and Prevention, National Center for Injury Prevention and Control (U49CE000520-01, 09/01/2005-08/31/2010). For additional information about the SHARE Study contact: Chiquita Rollins at rollinsconsulting@q.com or Annie Neal at annie.neal@multco.us. Reprinted by permission.

This simple-to-use questionnaire is a manageable assessment tool for primary care providers. Assessing for homelessness and housing instability promotes holistic care, essential to positive patient outcomes. While housing instability places individuals and families at risk, the consequences of homelessness are also far reaching; individuals lacking a regular residence are at risk for chronic health problems and communicable diseases, and have limited access to health care (O'Connell et al., 2010). Homeless adults are 3.5 times more likely to die when compared to housed adults, consistent with the widely understood phenomenon that premature mortality is one of the most serious consequences of chronic homelessness (O'Connell et al., 2010). Basic healthcare services are often unattainable for this population, and rates of health problems are significantly disparate (Seiler & Moss, 2012). An increase in various chronic health conditions has been observed, including but not limited to respiratory, neurological, gastrointestinal, vision, psychological, and infections conditions (Seiler & Moss, 2012).

Nurse practitioners are positioned well to provide holistic care for this population. The unique needs of these individuals are often poorly understood or underappreciated, creating challenges to providing optimum health services. Many homeless individuals are less likely to seek preventive care measures; instead they become high users of emergency healthcare services, creating cost and logistical challenges for the healthcare delivery system. A specific group of individuals commonly referred to as "rough sleepers" are homeless individuals who refuse to stay in shelters and, instead, prefer to sleep on the street (O'Connell et al., 2010). This population is more likely to use emergency services and less likely to access preventive care, therefore creating and perpetuating chronic health issues. Further, when practitioners have the opportunity to provide care for homeless persons, providers encounter the considerable challenges of rehousing. Even when homeless individuals are given stable housing, social networking and integration do not always improve (Tsai, Mares, & Rosenheck, 2012). For example, with supported housing, homelessness decreased considerably; however, individuals did not consistently engage in other forms of social integration, such as employment or connecting with social supports (Tsai et al., 2012). The results suggest the need for further research, such as examining how fostering empowerment and autonomy of choice might be effective in increasing social integration for formerly homeless populations (Tsai et al., 2012).

Developing a system to reduce homelessness and improve care among this population has been one of the country's most formidable challenges. One promising example of a city's response to the needs of the homeless is the effort of Boston's Health Care for the Homeless Program (BHCHP), a system providing care for over 12,000 homeless men, women, and children. BHCHP strives to remove treatment barriers, provide direct preventive and acute care, and reverse the health disparities within Boston's homeless population. Principles of the program can successfully be replicated if core components are emulated. One of BHCHP's important interventions was implementation of an electronic medical record (EMR) that allowed shelters to connect and communicate. This ensured documentation of existing and emerging health problems as well as the opportunity to monitor treatment outcomes (O'Connell et al., 2010). Boston's program allowed for the discovery and subsequent treatment of tuberculosis in 1985, and recently has been involved in identifying carriers of the H1N1 virus, profoundly affecting the city of Boston's health through intervention and prevention of communicable diseases.

Another innovative intervention of the BHCHP that has made great strides in delivering care to the homeless is the development of a delivery of care system known as "street medicine." As the name suggests, the program provides care to patients wherever they may be, including treatment in parks, alleys, and under bridges (O'Connell et al., 2010). The results of the program have been promising. For example, this population now has access to annual flu vaccinations, routine PPD screenings for tuberculosis, blood pressure monitoring, and even mammograms (O'Connell et al., 2010).

In addition, equally important components of BHCHP include efforts to evaluate and better understand the healthcare needs of this population. Forming a consumer advisory board (CAB) comprised of homeless (or formerly homeless) individuals, the organization can better address the barriers and obstacles to care delivery. For example, the CAB gathered a focus group—representing the aforementioned "rough sleepers"—to determine the optimal way to approach individuals on the street with the purpose of offering routine health assessments and treatment. The CAB also addressed the issue of "identification tags" that stigmatized patients who were part of the homeless program. After consultation, the ID cards were modified so that words such as *homeless* no longer appeared (O'Connell et al., 2010).

The BHCHP illustrates the promise of community partnerships to improve public health for the most at-risk populations. Nurse practitioners are a key component in the development of such programs, providing holistic and collaborative care as well as attending to the psychosocial complexities that complicate treatment outcomes (Seiler & Moss, 2012). Nurse practitioners treating the underserved and homeless populations have resources available such as the National Health Care for the Homeless Council. Providing resources and tools to healthcare providers working in the field, the organization offers treatment recommendations and adaptations that can be applied to the unique challenge of providing care for homeless patients as well as opportunities to connect with other providers (National Health Care for the Homeless Council, 2013).

Vicarious Traumatization

Lindsay is an 8-year-old female who has been residing in a group home since age 3 after being removed from her biological mother's care for issues of abuse and neglect. Mom was struggling with an opioid use disorder (actively using heroin intravenously). Lindsay had been physically abused and emotionally neglected by mom and experienced sexual abuse by mom's boyfriend. Initially, Lindsay was in the process of reunification with mom and both would present for medication management. One day, Lindsay attended the appointment without mom; instead, she arrived with a staff member from her group home. The previous night, Lindsay learned that mom had been admitted to a psychiatric facility after overdosing on heroin. A suicide attempt was suspected. What struck me about this crisis was Lindsay's reaction—resigned and completely unsurprised. When I assessed her internal state with age-appropriate questions, this 8-year-old girl responded with a shoulder shrug and the words, "Hope for the best, expect the worst, that's what they tell me to do." Although I had treated far more severe trauma cases over the years, this case evoked a profound sadness inside of me. I realized her resounding words echoed the frustrations I often encounter as a practitioner in child psychiatry.

Treating victims of trauma and chronic exposure to stories of violence, child abuse, and criminal acts takes its toll on clinicians. The term *compassion fatigue* was first coined by Joinson (1992; Tabor, 2011). Since then, other descriptors have been introduced, attempting to verbalize the emotional burnout that healthcare providers experience after treating victims of trauma. The term *vicarious traumatization (VT)* was used to describe such experiences. It is widely understood that VT "negatively alters personal feelings, beliefs, values, and judgments" (Tabor, 2011). Educating providers on the symptoms of VT—including disengagement from clients, reduced empathy, and isolation from peers (Tabor, 2011)—is an important step. Other signs that VT is beginning to cause deleterious effects include somatization, substance use, changes in self-esteem and/or level of objectivity or empathy, and poor life–work balance (Tabor, 2011). The acronym ACT—**A**cknowledge, **C**onnect, and **T**alk—is a simple intervention to prevent VT (Clark & Gioro, 1998; Tabor, 2011). Mental health providers with personal histories of trauma and victimization should be especially cautious in self-monitoring as personal experiences can increase the likelihood of developing VT (Tabor, 2011).

Risk Assessment

It is inevitable that psychiatric emergencies will emerge in both mental health and primary care settings. Crisis situations can take various forms: suicidal/homicidal patients, belligerent/dangerous patients, and delusional or psychotic patients, many of whom may be unsafe to leave the office.

> A nurse practitioner treats a patient for the first time who presents for a routine medication check. A 25-year-old male recently discontinued his antipsychotic medication several weeks ago. He presents as delusional, peering suspiciously around the room and making threatening comments to all the people who have been "looking at him hard." When assessing for dangerousness, he reports he has something in his bag to "take care of them all." Alarmed, the NP continues to assess the severity of delusion, psychosis, and dangerousness, gently attempting to extrapolate as much information as possible, including what type of weapon he is concealing in his large duffel bag. Due to the severity of his clinical presentation, the NP excuses herself from the room and places an emergency call to the police so the patient can be safely transferred to the emergency department for likely admission to an inpatient psychiatric facility. After calling the police, the NP continues the assessment. Worried that the patient is a flight risk, she chooses not to disclose the plan to the patient until emergency personnel arrive on scene. However, after a knock at the office door, she is told to leave the office immediately at which point three armed officers with an accompanying police K-9 enter the office. The patient, already paranoid, is in complete shock. He is compliant with the police; a search of his person and belongings reveals a small box cutter. He is transported to the emergency department, admitted to the psychiatric unit, and restarted on an antipsychotic medication.

This scenario exemplifies the unforeseen crises that can emerge during any routine office visit and the subsequent stress on both patient and provider. In this latest scenario, the level of potential dangerousness was appropriately prioritized; however, the therapeutic alliance was likely compromised. The philosophy of the patient–provider interview is built on the philosophy of respect and mutual decision making. Dangerous patients, severely psychiatrically ill patients, as well as suicidal patients often temporary lack the ability to make safe and appropriate decisions related to their care during periods of acute symptomatology. Determining when to admit a patient to a psychiatric facility is challenging; it becomes much more so when the NP and patient disagree on the plan. At this point, assessment of risk becomes key to appropriate planning and safe clinical care.

Suicide screening is a key component with any risk assessment. The statistics on suicide are staggering. The CDC reports suicide is the 10th leading cause of death in the United States with 90% of those people diagnosed with a psychiatric disorder (Bostwick & Rackley, 2012). In fact, according to the CDC, 1% of deaths in the United States are attributed to suicide. Most opportunities for suicide screening occur within the primary care setting. Recent studies show that individuals completing suicide had a visit with their primary care provider within a month of the suicidal act (Bostwick & Rackley, 2012). Two high-risk groups for suicidality—adolescent and geriatric populations—typically see their primary care provider at least once per year, suggesting that screening with both populations should be a part of routine office visits (Bostwick & Rackley, 2012). Consider the following clinical example.

> Marynelly is a 16-year-old female who recently moved to Massachusetts from Puerto Rico. Her English-speaking skills are limited, and she is experiencing difficulty with cultural integration. She has no previous history of depressive symptoms until moving to the United States 6 months ago, at which point she began to isolate socially. She continues to appear detached to family members, spending all day in her room; she exhibits marked irritability, hypersomnia, and has become school avoidant. Family denies any history of behavioral problems. Marynelly denies substance abuse, and this is confirmed by a negative toxicology screen. She denies any thoughts of self-harm. The NP prescribes fluoxetine for depression, and Marynelly is told to follow up in 2 weeks. The following day, the NP receives a call from the hospital with a report that Marynelly has overdosed on her mother's Vicodin. She is medically stable and awaiting transport to the inpatient psychiatric unit.

Adolescents are particularly vulnerable to suicide. Adolescent suicide attempts and completions have been identified as a major public health concern, yet routine suicide assessment in primary care settings is far from adequate (Fallucco, Conlon, Gale, Constantino, & Glowinski, 2012). National Vital Statistics reported that suicide is the second leading cause of death for individuals ages 10–24 (https://www.cdc.gov/nchs/data/nvsr/nvsr65/nvsr65_05.pdf). More adolescents die from suicide than from the combined mortality from cancer, pulmonary disease, HIV, and other infectious diseases (Bostwick & Rackley, 2012). The U.S. Preventive Task Force and the American Academy of Pediatrics have created guidelines for assessing and treating adolescent depression during routine office visits (Fallucco et al., 2012). Fallucco and colleagues (2012) conducted a study to assess the competency in suicide risk assessment among primary care providers. The study determined that suicide risk assessment during routine adolescent medical visits would be considerably improved pending additional training for the primary care providers. Providers in the study were given a seminar lasting 1 hour in length followed by a 1-hour training session where providers could begin using newly acquired assessment skills with simulated patients (Fallucco et al., 2012). The results showed that after a short training session, providers were more likely to screen adolescents for suicidality, diagnose depression, and assess for risk factors (i.e., access to weapons, history of violence) (Fallucco et al., 2012). Although guidelines are an important first step, implementation is equally important, and models for this type of routine assessment are not frequently offered in provider training curriculum (Fallucco et al., 2012). Training providers on risk assessment within the primary care setting and offering evidence-based models for intervention and implementation are critical to improving patient outcomes (Fallucco et al., 2012).

McDowell, Lineberry, and Bostwick (2011) discussed the importance of suicide risk assessment with particular attention to distinguishing between warnings signs and risk factors. *Warning signs* (anger, rage, impulsive behaviors, social isolation, changes in sleep patterns, lack of future orientation, suicidal thinking, planning, or gesturing) can typically be assessed in greater detail with various treatment modalities offered as interventions (pharmacotherapy, psychotherapy, referrals to social services). *Risk factors* (white, male, previous psychiatric diagnoses, history of psychiatric hospitalization, access to dangerous weapons, family history) are typically unalterable (McDowell et al., 2011). After determining the presence of warning signs providers can offer treatment and psychiatric services that can help prevent suicide attempts. Impulsive behaviors as well as acute anxiety are two of the most alarming warning signs as they are frequently associated with suicidal behaviors (McDowell et al., 2011).

A particularly promising treatment modality—the Collaborative Care Model—may increase the rate of successful treatment for depressive symptoms and reduce suicidal behaviors (McDowell et al., 2011). In 2009, the Prevention of Suicide in Primary Care Elderly: Collaborative Trial (PROSPECT) conducted a 24-month study, showing promise in suicide prevention and intervention. The model supports increasing education and support for care providers. The model also speaks to the importance of assigning a "depression care manager," a trained professional who offers patient support through educating, monitoring, and encouraging patient–provider communication, as well as promoting dialogue between the primary care and psychiatric providers (McDowell et al., 2011). The treatment successfully decreased the rate of suicide in patients aged 60 years and older (McDowell et al., 2011).

The mnemonic shown in **BOX 4-3** can be used to remember the key points when screening for depression (Carlat, 1998).

BOX 4-3 SIGECAPS: Mnemonic for Screening for Depression

SIGECAPS
Sleep disorder (either increased or decreased)*
Interest deficit (anhedonia)
Guilt (feelings of worthlessness,* hopelessness,* regret)
Energy deficit*
Concentration deficit*
Appetite disorder (either increased or decreased)*
Psychomotor retardation or agitation
Suicidality

Note: To meet the diagnosis of major depression, a patient must have four of the symptoms plus depressed mood or anhedonia, for at least 2 weeks. To meet the diagnosis of dysthymic disorder, a patient must have two of the six symptoms marked with an asterisk, plus depression, for at least 2 years.

Reproduced with permission from Carlat, D.J. (1998). The Psychiatric Review of Symptoms: A screening tool for family physicians. *American Family Physician, 58*(7), 1617-1624.

Additionally, the Patient Health Questionnaire (PHQ-9) is a validated and reliable measure to screen for depression within the primary care setting (Kroenke, Spitze, & Williams, 2001) (**EXHIBIT 4-3**).

Managing Bipolar Disorder in the Primary Care Setting

As seen in the previous chapter, managing depression has become routine practice for primary care providers. However, depression is not the only mental health diagnosis seen in primary care settings; recent research has shown that a large percentage of patients with bipolar disorder are treated by primary care providers, having never seen a psychiatry provider (Kilbourne, Goodrich, O'Donnell, & Miller, 2012). It is known that treating patients with bipolar disorder is the most costly of any psychiatric diagnoses (Kilbourne et al., 2012), occurring an estimated 70% of the total cost (Kilbourne et al., 2012). Bipolar depression is often mistaken for unipolar depression, resulting in inappropriate medication management. The reasons for this are twofold: First, depression is a common symptom of bipolar disorder, and without more extensive patient reporting, misdiagnoses are likely to occur. A second challenge is that patients often fail to recall manic episodes (Kilbourne et al., 2012). This is a complicated problem for the provider, requiring extensive face-to-face time for patient interviews and knowledge of differential diagnoses to first diagnose and then treat bipolar with psychopharmacology.

The Collaborative/Chronic Care Model (CCM) has been suggested as an appropriate method for managing bipolar disorder in the primary care setting. The CCM has been studied and found effective in managing chronic illnesses, including bipolar disorder, with minimal accrual of healthcare costs (Kilbourne et al., 2012). The CCM has six components: (1) confirming bipolar disorder diagnosis, (2) providing ongoing assessment of symptoms and side effects related to psychotropic medication, (3) soliciting resources from mental health clinicians to adhere to current treatment protocols, (4) seeking consultation with psychiatric specialists, (5) focusing on psychosocial issues likely to complicate treatment and symptom management, and (6) providing necessary referrals to community support services (Kilbourne et al., 2012).

For example, the use of case managers is critical for treatment progress. Case managers should have connections to psychiatric specialists for managing complex patient presentations as well as referral resources such as mental health clinicians (Kilbourne et al., 2012). Currently, most CCM implementation has not yet been adapted to smaller practices, and more research is needed to determine how to best implement this model across routine primary care settings (Kilbourne et al., 2012).

Understanding Scope of Practice

Most nurse practitioners, regardless of specialty or treatment setting, will routinely provide care for patients with psychiatric diagnoses. Unfortunately, there is no simple algorithm, biomarker, or treatment protocol available to determine when to diagnose and manage psychiatric symptoms in the primary care setting and when to refer to a specialist. A recent study in *Clinical Pediatrics* conducted a survey of

EXHIBIT 4-3 Patient Health Questionnaire (PHQ-9)

Patient Name ____________________ Date of Visit ____________________

Over the past 2 weeks, how often have you been bothered by any of the following problems?	Not at All	Several Days	More Than Half the Days	Nearly Every Day
1. Little interest or pleasure in doing things				
2. Feeling down, depressed, or hopeless				
3. Trouble falling asleep, staying asleep, or sleeping too much				
4. Feeling tired or having little energy				
5. Poor appetite or overeating				
6. Feeling bad about yourself—or that you're a failure or have let yourself or your family down				
7. Trouble concentrating on things, such as reading the newspaper or watching television				

(continues)

EXHIBIT 4-3 Patient Health Questionnaire-9 (PHQ-9) *(continued)*

Over the past 2 weeks, how often have you been bothered by any of the following problems?	Not at All	Several Days	More Than Half the Days	Nearly Every Day
8. Moving or speaking so slowly that other people could have noticed. Or, the opposite—being so fidgety or restless that you have been moving around a lot more than usual				
9. Thoughts that you would be better off dead or of hurting yourself in some way				
Column Totals		___ +	___ +	___
Add Totals Together				___

10. If you checked off any problems, how difficult have those problems made it for you to do your work, take care of things at home, or get along with other people?
☐ Not difficult at all ☐ Somewhat difficult ☐ Very difficult
☐ Extremely difficult

Developed by Drs. Robert L. Spitzer, Janet B.W. Williams, Kurt Kroenke and colleagues, with an educational grant from Pfizer Inc. No permission required to reproduce, translate, display or distribute.

pediatricians in Kentucky to gauge practice experience in assessing, diagnosing, and treating behavioral health problems in primary care (Davis et al., 2012). The results of the study are suggestive of the general climate, bearing similar results to previous surveys conducted across diverse geographical regions (Davis et al., 2012). Primary care providers often feel unprepared to deal with the complexities of psychiatric symptomatology. Clinical training varies widely across institutions, curricula, and residency programs, affecting providers' comfort level and confidence in managing certain conditions (Davis et al., 2012). One significant barrier is that providers often feel psychiatric specialists are unavailable for consultation and referral. When referrals are successful, providers complain that communication between primary care provider and psychiatric specialist is inadequate and this lack of dialogue creates barriers for optimal patient care (Davis et al., 2012).

Establishing strong connections with mental health specialists is critical in determining when a patient's presentation lies outside one's current scope of practice. Risk assessment is a key component of any patient interview, and learning to evaluate risk is necessary for safe clinical practice. On an individual level, it is also critical for providers to continue widening their knowledge base, in order to increase competency and confidence in managing psychiatric symptomatology. Globally, further research is needed to explore models of care that will improve mental health treatment within the primary care setting, such as the aforementioned Collaborative Care Model for managing bipolar disorder. This research is critical as management of mental health care continues to fall under the primary care provider's scope of practice.

The NP Role in Caring for Vulnerable Populations

Nurse practitioners caring for vulnerable populations are responsible for thorough assessment and holistic care of the whole person. In most cases, vulnerability exists in a complex paradigm with multiple layers of risk factors. In an average clinic, homelessness, substance use disorders, and trauma reactivity are compounded, perpetuating chronic physical and mental health conditions. Lack of education, lack of access, and distrust of the healthcare system create further barriers to accessing care. Consider the following clinical example that illustrates both this complicated paradigm and the pivotal position of the nurse practitioner.

MARVIN'S STORY

Marvin is a 38-year-old African-American male who has been my patient for the past 4 years. He is certainly one of my most nonadherent patients, but I am ever hopeful and allow him a lot of leeway due to his life circumstances.

Marvin is the youngest of four brothers and two sisters. Two of his older brothers were murdered in gang-related activity. He has one sister that lives in the same town and has tried to be helpful, but it has been difficult for her. Marvin never learned how to read or write, and cannot remember what grade he finished. He landed in jail at age 18, and spent time in and out of the prison system until I met him at age 34 years. Somewhere along the way he was infected with HIV; his belief is that it was through unprotected sex. Finding out all of this information took many visits, as it was probably the fourth or fifth visit to the clinic waiting room with a case manager before he actually made it to an examination room.

The first time we met in the exam room it was basically for him to assess whether or not I was someone he wanted to take care of him. We kept our spatial boundaries and did preliminary introductions. I assured him we would be working together on his care plan and requested he get some blood work done, and to bring me his medical records from his incarceration, as they are frequently the best source of information available to me regarding his HIV and health maintenance status.

It took many visits and quite a lot of reassurance from me until our relationship started building some level of trust. Once Marvin realized I just wanted to help him avoid dying from some opportunistic infection, we were able to start trying medications. When he kept returning without an appointment (much to the front staffs' chagrin) with pills and pill boxes all askew, I gently asked him if he could read. He told me he could not. So, he would walk in weekly (never at the correct appointment time) for me to fill his pill box and review our plans. When he met a girlfriend, he brought her in to me to talk about HIV and how to protect her, and many other personal issues. When she broke up with him, he showed up distraught and cried once I closed the exam room door. He also confided he had been sexually assaulted in prison, and believes that is where he was infected with HIV.

Since that time, I have moved to another clinic across town. Marvin followed me there, still shows up without appointments because he knows I am there on Thursdays. The front staff is still irritated despite my short lectures on caring for the disenfranchised. Many attempts to get visiting nurses are unsuccessful because of Marvin's distrust of the "system." Unfortunately, his reluctance to take medications has led him to an extremely low CD4 count, and he recently came in with cerebral toxoplasmosis. Now there are an enormous amount of pills to take, numerous times per day. I continue to request visiting nurse services, as well as instructing the support and nursing staff to let him be seen whenever he comes in so I can try to get him adherent to medications to prolong his life as long as possible. I know most everyone else has given up on Marvin, and he knows that too. He knows I care, and although I have so much more to offer as his healthcare provider, it might be too late for Marvin. He certainly didn't choose to be born into a chaotic and violent family, and he tries very hard to believe he has the ability to choose a better life now, but we as a society have to provide so many support services for an individual such as Marvin.

During these years of cuts to healthcare and support service agencies, and funding from Ryan White at risk for more major cuts, people such as Marvin have little chance for success without healthcare providers willing to take the time and effort to provide holistic care for them. Nurse practitioners are equipped with the tools and skills to care for these vulnerable people needing health care.

Nurse practitioners are responsible for the care of vulnerable populations—care that requires specialized attention to the psychosocial factors that contribute to health disparities and prevent positive treatment outcomes. The importance of recognizing and responding to the needs of these populations in a time-sensitive, clinically effective manner should be prioritized within clinical practice. While further research is still greatly needed, the current literature has paved the way for nurse practitioners, laying the foundation for future practice goals. With increased emphasis on routine screening, comprehensive assessment, collaborative care, and early identification and referral, nurse practitioners can continue to offer services and holistic care that will help stabilize and empower the most vulnerable members of our society.

Seminar Discussion Questions

1. What are the most common mental health issues in your clinical setting?
2. Reflect on your own biases related to dealing with patients suffering from substance abuse and/or mental health problems. Identify two methods for helping you to deal with these biases.
3. Practice interviewing psychosocial histories with other students. Identify areas that cause you discomfort and develop a more comfortable approach to this portion of history-taking.
4. Locate local agencies to refer patients
   a. Who are in psychiatric crisis
   b. Who need social support for family problems
   c. Who need hotline numbers for relieving stress due to flashbacks from childhood sexual abuse
   d. Who ask about Alcoholics Anonymous or Narcotics Anonymous

CASE STUDY

A 26-year-old male presents to your office requesting a refill for Seroquel 50 mg which he reports is needed for sleep and Adderall XR 30 mg for symptoms of ADHD. He recently moved from Florida and has no refills remaining. Upon assessment, he discloses that he has a history of cocaine and opioid abuse (prescription painkillers). He then reports that he is living with his mother but that she recently asked him to leave. He reports that he has been "irritable and arguing with her about everything." His medical history is nonremarkable. His psychiatric history includes four prior detoxification programs, each lasting approximately 7 days. He reports a psychiatric admission 2 years ago for suicidal ideation. You are practicing in a rural area where few psychiatric specialists are accepting new patients. You are certain that the waiting list for a referred patient will be at least 3 months long.

Discussion Questions

1. What further assessments would you perform on this patient?
2. How would you respond to the patient's request for a refill of Seroquel and Adderall?
3. What laboratory tests would you request?
4. What is your differential and/or rule-out diagnosis?

References

American Psychiatric Association. (2000). *Diagnostic and statistical manual of mental disorders* (4th ed., Text Rev.). Washington, DC: Author.

Anda, R. F., Brown, D. W., Felitti, V. J., Bremner, J. D., Dube, S. R., & Giles, W. H. (2007). Adverse childhood experiences and prescribed psychotropic medications in adults. *American Journal of Preventive Medicine, 32*(5), 389–394.

Baglivio, M. T., Wolff, K. T., Piquero, A. R., Greenwald, M. A., & Epps, N. J. (2017). Racial/ethnic disproportionality in psychiatric diagnoses and treatment in a sample of serious juvenile offenders. *Journal of Youth and Adolescence, 46*(7), 1424–1451. doi:10.1007/s10964-016-0573-4

Barrio, C., Yamada, A. M., Hough, R. L., Hawthorne, W., Garcia, P., & Jeste, D. V. (2003). Ethnic disparities in use of public mental health case management services among patients with schizophrenia. *Psychiatric Services, 54*, 1264–1270.

Boston Health Care for the Homeless Program. Retrieved from https://www.bhchp.org/

Bostwick, J. M., & Rackley, S. (2012). Addressing suicidality in primary care settings. *Current Psychiatry Reports, 14*(4), 353–359.

Carlat, D. J. (1998). The psychiatric review of symptoms: A screening tool for family physicians. *American Family Physician, 58*(7), 1617–1624.

Carpenter-Song, E., Whitley, R., Lawson, W., Quimby, E., & Drake, R. E. (2011). Reducing disparities in mental health care: Suggestions from the Dartmouth-Howard collaboration. *Community Mental Health Journal, 47*(1), 1–13.

Carroll, K. M. (2005). Recent advances in the psychotherapy of addictive disorders. *Current Psychiatry Reports, 7*(5), 329–336.

Centers for Disease Control and Prevention. Retrieved from https://www.cdc.gov/nchs/data/nvsr/nvsr65/nvsr65_05.pdf

Chen, S. M., Creedy, D., Lin, H. S., & Wollin, J. (2012). Effects of motivational interviewing intervention on self-management, psychological and glycemic outcomes in type 2 diabetes: A randomized controlled trial. *International Journal of Nursing Studies, 49*(6), 637–644.

Choi, J., Jeong, B., Polcari, A., Rohan, M. L., & Teicher, M. H. (2012). Reduced fractional anisotropy in the visual limbic pathway of young adults witnessing domestic violence in childhood. *NeuroImage, 59*(2), 1071–1079.

Clark, M. L., & Gioro, S. (1998). Nurses, indirect trauma, and prevention. *Image—The Journal of Nursing Scholarship, 30*(1), 85–87.

Corsino, L., Rocha-Goldberg, M. P., Batch, B. C., Ortiz-Melo, D. I., Bosworth, H. B., & Svetkey, L. P. (2012). The Latino Health Project: Pilot testing a culturally adapted behavioral weight loss intervention in obese and overweight Latino adults. *Ethnicity & Disease, 22*(1), 51–57.

Davis, D. W., Honaker, S. M., Jones, V. F., Williams, P. G., Stocker, F., & Martin, E. (2012). Identification and management of behavioral/mental health problems in primary care pediatrics: Perceived strengths, challenges, and new delivery models. *Clinical Pediatrics, 51*(10), 978–982.

Fallucco, E. M., Conlon, M. K., Gale, G., Constantino, J. N., & Glowinski, A. L. (2012). Use of a standardized patient paradigm to enhance proficiency in risk assessment for adolescent depression and suicide. *Journal of Adolescent Health: Official Publication of the Society for Adolescent Medicine, 51*(1), 66–72.

Felitti, V. J., Anda, R. F., Nordenberg, D., Williamson, D. F., Spitz, A. M., Edwards, V., . . . Marks, J. S. (1998). Relationship of childhood abuse and household dysfunction to many of the leading causes of death in adults. The Adverse Childhood Experiences (ACE) Study. *American Journal of Preventive Medicine, 14*(4), 245–258.

Golin, C. E., Earp, J. A., Grodensky, C. A., Patel, S. N., Suchindran, C., Parikh, M., . . . Groves, J. (2012). Longitudinal effects of SafeTalk, a motivational interviewing-based program to improve safer sex practices among people living with HIV/AIDS. *AIDS and Behavior, 16*(5), 1182–1191.

Heron, M. (2014). Deaths: Leading causes for 2014. *National Vital Statistics Reports, 65,* 5.

Joinson, C. (1992). Coping with compassion fatigue. *Nursing, 22*(4), 116, 118–120.

Kilbourne, A. M., Goodrich, D. E., O'Donnell, A. N., & Miller, C. J. (2012). Integrating bipolar disorder management in primary care. *Current Psychiatry Reports, 14*(6), 687–695.

Kroenke, K., Spitzer, R. L., & Williams, J. B. (2001). The PHQ-9: Validity of a brief depression severity measure. *Journal of General Internal Medicine, 16*(9), 606–613.

McDowell, A. K., Lineberry, T. W., & Bostwick, J. M. (2011). Practical suicide-risk management for the busy primary care physician. *Mayo Clinic Proceedings, 86*(8), 792–800.

Miller, W. R., & Moyers, T. B. (2017). Motivational interviewing and the clinical science of Carl Rogers. *Journal of Consulting and Clinical Psychology, 85*(8), 757–766. doi:10.1037/ccp0000179

Miller, W. R., Benefield, R. G., & Tonigan, J. S. (1993). Enhancing motivation for change in problem drinking: A controlled comparison of two therapist styles. *Journal of Consulting and Clinical Psychology, 61,* 455–461.

National Association of Mental Illness. (2003). *Dual diagnosis and integrated treatment of mental illness and substance abuse disorder.* Retrieved from http://www.nami.org/Template.cfm?Section=By_Illness&Template=/TaggedPage/TaggedPageDisplay.cfm&TPLID=54&ContentID=23049

National Health Care for the Homeless Council. (2013). *Clinical practice and administration resources.* Retrieved from http://www.nhchc.org/resources/clinical

O'Connell, J. J., Oppenheimer, S. C., Judge, C. M., Taube, R. L., Blanchfield, B. B., Swain, S. E., & Koh, H. K. (2010). The Boston Health Care for the Homeless Program: A public health framework. *American Journal of Public Health, 100*(8), 1400–1408.

Ouellet-Morin, I., Odgers, C. L., Danese, A., Bowes, L., Shakoor, S., Papadopoulos, A. S., . . . Arseneault, L. (2011). Blunted cortisol responses to stress signal social and behavioral problems among maltreated/bullied 12-year-old children. *Biological Psychiatry, 70*(11), 1016–1123.

Pliszka, S. R. (2009). *Treating ADHD and comorbid disorders: Psychosocial and psychopharmacological interventions*. New York, NY: Guilford Press.

Prins, A., Ouimette, P., Kimerling, R., Cameron, R. P., Hugelshofer, D. S., Shaw-Hegwer, J., . . . Sheikh, J. I. (2004). The primary care PTSD screen (PC-PTSD): Corrigendum. *Primary Care Psychiatry, 9*, 151. PC-PTSD is in the Public Domain and available at www.ptsd.va.gov

Rollins, C., Glass, N. E., Perrin, N. A., Billhardt, K. A., Clough, A., Barnes, J., . . . Bloom, T. L. (2012). Housing instability is as strong a predictor of poor health outcomes as level of danger in an abusive relationship: Findings from the SHARE Study. *Journal of Interpersonal Violence, 27*(4), 623–643.

Santucci, K. (2012). Psychiatric disease and drug abuse. *Current Opinion in Pediatrics, 24*(2), 233–237.

Seiler, A. J., & Moss, V. A. (2012). The experiences of nurse practitioners providing health care to the homeless. *Journal of the American Academy of Nurse Practitioners, 24*(5), 303–312.

Skinner, H. A. (1982). The drug abuse screening test. *Addictive Behaviors, 7*(4), 363–371.

Stewart, W. F., Ricci, J. A., Chee, E., Hahn, S. R., & Morganstein, D. (2003). Cost of lost productive work time among US workers with depression. *Journal of the American Medical Association, 289*(23), 3135–3144.

Substance Abuse and Mental Health Services Administration. (n.d.). *National outcome measures.* Retrieved from http://www.samhsa.gov/co-occurring/topics/data/nom.aspx

Suchman, N. E., McMahon, T. J., Zhang, H., Mayes, L. C., & Luthar, S. (2006). Substance-abusing mothers and disruptions in child custody: An attachment perspective. *Journal of Substance Abuse Treatment, 30*(3), 197–204.

Tabor, P. D. (2011). Vicarious traumatization: Concept analysis. *Journal of Forensic Nursing, 7*(4), 203–208.

Teicher, M. H., Anderson, C. M., & Polcari, A. (2012). Childhood maltreatment is associated with reduced volume in the hippocampal subfields CA3, dentate gyrus, and subiculum. *Proceedings of the National Academy of Sciences of the United States of America, 109*(9), E563–E572.

Tsai, J., Mares, A. S., & Rosenheck, R. A. (2012). Does housing chronically homeless adults lead to social integration? *Psychiatric Services (Washington, D.C.), 63*(5), 427–434.

U.S. Department of Health, Human Services, Substance Abuse, Mental Health Services Administration, Center for Mental Health Services. (2001). *Mental health: Culture, race, and ethnicity*. Rockville, MD: U.S. Department of Health, Human Services, Substance Abuse, Mental Health Services Administration, Center for Mental Health Services.

Wells, K., Klap, R., Koike, A., & Sherbourne, C. (2001). Ethnic disparities in unmet need for alcoholism, drug abuse, and mental health care. *American Journal of Psychiatry, 158*, 2027–2032.

Yudko, E., Lozhkina, O., & Fouts, A. (2007). A comprehensive review of the psychometric properties of the drug abuse screening test. *Journal of Substance Abuse Treatment, 32*, 189–198.

CHAPTER 5

Cultural Sensitivity and Global Health

Michelle A. Cole and Christina B. Gunther

Introduction

One of the most noted fundamental teachings in many of the world's religions is commonly referred to as the Golden Rule. The Golden Rule, "Do unto others as you would have them do unto you," is likely the most familiar moral value in Western culture (Stanglin, 2005). The rule has a strong connection to many religions including Christianity, Buddhism, Judaism, and Islam. Despite the origin, the tenet of the Golden Rule guides us to treat others as we would like to be treated. Its foundation is the reciprocity of kindness and human giving. The Golden Rule must be used with caution; it is when our best intentions to treat others with the compassion, respect, and care while following the fundamental underpinnings of the Golden Rule that we may have unintended outcomes (Corazzini et al., 2006). The general principles that often drive the day-to-day decisions and actions of nurse practitioners (NPs) need reconsideration for the diverse and unique populations in their care.

There is an assumption that people who resemble us or speak our language are the same and should be treated as we would like to be treated. As the providers of direct care to individuals and populations, NPs must consider how those they provide care for want to be treated. This consideration differs from the Golden Rule, in which we treat others in a manner that is acceptable to our standards and beliefs without consideration of the individual's preferences. Stepping away from viewing circumstances from our own perspective to the patient's perspective is a critical step in the care of others in a diverse world. Putting aside an imperialistic attitude of thinking one knows what is best for others, and taking the time to know what is significant to individuals and communities, is an important step in developing a successful patient–NP relationship (Ott & Olson, 2011).

As the United States is becoming more diverse, healthcare providers are caring for individuals and groups who have varied perspectives; many are distinct from the mainstream healthcare system. Many healthcare providers, including NPs, do not identify themselves with any one particular culture; however, they often do view their patients and families to have cultural traits (Matteliano & Street, 2012). The notion that our own cultural and societal norms can be applied to the general population can create obstacles and barriers in caring for patients. These beliefs are a result of personal, professional, and educational socialization. Ethnocentrism impedes the delivery of culturally competent nursing care (Dayer-Berenson, 2014). Not understanding others, or having limited information about another group, can lead primary care providers to make false assumptions that could potentially be harmful, hurtful, and destructive. Believing that the culture one is most familiar with is the cultural standard does not afford providers the opportunity to comprehend and appreciate the needs of others. Critical to understanding the perspective of others is the willingness of NPs to acknowledge their own beliefs and recognize that other individuals' values are cogent despite being different from their own (Dayer-Berenson, 2014). Considering the viewpoint of others is the first step to comprehending the ideals from the eyes of others and the avoidance of unfounded assumptions and biases.

Global Diversity

The world is becoming increasingly more diverse. Globalization brings diversity and affects societies as cultures, values, and traditions transcend into new territory. The U.S. population is becoming increasingly more ethnically and socioculturally varied. In the United States between 2000 and 2010, a large increase in the Hispanic population accounted for more than half of the growth in the total U.S. population, while growth of the Asian population grew more rapidly than any other main race group (Census Bureau, 2011). The data highlight the changes in population and increasing diversity of the United States. Considering the United States as a "melting pot" or the blending together of various cultures to form one, is not considering the unique qualities of the various cultures of the population. Instead, looking at the U.S. society as a "tossed salad," where the diversity of the culture is valued for what it contributes to the whole, embraces a more culturally aware viewpoint. As advanced practice nurses, NPs are challenged to respond to this "tossed salad" culture by providing care for the health and wellness needs of the population. In 2009, a study commissioned by the Joint Center for Political and Economic Studies indicated the estimated combined cost of health disparities and subsequent deaths due to inadequate and/or inequitable care at $1.24 trillion (LaVeist, Gaskin, & Richard, 2009). Clearly, this is unacceptable, and healthcare providers and organizations need to work on reducing health disparities.

Leininger's theory on diversity and universality implies that for a caregiver's work to be meaningful and relevant, transcultural knowledge and competencies are imperative to guiding decisions and actions for effective and successful outcomes (Tomey & Alligood, 2002). Leininger's theory is suitable for application to the care of diverse populations. Her theory states that the provision of care needs to be harmonious with an individual's or group's cultural beliefs, practices, and ideals (Sitzman & Eichelberger, 2004). With the impact of globalization, primary care providers must possess sensitivity, compassion, and competence to care for individuals and communities from diverse cultural backgrounds. To effect positive health promotion activities and influence positive healthcare outcomes of individuals and communities, healthcare providers must understand and appreciate the importance of culturally competent care (Sitzman & Eichelberger, 2004). NPs are charged with integrating cultural care into practice through a comprehensive clinical approach, role modeling, policy development, performance, evaluation, and use of the advanced nursing process (McFarlane & Eipperle, 2008). The advanced practice NP has an obligation to develop the skills necessary to be a culturally competent practitioner.

Cultural Competency and Clinical Education

Cultural competency is an essential component to be infused into professional practice. Professional nursing organizations recognize the need for nurses, at all levels, to respond to the diversity in the population. The American Association of Colleges of Nursing (AACN), in the *Essentials of Baccalaureate Education for Professional Nursing Practice*, states, "The professional nurse practices in a multicultural environment and must possess the skills to provide culturally appropriate care" (2008, p. 6). The *Essentials of Master's Education of Advanced Practice Nurses* includes cultural competence as an essential component of the advanced practice nurse's educational preparedness (AACN, 1994). Cultural sensitivity and awareness are concepts guiding the practice of the Doctorate of Nursing Practice prepared nurse (AACN, 2006). Cultural competency is an essential component of the educational preparedness of nurses; and the inclusion of cultural sensitivity and awareness into the curriculum will promote cultural competency within the profession of nursing.

Medical and nursing academics are infusing cultural competence preparation into their educational curricula. Over 90% of medical schools' curricula in the United States include cultural competence training (Boutin-Foster, Foster, & Konopasek, 2008). The AACN essentials outline the required curriculum requirements and student learning outcomes, which include cultural competency. Nursing and medical faculty are charged to develop teaching strategies to achieve the set standards over the curriculum recognizing that cultural competence is a developmental process. In an effort to design the graduate nursing curriculum to meet these expectations, faculty have collaborated with community leaders to develop recommendations for the development of competencies for graduate nursing curricula (Axtell, Avery, & Westra, 2010). Five student themes emerged: (1) self-awareness, (2) basic knowledge of culture and identity, (3) attitudes that promote intercultural communication, (4) cross-cultural clinical skills, and (5) advocacy skills. The inclusion of the community to assist in the development of the graduate nurse was viewed as a positive strategy in the development and projected outcomes of the identified objectives (Axtell et al., 2010). Caring for individuals necessitates understanding the influence of culture on their healthcare situation. Approach the individual without preconceived assumptions to avoid treating persons with common backgrounds the same. Each individual should have input into their healthcare choices, incorporating their cultural preferences.

"Assume every encounter is a cross-cultural encounter. This refers to the fact that even when a care provider and care recipient may appear to have a common background, they most likely do not view health care situations in the same way, so it is important to ask questions, discuss relevant issues, and avoid making assumptions in all clinical encounters." (Axtell, S., Avery, M., & Westra, B., *Journal of Transcultural Nursing 21*(2), p. 187,

The NP must be aware of the secondary elements of diversity in these situations that are not typically considered to be a cultural encounter. Loden and Rosener (1991) first developed the "dimensions of diversity" model to incorporate elements of diversity such as religion, sexual orientation, education, gender, age, and socioeconomic class, among others. Asking questions that incorporate the broader elements of diversity will make the patient encounter and healthcare outcomes more successful.

Cultural Awareness

"We don't see the world the way it is. We see the world the way we are."

—Anais Nin

Cultural awareness is being knowledgeable about one's own thoughts, feelings, and sensations, as well as the ability to reflect on how these can affect one's interactions with others (Giger et al., 2007). One's perceptions of "what is" are connected to our interpretation of the world, our experiences, values, and beliefs. To deliver care that is culturally sensitive the NP needs to have an appreciation of the culturally relevant facts about a client and the provision of care. Giger and Davidhizar's "transcultural assessment model" includes six cultural phenomena that influence healthcare delivery (Giger, 2017).

Communication

Language or communication patterns are a significant part of how information is transferred in the healthcare setting. Communication, however, extends beyond linguistics and includes the process of communication. "Nurses need to have not only a working knowledge of communication with clients of the same culture, but also a thorough awareness of racial, cultural, and social factors that may affect communication with persons from other cultures" (Giger, 2017, p. 20).

Space

Personal space is the area that surrounds an individual and his or her level of comfort, which may vary from one individual to another. Space should consider sensory aspects including olfactory, sensory, auditory and visual, all of which can have cultural implications.

> After discussing the pathology report, the NP reached out and embraced the young female patient. The NP, feeling her embrace was not welcomed, later reflected on the gesture. The gesture, intended to be a measure of comfort, was not positively received by the client. The client, from a culture where touch is limited, felt that the NP was intrusive, especially when distressing news was recently discussed.

Social Organization

Social organizations are structured groups that have a pattern of behaviors and set norms, beliefs, and values that influence the persons within the group. Examples include family, religious groups, communities, and organizations. Race and ethnicity may also be considered a social organization.

Time

The concept of time can have different implications based on a person's cultural view. Culture can impact one's relationship to time—past, future, or present orientation. Future orientation considers the future in present-day terms, past orientation has a connection to the past. New changes are based on what was considered in the past. Present orientation is focused on the current time. Understanding a client's orientation to time can be helpful in determining possible reasons for motivation, compliance, and participation.

> The toddler came into the office with several layers of clothing. The day was warm and comfortable. The mother stated, "My baby has a cold." Believing that the source of the cold was from the cool evening air that the infant was exposed to was a literal belief that the mother held from her past; the "chill was caught."

Environmental Control

The relationship between a person, the environment, and health and wellness determines the person's environmental control. Considerations of environmental control include the locus of control. *The client verbalized that the illness was in God's hands and they did not have any control.* Alternative therapies are more frequently considered in Western medicine. In 2007, approximately 38% of adults and approximately 12% of children were using some form of complementary and alternative medicine (CAM) (National Center for Complementary and Integrative Health [NCCIH] and the National Center for Health Statistics, 2008).

> The scent of lavender was present in the hospital room. The patient applied the essential oil to her temples to relieve the tension headache she was experiencing.

Biological Variations

Biological variations exist among different racial groups and should be considered when caring for individuals and groups. A person's shape, size, and skin color are variable and have genetic and ethnic connections. Genetics (the study of heredity) and genomics (the study of genes and their functions) are part of the NP's practice. Some genetic conditions are more likely to occur in a particular group; however, one cannot assume that a biological variation exists based on an individual's culture or ethnicity. For example, in the United States, sickle cell anemia is most prevalent in the African-American population.

> A young African-American mother brought her toddler in for a physical exam. She reported her daughter was pale and she expressed concern that her daughter might have sickle cell disease, like her brother. She was told as a young child their family had "bad cells" and her fear of her daughter

having the disease was frightening. Upon further examination of the child, it was determined she had iron deficiency anemia, a condition common in toddlers who consume excessive amounts of cow's milk, and not sickle cell disease caused by a genetic mutation.

Hofstede's Cultural Dimensions Theory

Geert Hofstede developed a framework for cross-cultural communication that describes the effects of a society's culture on the values of its members. Understanding the culture's values can provide a clearer understanding of how to relate to the culture. Although Hofstede's work focused on the influence of culture on the values in the workplace, the information obtained can be applied to other settings. Applying Hofstede's model on national culture to the healthcare industry equips the provider with insight about culture and fosters opportunities to recognize the uniqueness of another culture through a comparison perspective. (Hofstede's model on national culture can be found at https://geert-hofstede.com/national-culture.html.)

Cultural Humility

Culture has many different components that shape who we are and how we interact with the world. It is dynamic and multifaceted. Each of us has our own personal culture evolving from not only our own ethnic background but also our gender, age, socioeconomic status, life experiences, and so on (California Health Advocates, 2007; Office of Minority Health [OMH], 2011b; Tervalon & Murray-Garcia, 1998). Reading and learning about other cultures is a worthwhile endeavor; however, it is unlikely that one can become competent in every culture. Being aware of this limitation, the concept of "cultural humility" is perhaps a better term to assist the NP in improving meaningful relationships with patients, coworkers, and others.

In the *Handbook of Humility: Theory, Research, and Applications* (2016), Mosher and colleagues describe cultural humility as placing a priority on "developing mutual respect and partnership with others" (p. 91). This requires self-awareness and reflection as a lifelong process to develop a respectful relationship with patients. It also requires the provider to be flexible and humble in order to be open to the cultural dimensions of each patient encounter. Values associated with cultural humility include openness, appreciation, and acceptance, in addition to flexibility (Luluquisen, Schaff, & Galvez, n.d.).

Further, it is important for the NP to focus on both interpersonal and intrapersonal components of cultural humility—realizing one's own limitations in understanding cultural backgrounds and being open to the "other" (Mosher et al., 2016). One needs to be acutely aware of the potential power imbalances that can occur in the healthcare expert–patient interaction. By continually working to be open, flexible, appreciative, and accepting of their patients, in addition to striving to avoid any imbalance of power, NPs can create meaningful partnerships with patients and communities to develop treatment plans, and individual and community goals to improve health. Practicing lifelong self-awareness and reflection will assist the NP to be a culturally sensitive healthcare provider.

In an effort to educate healthcare providers (NPs, physicians, PAs) about delivering culturally sensitive care, *A Physician's Guide to Culturally Competent Care* was developed by the U.S. Department of Health and Human Services, Office of Minority Health (OMH, n.d.b). It contains nine Cultural Competency Curriculum Modules (CCCMs), including Standards for Culturally and Linguistically Appropriate Services in Health Care (CLAS standards), which are available for free at https://cccm.thinkculturalhealth.hhs.gov/. CME credits can be earned.

The objectives for this educational program are for NPs, PAs, and physicians to:

- Define issues related to cultural competency in medical practice.
- Identify strategies to promote self-awareness about attitudes, beliefs, biases, and behaviors that may influence the clinical care.
- Devise strategies to enhance skills toward the provision of care in a culturally competent clinical practice.
- Demonstrate the advantages of the adoption of the CLAS standards in clinical practice.

In many of the modules are patient cases and scenarios that require the healthcare provider to reflect upon what is being presented by the case, as well as how the reader feels about the situation. The fictional practice setting includes a profile of the community and the patients that are seen at the setting. The vast majority of the populations are white, non-Hispanic, who have at least a high school education; however, there are many migrant farm workers who use the practice, as well as Native Americans. The providers and support staff come from a variety of ethnic backgrounds and take different approaches to their practice. The practice setting is in need of much improvement, to work more efficiently and to provide culturally competent care to their patients. Through the learning modules, the healthcare provider is encouraged to consider what the patient's perspective is, to be more sensitive to one's own attitudes, including biases and the behaviors they may have displayed that affect patient care. **BOX 5-1** represents eight essential elements to consider in developing a culturally competent healthcare provider.

BOX 5-1 Eight Elements of Cultural Competence for Primary Healthcare Providers

1. Examine your values, behaviors, beliefs, and assumptions.
2. Recognize racism and the institutions or behaviors that breed racism.
3. Engage in activities that help you to reframe your thinking, allowing you to hear and understand other worldviews and perspectives.
4. Familiarize yourself with core cultural elements of the communities you serve.
5. Engage clients and patients to share how their reality is similar to, or different from, what you have learned about their core cultural elements.
6. Learn, and engage your clients to share, how they define, name, and understand disease and treatment.
7. Develop a relationship of trust with clients and co-workers by interacting zwith openness, understanding, and a willingness to hear different perceptions.
8. Create a welcoming environment that reflects the diverse communities you serve.

Reproduced from Nova Scotia Department of Health. (2005). *A cultural competence guide for primary health care professionals in Nova Scotia*. Halifax, Nova Scotia: Author.

▸ Cultural Competence and the Clinician

Nurse practitioners are poised to lead initiatives to implement the strategies to meet the challenge of fulfilling national standards of cultural competence in health care. Since there are hundreds of ethnic groups in our society with diverse needs, there is no one specific intervention for each health issue. To improve the health and well-being of individuals and communities, there are some general principles that can be practiced when delivering care to clients with a different culture than our own (Bomar, 2004). Reflecting on one's own culture, seeking knowledge about local cultures, understanding political issues of culturally diverse groups, and using culturally sensitive and linguistically appropriate resources are among the few (Bomar, 2004). Schools of nursing and organizations recognize the need to promote cultural awareness and sensitivity and provide opportunities for enhancing the practice of nursing (AACN, 2009). The American Association of Colleges of Nursing (2009) calls for the need for cultural competence education in graduate nursing to address the diverse needs of patients and minimize disparities in health. Once healthcare providers identify their own need for cultural growth, they can engage themselves in a variety of actions to increase their cultural competence on an individual level. This engagement calls for self-reflection and acknowledgement that their own beliefs, values, and attitudes may affect the care they provide to others. The NP can take a "cultural approach," being cognizant of "cultural variations" that will be advantageous to the patient as a management plan is developed for the individual. Each encounter should be approached as unique. Clustering values, beliefs, and behaviors from a cultural group and applying them to all persons of that culture does not consider the multiple variables that may influence an individual's cultural uniqueness. The following example demonstrates misinterpretation of communication style.

> Elsu, a 76-year-old Native American male, arrived to the clinic for reevaluation of hypertension. The nurse assessing the patient felt that Elsu was "not truthful." The nurse expressed the concerns to the practitioner in charge of his care. Upon entering the room, the practitioner noticed that Elsu avoided eye contact and participated minimally in conversation. The nurse who initially encountered the patient viewed his behaviors as untrusting. Elsu, being a Native American, is quiet and reserved when meeting new people. Eye contact, for the Native American, is considered a sign of disrespect and hence is avoided. The nurse assumed that Elsu's communication style had a different and undesirable meaning.

Patterns of culturally incompetent care from providers affects patient care outcomes and may widen the healthcare disparities gap (Doorenbos, Schim, Benkert, & Borse, 2005). Health disparities are linked to social, economic, and environmental disadvantages causing a difference in one's well-being (Office of Disease Prevention and Health Promotion, 2010). *Healthy People 2020* identifies populations who experience barriers to health care at higher rates than the general population; these groups include Hispanics, African-Americans, those with low levels of education, and the poor. The American College of Physicians (2010) in a position paper, *Racial and Ethnic Disparities in Health Care,* discuss the disparities and poor health care that exist among racial and ethnic groups. The American College of Physicians

(2010) makes several recommendations to reduce the disparities that affect health and wellness. Culturally competent care providers can influence the health of the population by reducing the barriers that negatively impact health. Cultural sensitivity and awareness are important steps to understanding the complex issue of racial and ethnic health disparities.

Culture Awareness and Cultural Sensitivity

According to the American Nurses Association (ANA, 2012), "diversity awareness" can be defined as the acknowledgement and appreciation of the existence of differences in attitudes, beliefs, thoughts, and priorities in the health-seeking behaviors of different patient populations. Cultural awareness is having the knowledge or information about what is unique or the same among various cultures. In contrast, cultural sensitivity is the individual's attitude about themselves or others and their desire to learn about the cultural aspects of others (Schim, Doorenbos, Benkert, & Miller, 2007). In an effort to meet the needs of communities and populations, we need to be open to learning about the unique characteristics they possess. Being aware and sensitive will allow us the ability to see beyond what is the accepted norm within our society. Cultural sensitivity is when we are able to appreciate the situation from another's perspective and value the viewpoint of others, despite it being different from our own.

What Determines Cultural Competence?

Many theoretical and methodological models exist that attempt to determine cultural competence. Schim, Doorenbos, Miller, and Benkert (2003) describe a theoretical model of cultural competence with three components: the circumstance in which the clinician incorporates the cultural diversity experience; the clinician's awareness of his or her reactions to people who are different; and lastly, examining attitudes and cultural bias toward other sociocultural groups. Based on this description and the cultural competence model developed by Schim and Miller (as cited in Schim et al., 2003), the Cultural Competence Assessment (CCA) was developed. The CCA tool is a method of measuring cultural competence behaviors (CCB) and cultural awareness and sensitivity (CAS).

In contrast, the *Purnell Model for Cultural Competence* (Purnell, 2002) uses a methodological approach to determine cultural competence. The basic assumptions of the model derive from multidisciplinary theories including organizational, administrative, communication, and family development as well as anthropology, sociology, psychology, and several others. The model has evolved to include 12 domains in a framework that assist the NP in developing cultural competence abilities.

TABLES 5-1 and **5-2** feature other theoretical and methodological models. None of the models are without limitation. Constraints vary from lack of measurement of healthcare outcomes to the abstract nature, making the models difficult to put into practice. One model that lies outside of the healthcare realm describes a more concrete approach to cultural competence.

International education scholar Darla Deardorff developed the Pyramid Model of Intercultural Competence (2006, 2009) which includes requisite attitudes necessary to develop cultural competence. These attitudes include respect, openness, and curiosity and discovery. Respect includes valuing other cultures and cultural diversity; openness

TABLE 5-1 Theoretical Models of Cultural Competence

Authors year	Model Name	Components of Constructs or Domains	Sources	Assessment Instrument Linkage	Validation
Campinha-Bacote, 20026	Culturally competent model of care	Five constructs within the cultural content of individual, family, and community (cultural awareness, knowledge, skill, encounters and desire [cultural desire added in 1998])	Lelninger's (1991) transcultural nursing theory; Pedersen's (1998) multicultural development theory (as cited in Campinha-Bacote, 2002b)	Inventory for assessing the process of cultural competence among healthcare professionals, revised (IAPCC-R)	Yes
Papadopoulos et al.,	Model for the development of culturally competent health practitioners	Four components (cultural awareness, cultural knowledge, cultural sensitivity, cultural competence)		Cultural competence assessment tool (CCA Tool), 2004 (40 items) based on Papadopoulos et al's 1998 model	Yes
Kim-Godwin, et al, 2001	Culturally competence community care model	Three constructs (cultural competence, health care system, and health outcomes) with four dimensions (caring, cultural sensitivity, cultural knowledge, and cultural skills)	Concept analysis	Cultural competence scale to test the 3 dimensions of cultural sensitivity. Knowledge, and skills	Yes

TABLE 5-1 Theoretical Models of Cultural Competence *(continued)*

Authors year	Model Name	Components of Constructs or Domains	Sources	Assessment Instrument Linkage	Validation
Jeffrey's, 2010a	Cultural competence and confidence model	Transcultural nursing skills in cognitive, practical, and affective dimensions, transcultural self-efficacy, and culturally congruence care	Lelninger's transcultural nursing theory; Bandura's (1986) self-efficacy theory in psychology	Transcultural self-efficacy coal (TEST)	Yes
Schism & Doorknobs, 2010; Schism Doarenbes, Bunkers, & Miler, 2007; Schism, Docrenbes, Miller &, Bunker, 2003	3-D model of culturally congruent care	Three dimensions of provider level (cultural diversity, cultural awareness, cultural sensitivity, and cultural competence behaviors), client level (patient, family, and community bellies, and behaviors) and culturally congruent care as outcome layer (when provider and client levels for well together)	Lelninger's transcultural nursing theory	Cultural competence assessment (CCA)	Yes
Campinha-Bacote, 2005	Biblically based cultural competence model	Eighteen intellectual and moral virtues (love, caring, humility, love of truth, teachabilness, intellectual honesty, inquisitiveness, wisdom, discernment, judgment, prudence, attentiveness, studiousness, practical and compassion) incegraced into the five constructs (cultural awareness, cultural knowledge, cultural desire, cultural skill and cultural encounters)		Inventory for assessing a biblical worldview of cultural competence (IABWCC) among healthcare professionals	

(continues)

TABLE 5-1 Theoretical Models of Cultural Competence *(continued)*

Authors year	Model Name	Components of Constructs or Domains	Sources	Assessment Instrument Linkage	Validation
Pepadopoulos & Lees, 2008	Model for the development of culturally competent researchers	Four components (cultural awareness, cultural knowledge, cultural sensitivity, cultural competence) with culture-generic and cultures-specific competence as the two layers of cultural competence			
Wills, 1999	Framework for cultural competence	Seven-step progression (knowledge of one's own culture, knowledge of others culture, cultural interaction, cultural tolerance, cultural induction, cultural appreciation acceptance, cultural competence)			
Wills, 2000	Cultural development model (for individual and institutional cultural competence development)	A continuson of six stages in two phases (cultural incompetence, cultural knowledge, and cultural awareness as the cognitive phase; cultural sensitivity, cultural competences, and cultural proficiency as the affective phase)	Cross et al. 1989' Orinda 1992		

TABLE 5-1 Theoretical Models of Cultural Competence *(continued)*

Authors year	Model Name	Components of Constructs or Domains	Sources	Assessment Instrument Linkage	Validation
Burchum, 2002	Model for cultural competence	Six attributes (cultural awareness, knowledge, understanding , sensitivity, interaction, and skill) a nonlinear, expensive process of becoming culturally competent	Concept analysis		
Pacqutao, 2012	Culturally competent model of ethical decisions	Three competence cultural context compassions advocacy for social justice and human rights protection for culturally congruent healthcare for wearable populations and culturally competent healthcare by real station of cultural patterning	Lelninger's transcultural nursing theory and principles of culturally congruent healthcare as a basic human right		
Suh, 2004	Model of cultural competence	Four domains as antecedence cognitive (cultural awareness, knowledge), effective (sensitivity), behavior (skills) and environmental (encounters); three attributes of cultural competence (ability, openness, flexibility); and three variables (receiver-based, provider-based, and health outcomes)	Concept analysis		

Reproduced from Shen, Z. (2015). Cultural competence models and cultural competence assessment instruments in nursing: A literature review. *Journal of Transcultural Nursing, 26*(3), 308–321.

TABLE 5-2 Methodological Models of Cultural Competence

Authors	Model Name	Components/Constructs/Domains	Sources	Assessment Instrument Linkage	Validation
Giger & Davidhizar, 2004, 2008	Transcultural assessment model	Six cultural phenomena (communication, space, social organization, time, environment control, and biological variations)	Leininger (1991); Spector (1996); Orque, Bloch, & Monrroy (1983); as cited in Giger & Davidhizar (2004, 2008)	Tested Smith (1998b) with three scales CAS by Bonaparte [1997, 1979]; CSES by Bernal & Froman [1987, 1993]; and Rooda's [1990, 1992] knowledge-based questions on cultural competence); also as cited in Giger & Diwidhizar, 2002	yes
Spector, 2004s, 2009	Health traditions model	Five respects of heritage consistency (culture, ethnicity, religion, [acculturation and socialization, 2009]) interrelated with six cultural phenomena (communication, space, social organization, time, environmental control, and biological variation) to maintain, process, and restore the health of the body, mind, and spirit.	Giger & Davidhizar's (1999, 2002, 2004, 2008) model; Ester & Ziow's theory (as cited in Spector, 2013)	Heritage assessment tool with 29 questions, Spector (2004b)	
Orque, 1983	Ethnief cultural system framework	Eight components applicable to nurses and clients (diet, family life processes, healing beliefs and practices, language and communication process, social groups' interactive patterns, value orientations, religion, art land history) along with two models (intercultural communication model and model of biological, sociological and psychological systems)	Nursing, sociology	Bloch's (1983) assessment guide for ethniefcultural variations	

TABLE 5-2 Methodological Models of Cultural Competence *(continued)*

Authors	Model Name	Components/Constructs/Domains	Sources	Assessment Instrument Linkage	Validation
Leininger, 1991	Sunrise model	Six domains (culture values and lifeways; religion, philosophical, and spiritual beliefs; economic factors; educational factors; technological factors; kinship and social ties; and political and legal factors) and three modalities (cultural care preservation and maintenance; cultural care accommodation and negotiation; and cultural care repatterning and restructuring)	Nursing, anthropology		
Purcell, 2003, 2008	Purcell model for cultural competitions	Twelve cultural domains (overview, inhabited localities, and Logography, communication, family roles and organization, work influence issues; bicultural ecology; high-risk health behavior nutritious pregnancy and childbearing practices; death rituals spiritually; healthcare practices and healthcare practitioners)	Organizational administrative, communication, and family development theories		
Andrews & Boyish 2008	Transactional nursing assessment guide for individuals and families	Twelves categories of cultural knowledge (cultural affiliations, values concentration, communication, health rebuild beliefs and practice, nutrition, social economic considerations, organizations providing cultural supports education, religion, cultural aspects of disease incidence biocultural variations, and developmental considerations across the life aspan p. 35)	Feininger's transcendental nursing theory		

Reproduced from Shen, Z. (2015). Cultural competence models and cultural competence assessment instruments in nursing: A literature review. *Journal of Transcultural Nursing, 26*(3), 308–321.

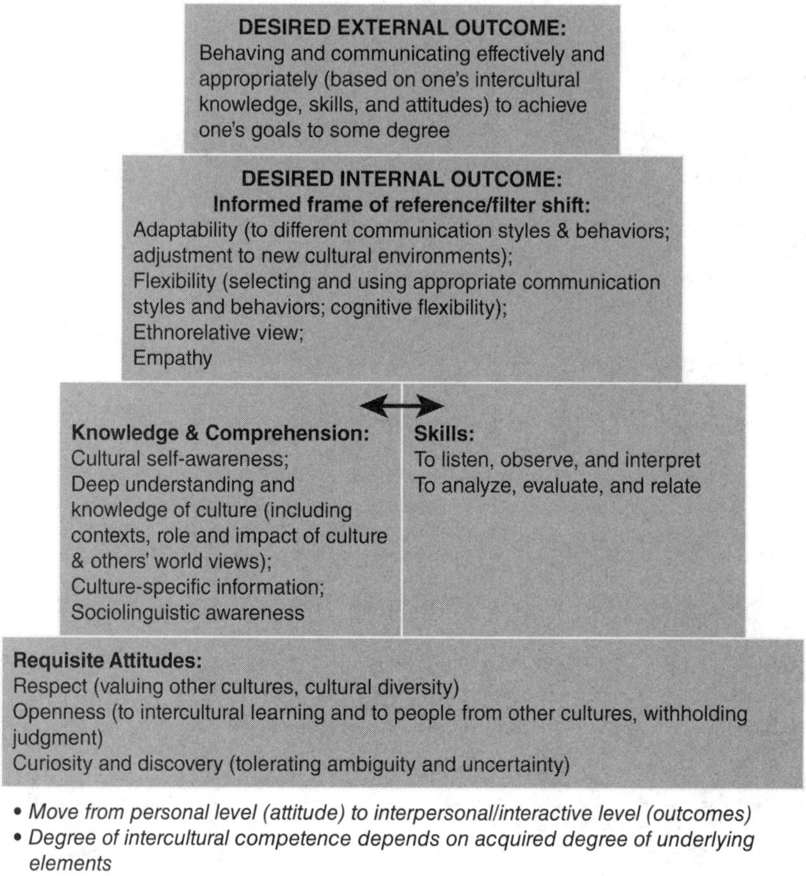

DESIRED EXTERNAL OUTCOME:
Behaving and communicating effectively and appropriately (based on one's intercultural knowledge, skills, and attitudes) to achieve one's goals to some degree

DESIRED INTERNAL OUTCOME:
Informed frame of reference/filter shift:
Adaptability (to different communication styles & behaviors; adjustment to new cultural environments);
Flexibility (selecting and using appropriate communication styles and behaviors; cognitive flexibility);
Ethnorelative view;
Empathy

Knowledge & Comprehension:
Cultural self-awareness;
Deep understanding and knowledge of culture (including contexts, role and impact of culture & others' world views);
Culture-specific information;
Sociolinguistic awareness

Skills:
To listen, observe, and interpret
To analyze, evaluate, and relate

Requisite Attitudes:
Respect (valuing other cultures, cultural diversity)
Openness (to intercultural learning and to people from other cultures, withholding judgment)
Curiosity and discovery (tolerating ambiguity and uncertainty)

- *Move from personal level (attitude) to interpersonal/interactive level (outcomes)*
- *Degree of intercultural competence depends on acquired degree of underlying elements*

FIGURE 5-1 Pyramid Model of Intercultural Competence

Reproduced with permission of SAGE Publications, Inc. from Deardorff, D. (2006). Identification and assessment of intercultural competence as a student outcome of internationalization. *Journal of Studies in International Education, 10*(3), 241–266. Permission conveyed through Copyright Clearance Center, Inc.

is a measure of withholding judgment of other cultures and diversity; curiosity and discovery allow for tolerating ambiguity and uncertainty. See **FIGURE 5-1**.

Measuring our cultural competency aids in our understanding and responsiveness to the components of care crucial for meeting the needs of the diverse populations that NPs serve. Using a tool such as the CCA will enable educators, mentors, and primary care providers the opportunity to evaluate their progress or journey of cultural competency.

A personal self-assessment tool for the primary healthcare provider can provide insight into the cultural competence of the care provider (see **BOX 5-2**). This quantitative tool requires the clinician to reflect on various areas of the cultural provision of care. Although there are no right or wrong answers, responding that "I rarely or never do" may suggest limitations in the ability to "demonstrate beliefs, attitudes, values, and practices that promote cultural competence within healthcare delivery programs" (Nova Scotia Department of Health, 2005, p. 19).

BOX 5-2 Promoting Cultural Competence in Primary Health Care

I. Physical Environment, Materials, and Resources
   A. I ensure the printed and posted information in my work environment reflects the diversity and literacy of individuals or families to whom I provide service.

II. Communication Styles
   A. When interacting with individuals and families who do not have spoken English proficiency, I always keep in mind that:
      1. Spoken English proficiency does not reflect literate English proficiency or language of origin proficiency or literacy.
      2. Limited ability to speak the language of the dominant culture has no bearing on ability to communicate effectively in one's mother tongue.
      3. Limitations in English proficiency do not reflect mental ability.
   B. I use bilingual and/or bicultural staff trained in medical interpretation when required or requested.
   C. For individuals and families who speak languages other than English, I attempt to learn and use key words in their language so I am better able to communicate with them during assessment, treatment, or other interventions.
   D. I understand the cultural context for naming disease and try to be respectful of this in my interactions. (In some cultures, there is stigma associated with terminal disease, sexually transmitted disease, and/or communicable diseases. In some cultures, this stigma is avoided by naming the disease by its attributes, rather than its medical name (e.g., AIDS is sometimes named "the sleeping sickness").
   E. I can provide alternatives to written communication if required or preferred.

III. Social Interaction
   A. I understand and accept that family is defined in a variety of different ways by different cultures (e.g., extended family members, kin, godparents).
   B. Even though my professional or moral point of view may differ, I accept individuals and families as the ultimate decision makers for services and supports affecting their lives.
   C. I understand that age, sex, and life-cycle factors need to be considered in interactions with individuals and families. For instance, a high value may be placed on the decisions of elders, the role of eldest male or female in families, or roles and expectations of children within the family.
   D. I accept and respect that male–female gender roles may vary among different cultures and ethnic groups (e.g., which family member makes major decisions for the family).

IV. Health, Illness, and End-of-Life Issues
   A. I understand that the perceptions of health, wellness, and preventive health services have different meanings to different cultural or ethnic groups.
   B. I intervene in an appropriate manner when I observe other staff or clients within my program or agency engaging in behaviors that are not culturally competent.
   C. I screen resources for cultural, ethnic, or racial stereotypes and/or inclusion before sharing them with individuals and families served by my program or agency.

(continues)

BOX 5-2 Promoting Cultural Competence in Primary Health Care *(continued)*

D. I am aware of the socioeconomic and environmental risk factors that contribute to the major health problems of culturally, ethnically, and racially diverse populations served by my program or agency.
E. I avail myself to professional development and training to enhance my knowledge and skills in the provision of services and supports to culturally, ethnically, racially, and linguistically diverse groups.
F. I advocate for the review of my program or agency's mission statement, goals, policies, and procedures to ensure that they incorporate principles and practices that promote cultural and linguistic competence.

Reproduced from Nova Scotia Department of Health. (2005). *A cultural competence guide for primary health care professionals in Nova Scotia.* Halifax, Nova Scotia: Author.

Cultural Immersion Experiences

Cultural competency, infused into the skill set of all NPs, is a starting point for the reduction of disparities that exist within our healthcare system. Increasing cultural competence among providers will facilitate the goal of decreasing the healthcare disparities gap (Doorenbos et al., 2005). Cultural immersion experiences have been cited as a method to increasing cultural awareness and sensitivity (Green, Comer, Elliott, & Nuebrander, 2011; Johns & Thompson, 2010; Jones, Ivanov, Wallace, & VonCannon, 2010; Larson, Ott, & Miles, 2010). When individuals interact with various culturally diverse groups, their own beliefs regarding a cultural group will be affected and thus prevent stereotyping (Campinha-Bacote, 2003). A substantial portion of the literature on cultural immersion experiences affecting cultural awareness and sensitivity relates to students within the educational setting. Inclusion of service learning activities that increase the cultural sensitivity and awareness of students is a means to addressing the needs of our society. Students are likely to gain global attitudes and perspectives when schools of nursing include global experiences in their curriculum (Riner, 2011). This preparation will develop a sensitivity to and appreciation of cultures in an effort to provide high-quality care across various settings. The following is a reflection of a graduate student who participated in a clinical immersion experience in Central America:

> One of the things that really affected me while we were in Guatemala was seeing the number of children that were unable to go to school because they had to work to help support their families. Growing up in the United States, our culture prides itself on education for all children. However, going to Guatemala and speaking with children who actually cannot go to school because they have to work really struck a chord with me. It is so easy for Americans to live in their little bubble because many have no idea what it is like to not have that option. In other words, we can complain about school because there is little risk that school won't be there for us. We see it as our inherent "right." Then there are the kids in Guatemala that are longing to go to school who are denied because their family needs them to help put food on the table. Kids who are 6, 7, and 8 years old, who, in America, would be

> doing homework, are instead out on the street selling bracelets at 10 pm at night in order to help their families. Talk about perspective! It really helps me to appreciate all the educational opportunities I have been and still am being given. (Regina, graduate student)

Cultural awareness and sensitivity improvements can be directed toward practicing providers within the healthcare setting. Communication and cultural awareness education can infuse a healthcare provider's communication skills with empathy, a nonjudgmental approach to patients, enhanced awareness of self, and awareness of his or her own nonverbal communication (Thomas & Cohn, 2006). To care for the population in a culturally competent manner, NPs should see themselves on a journey growing and cultivating distinctive experiences, which will lead toward achieving cultural competence (Campinha-Bacote, 2003). This journey provides the opportunity to learn and appreciate the uniqueness of culture. In the following excerpt a nurse educator speaks about her journey to develop cultural competency:

> As an educator I prided myself in having knowledge to share with others. Reflecting on years of direct patient care, caring for individuals and groups of various cultural and ethnic backgrounds, I was humbled by what I still did not know. It is when I examined my cultural competence that I began to realize that I will not "achieve" cultural competence but will be on a journey forever to reach competency. Each interaction I have with others will increase my understanding, my sensitivity, and my awareness. I will approach others with openness and nonjudgment as I persist in my efforts along the journey. (Carolina, nurse faculty)

Demystifying the Cultural Competence Puzzle

Cultural awareness training may be helpful in increasing cultural awareness, yet it is not an easy fix to improving outcomes for disparate populations. Sequist and colleagues (2010) in a randomized control study noted that primary care clinicians had increased awareness of racial disparities after an intensive 12-month program consisting of cultural competency training and race-stratified performance feedback. This training did not improve important aspects of disease control for black diabetic patients in the program, suggesting a need for further interventions (Sequist et al., 2010). Awareness of cultural aspects of a particular group can be insightful, aiding in increased understanding, but it is not until the provider recognizes the influence of culture on a person's existence that it is significant. A partnership between a NP and client could assist in developing a greater understanding and appreciation of the culturally specific needs of the client in the context of his or her population. As expressed by the graduate student below, having one piece of the cultural competence puzzle is not enough:

> We talked about various cultures in the cultural nursing course, but it had little meaning to me. I am a NP student who has not encountered much diversity in my life. As a future NP, I know I need cultural skills to be effective in my role. But is having the knowledge I learned in class enough?

In a 2010 qualitative study, Erwin et al. (2010) examined the barriers and opportunities of Latino women to obtain health screenings and interventions. The study found that country of origin and their current geographical location affected their experiences with healthcare systems and access to services. Several cultural themes emerged including the influence of "machismo" and putting the family before themselves. The effects of these culturally based influences can present as barriers to women obtaining healthcare services (Erwin et al., 2010). Cultural influences, such as the (American/U.S.) approach where women are encouraged to care for themselves and seek health promotion services, may be regarded as a method of empowerment in one culture, yet perceived as a barrier in other cultures.

For the Latino woman who depends on the input of her husband to receive care, it is in the best interest of the woman to involve her husband in the decision-making process regarding care decisions. By considering the Latino family's views as the preferred approach to health care, the healthcare team may have greater success in meeting the family's healthcare needs.

The following case study is representative, in that it involves a Guatemalan male in the implementation of care for his infant child:

> Ana, a mother who walked 90 minutes to the clinic in a developing country, brought her 3-month-old baby, Alessandra, to the clinic our team sponsored. The mother reported she was told to bring her baby home to die; the doctors in her country could not help her. When Alessandra arrived at the clinic she was just over 3 pounds, nearly 2 pounds less than her birth weight. The team, after assessing the baby, determined that she was drinking cow's milk and had severe gastrointestinal and cutaneous symptoms. The team developed a feeding plan utilizing soy-based formula. When the team discussed the plan with the mother, it was apparent that the father of the baby needed to consent to the outlined plan. Ana was not able to make the decision for her baby. A community leader, who served as the liaison between team and family, facilitated the communication of the plan to the father, who consented. It was through the use of the community leader and a nonjudgmental approach, incorporating cultural considerations into the plan, that a successful plan was created for Alessandra. (Ellen, public health nurse)

In a article describing the fasting practices of women during pregnancy and breastfeeding, the differences between some practicing Muslim women and U.S. standards were discussed (Kridli, 2011). In a culture where pregnant women are encouraged to "eat for two," caregivers may find that the practice of fasting during pregnancy or breastfeeding is strange or wrong. It is important for the NP to take the time to understand the significance of fasting in the spiritual life of the Muslim woman. It is when healthcare providers can accept and appreciate the cultural uniqueness of an individual that they can then adapt the provision of care to meet the needs of the patient. The following case scenario is an example of how the nurse practitioner helped the patient with strong religious beliefs navigate his care in a complex health system:

> As a nurse practitioner I often need to reassess my own ability to reframe the ability to accept my patients' beliefs regarding healthcare treatments as well as their spirituality. It is sometimes difficult when we feel strongly that current practices are the only viable option for patients to choose, particularly when their choice is almost always one that will significantly alter the

ability to survive. Religious beliefs can stir up much passionate argument for insisting patients do things "our" way. I will touch upon this in my short story.

George was a middle-aged gentleman who came in yearly for his physical examination. He was doing very well in keeping his cholesterol in check with diet and a low dose statin, and was up to date with immunizations. Until one recent visit, there were no other significant healthcare-related issues. At that visit George described feeling so fatigued he could hardly get through his workday as a manager for a large home goods store. He said he was bruising easily, and was very concerned, as was I. I knew that George was a Jehovah's Witness, and we had in his file his official document regarding no blood transfusions. I have some members of my family who are also Jehovah's Witnesses, so I was well aware of all the details and scriptural support for this belief. Unfortunately, his blood work returned showing a severe pancytopenia. I convinced him to go for the consultation with the hematologist we worked closely with, assuring him I would be his advocate for him to be the main director of his own healthcare treatment plan once he was fully assessed and treatment options were discussed. Being an advocate, I also had to speak with the hematologist before George went there so he could understand what issues could cause tension within their patient–physician relationship during this time of turmoil. Unfortunately, it did appear that George had aplastic anemia.

We are working to find the cause, and he has opted to use complementary and alternative therapies instead of blood transfusions. The hematologist made George sign a document that released him from liability regarding George's decisions; however, he is still working with us for the time being. George is well aware of the possibility of dying without getting transfused, and he strongly holds to his belief system. As his primary care provider, I try to be supportive, as well as honest, when discussing his current status and his options. I have found that I am often being an advocate for George among the staff and other providers, using opportunities to correct inaccurate understanding regarding Jehovah's Witnesses.

Incorporating a cultural assessment or the collection of relevant cultural data relating to a patient's diagnosis or health concern is vital in the care of diverse populations (Campinha-Bacote, 2003). It is important to consider the biological, physical, and physiological cultural variations that may influence the physician's ability to conduct an appropriate and correct physical evaluation (Purnell, 1998, as cited in Campinha-Bacote, 2003). Significant cultural data should be gathered, adapted prior to and during the evaluation, and used in the planning and implementation of care. Goldbach, Thompson, and Hollaren Steiker (2011) discuss the importance of cultural consideration in the care of Latinos with substance abuse. The Latino culture values family orientation, *familismo*, and respect, *respeto*, in their lives. The inclusion of culturally specific aspects of care, along with acculturation, were identified as considerations when treating adolescents with substance abuse (Goldbach et al., 2011). Current strategies or approaches that do not include culturally specific strategies may be ineffective in meeting the unique needs of a specified population. To care for the adolescents, the practitioner must care for the family, use respect, and understand the psychosocial adjustment to the society in which the adolescent lives.

To understand health, it must be examined from the viewpoint of the individual or family. Health must not be gauged by others; the information must come directly from the person or community and be related to their specific circumstances (Kagan, 2008). To be effective practitioners caring for individuals, communities, and populations of need it is important to use awareness and sensitivity, authentic listening, trust, partnerships, and commitment. It is when we strive for cultural competence that we are able to improve the lives of others.

Language and Communication

The Institute of Medicine (IOM, 2003) report, *Unequal Treatment: Confronting Racial and Ethnic Disparities in Health Care,* illustrates the importance of cross-cultural communication. Effective culturally sensitive communication will lead to patient satisfaction, leading to adherence, and thus favorable patient outcomes, as seen in **FIGURE 5-2**. Faulty communication and a lack of consideration of the sociocultural factors will lead to poor patient outcomes and racial and ethnic disparities in care (IOM, 2003). To be an effective communicator, the NP must possess curiosity, empathy, respect, and humility (IOM, 2003) during interactions with individuals and communities. It is when providers ask questions and listen to the response that assumptions can be avoided.

The Office of Minority Health (OMH) was established in 1986 in response to the increased awareness regarding poor health outcomes in racial and ethnic minority populations in the United States (OMH, 2011a). CLAS standards were developed by the OMH for healthcare systems to use in order to provide the best care possible for the diverse patient populations seeking care in the United States. These standards were recently enhanced, and the goals are to (1) advance health equity, (2) improve quality, and (3) help eliminate healthcare disparities. Providing services that are adapted to an individual's cultural and language preference can aid in positive patient outcomes. The 14 CLAS standards guide the NP and other healthcare providers to the recommended language and communication processes in healthcare settings that will enhance patient care outcomes (OMH, n.d.a). For example, the NP should know the qualifications of the interpreter, interpreters must be trained in their role, and the clinician should speak directly to the patient and not the interpreter. The Think Cultural Health initiative contains educational resources to aid in the development of healthcare providers and organizations (https://www.thinkculturalhealth.hhs.gov/index.asp).

Listening

An important element of communication must not be overlooked: listening. Listening is an important yet underused skill. Patients express a desire to be listened to by their

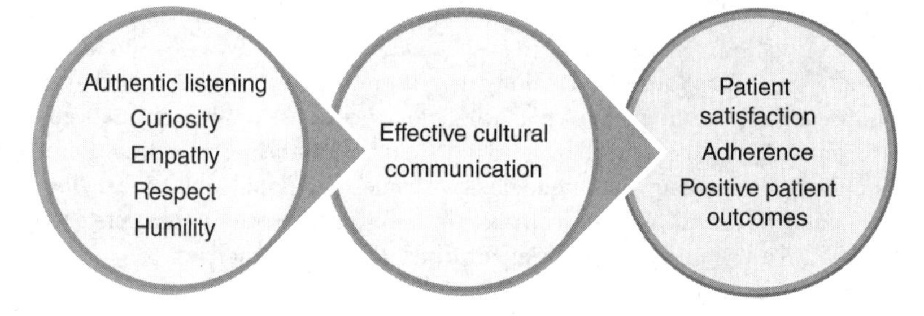

FIGURE 5-2 Communication Model

healthcare providers more than anything else (Berman & Chutka, 2016). Listening is an essential part of the appreciation and awareness of the viewpoints and feelings of others and is inherently connected to quality of life (Kagan, 2008). It is especially beneficial to employ therapeutic listening when working with individuals or groups from other cultures.

One study illustrated the benefit of listening and gaining insight into the lives of immigrant women (Belknap & VandeVusse, 2010). Using active listening, the researchers were able to identify emerging themes related to the lived experience of the women. Interventions and support related to the themes can be developed based on the knowledge obtained from listening sessions. The NP must become familiar with culturally competent organizations in the community to assist families. Partnering with the community and listening to their needs can assist the NP with the assessment, development, and implementation of interventions for the specified community. The listener, by providing a safe environment, allows the individual or group to feel secure to voice their expression. It is essential for the listener to be nonjudgmental, accepting, and negate all preconceived ideas, prejudices, and negative attitudes (Shipley, 2010). It is through active listening that the provider is receptive to discovering the needs and desires of others. NPs are often seen as the care providers that hear the patient; NPs often have the ability to truly listen to the patient's voice, and this has significant implications in the cultural considerations of care.

The ETHNIC mnemonic represented in **BOX 5-3** has been identified as a tool to assist the primary care provider in obtaining a history that encourages the inclusion of the patient's cultural perspective.

Trust

There is mistrust of the healthcare system by minority patients. Their mistrust is connected to treatment refusal for a variety of reasons including discontentment with the patient–provider relationship (Baldwin, 2003). As part of the most trusted profession (ANA, 2016), NPs are in a position to establish trusting and meaningful relationships with individuals, groups, and communities. Many of the skills necessary to build cultural awareness and sensitivity are instrumental in establishing trust: empathy, respect, listening, and a nonjudgmental approach. Taking time to build a rapport will aid in the development of trust and build relationships between the provider and the patient community. The following below displays examples of a trusting relationship between an NP and a high-risk patient:

> Jana is an African-American mother of a 2-year-old, recently paralyzed child. The child suffered the injuries during a motor vehicle accident in which her maternal grandmother was under the influence of an illegal substance. Jana herself is a recovering drug addict and prostitute who is starting to make great strides in her life. She is working and independently living in a small apartment with her daughter. As the NP overseeing her care in the hospital setting, I have the tremendous responsibility of working with the mother with the mutual goal of discharging the daughter home.
>
> The initial discharge was complex. There were many considerations: ventilator, G-tube feedings, wheelchair, and nursing, to highlight several. As I discussed the plan with the discharge coordinator, we were encountering obstacle after obstacle to meeting our goal. Was the home accessible? Was it safe? Did the mother have adequate support? We updated the mother frequently with the progress (or lack of progress). One morning the mother was angry

BOX 5-3 The ETHNIC Mnemonic

E: *Explanation*
What do you think may be the reason you have these symptoms? What do friends, family, or others say about these symptoms? Do you know anyone else who has had or who has this kind of problem? Have you heard about/read/seen it on TV/radio/newspaper? (If patient is unable to offer an explanation, ask patient what is most concerning about the problem.)

T: *Treatment*
What kinds of medicines, home remedies, or other treatments have you tried for this illness? Is there anything you eat, drink, or do (or avoid) on a regular basis to stay healthy? Tell me about it. What kind of treatment are you seeking from me?

H: *Healers*
Have you sought any advice from alternative/traditional or folk healers, friends, or other people (nondoctors) for help with your problems? Tell me about it.

N: *Negotiate*
Negotiate options that will be mutually acceptable to you and your patient and that do not contradict, but rather incorporate, your patient's beliefs.

I: *Intervention*
Determine an intervention with your patient. This may include incorporation of alternative treatments, spirituality, and healers, as well as other cultural practices (e.g., foods eaten or avoided both in general and when sick).

C: *Collaboration*
Collaborate with the patient, family members, other healthcare team members, healers, and community resources.

Adapted, Displayed, and Reproduced with permission from *Patient Care: The Practical Journal for Primary Care Physicians. Special Issue: Caring for Diverse Populations: Breaking Down Barriers, 34*(9), 189. Patient Care is a copyrighted publication of Advanstar Communications Inc.

> and started to voice her concerns in a loud and disruptive manner; she said she "had it" with "all of you." After calming her and listening to her concerns it was apparent that she did not trust that we were truly trying to discharge her daughter to home. She felt the obstacles were hiding what she felt we considered the "true" issue: that she was unfit, due to her past history, to provide care to her daughter. Despite displaying the skills and behaviors that could support her daughter's needs, Jana felt that the staff saw her as an unfit parent. I was shocked. I thought we had a professional relationship that fostered trust, but what I did not understand was how Jana's life events affected her ability to trust us and voice her concerns. I learned, after caring for Jana and her daughter, that experiences can affect a person's perception and reaction. As an NP, I need to ensure that patients and their families are able to trust me as their care provider. I need to find ways to better understand them and their experiences.

Trust and privacy were major themes that emerged in a 2012 study examining the provision of health-related services to bisexual men (Dodge et al., 2012). Perception of others, confidentiality, and trusting relationships influenced their likelihood of seeking healthcare services. Fearing that their privacy and trust will be violated, many marginal groups may distance themselves from the healthcare services they require. This separation leads to continued disparities in the provision of care and negatively affects their health and well-being.

Global and race-based medical mistrust were high among black women who have sex with black women in a recent study (Brenick, Romano, Kegler, & Eaton, 2017). Individuals with mistrust have less engagement in health care, which is of concern for the health and well-being of this identified population. Stigma from race or sexual orientation, although low in the study, should be considered to reduce disparities and promote engagement in health care.

Trust can influence health. Another study examining the relationship of trust between patients with type 2 diabetes and their physicians demonstrated that trust was related to patient outcomes. The authors concluded that "trust in physicians could contribute to improvements in patient outcomes over time" (Lee & Lin, 2011, p. 411). When caring for populations, trust is essential to building a caring relationship, and having trust in a relationship is an important aspect of care that can improve health outcomes. If a provider is culturally competent, it will positively impact the treatment adherence of the patient and the quality of care (Davey, Waite, Nuñez, Niño, & Kissil, 2014).

Nurse practitioners are viewed as being skillful in developing trusting relationships with patients. The trust is developed by learning about the patient's family, culture, and socioeconomic needs; developing and using cultural tools; and incorporating nursing tenets from professional training.

Community Partnerships

When providing care to marginalized or culturally based populations, establishing a relationship with the community is essential. Partnership, defined as two or more individuals or groups working together for a shared goal, is a key element to community engagement. Meade, Meanard, Therival, and Riveria (2009) discuss the importance of community partnerships in the development and adaptation of sustainable breast education and outreach programs for Haitian women. The partnership worked on the unique needs of the community and included cultural, educational, and literacy considerations. The development of a partnership affords the ability to determine factors that affect health and to develop approaches to maximize health and wellness. Partnerships with community leaders and community gatekeepers are essential features to the success of outreach initiatives (Meade et al., 2009).

An example of a lack of partnerships within the healthcare setting was presented in a 2009 study examining the use of CAM in the treatment of autism spectrum disorder (ASD) in the United States and China. An interesting finding from this study revealed that only 22.4% of respondents informed their doctors about CAM use to treat ASD. The study suggests that the participants did not inform their physician of the CAM use because they felt that the Western physician would not allow CAM nor believe its effectiveness (Wong, 2009). Lack of trusting partnerships can lead to continued healthcare disparities.

In a study exploring the influence of NPs on the delivery of culturally competent care, NPs stated that collaborating with other members of the healthcare team, as well as patients, was effective in the delivery of culturally competent care. Working with patients to meet their identified needs was a priority for the NP, as well as for the patient. Addressing other impending concerns was completed by negotiation and partnering.

In a 2011 study of Native American men and HIV, barriers to HIV/AIDS care were presented. Many of the barriers were related to and contributed to the disparity in the provision of care to Native American men. The participants in this study identified that using indigenous outreach workers would be an effective approach to the prevention and intervention efforts (Burks, Robbins, & Durtschi, 2011). They also expressed the importance of inclusion of traditional healing practices into the provision of HIV/AIDS services. Establishing partnerships with community leaders and outreach workers could improve the health of the community by addressing their needs with a culturally focused approach.

In addition, Saha and colleagues (2013) found that minority HIV patients who had a provider who scored toward the middle or high ranges of cultural competence were more likely to be on antiretrovirals than patients who had a provider who scored low in cultural competence. Again, this study shows that the cultural competence of the healthcare provider is connected to healthcare quality and outcomes of patients.

Pulling It All Together

Caring for patients and addressing and adapting care to meet the cultural needs of patients takes a holistic approach. When care is provided in a culturally sensitive manner, it extends beyond the medical concerns presented. The inclusion of social, spiritual, lifestyle, societal, and familial aspects of the individual is imperative to determining and responding to the patient's needs. Having a holistic approach is to look at the patient's complete life, not solely focusing on illness.

The LIAASE, a general cultural competence tool, is a helpful structure to guide the provider in providing care that is sensitive to the individual's culture and preferences (see **BOX 5-4**).

In the following case scenario, the NP uses components of the LIAASE tool as she develops a culturally competent plan of care for the patient.

Using the LIAASE Tool to Provide Culturally Sensitive Care

While working in a busy OB/GYN clinic as a new FNP, I was quickly moving my novice skill level to advanced due in part to the resident physicians' avoidance of the clinic. It was also a wonderful place to provide culturally sensitive care. We had a large number of patients from Haiti and Guatemala, in addition to almost every other country. One day I went into an examination room and found a pleasant young couple waiting for a new OB examination. The woman was covered in a very colorful sari and was smiling, but quiet and deferential to her equally pleasant husband.

He very nicely told me that since I was the only female provider in the clinic that day that they had requested I do her initial intake and examination. I loved doing the new OB visits, so that was not the challenge—the challenge was in trying to do a pelvic exam and get a PAP smear and ultrasound with all that clothing. Saris can be worn in different colors to represent different meanings; for instance, yellow can typically be worn for the first 7 days postpartum, and paisley can be worn as a symbol of fertility. The couple was pleased that I managed to get all the necessary portions of the examination done while maintaining the woman's privacy. We developed a mutually understanding and respectful partnership during a time of joy for this newly pregnant couple in what could have been disastrous if the provider who attended to them was not culturally sensitive.

BOX 5-4 The LIAASE: A General Cultural Competence Tool

Learn Read literature from other cultures. Identify your own biases and stereotypes.	**Avoid Polarization** Solicit other options or points of view. Ask what perspective a person from a different background would have.
Inquire Ask questions to clarify and understand information. Dig deeper to find reasons for behaviors or attitudes. Frame inquiries as searches for answers, showing a willingness to learn. Do not judge or interpret actions or speech; verify that what you understand is correct. Speak clearly; avoid slang, colloquial expressions, and large, complex words.	**Avoid Arguing and Defending** Curb the impulse to defend your point of view or opinion. Agree to disagree on differences in values. **Show Empathy** Listen not just to the words, but to the feelings behind the words. Acknowledge and validate powerful emotions when expressed.
State Your Needs and Expectations It is important to set a respectful tone for the interaction. Let people know what you want and what you consider unacceptable behavior. In this way assumptions, conflict, and/or resentment can be avoided.	

Reproduced from Nova Scotia Department of Health and Wellness. (2005). *A cultural competence guide for primary health care professionals in Nova Scotia*. Retrieved from http://www.healthteamnovascotia.ca/cultural_competence/Cultural_Competence_guide_for_Primary_Health_Care_Professionals.pdf. Used by permission of Nova Scotia Department of Health and Wellness.

Evaluation

When working with individuals or groups, there is a need to evaluate the outcomes of the interventions, including the evaluation of those we partner with. Outcome evaluations should be culturally sensitive; they should use wording and terms that the community or individual would understand within the context of their culture. It is important to receive feedback from the community or individual on whom the intervention focused. Do they perceive the intervention as useful or beneficial? After using focus groups to determine the best interventions to use in a community-based intervention program for Mexican American women, Ingram et al. (2012) used a participatory evaluation process to adapt to the needs of the women in the community. The authors, using the women's responses, were able to understand the behavioral and knowledge changes as a result of the program's interventions. Their responses revealed why they adapted their behaviors and the barriers they encountered when following the intervention recommendations (Ingram et al., 2012). Their input was valuable to gaining their perspective on the significance of the interventions as well as their perceived barriers, thus contributing an important aspect of program evaluation. When examining the outcomes of a program or intervention, cultural influences must be considered when applying meaning to the results (Issel, 2009).

Evaluation is the ability to reflect on our care as NPs in an effort to gain greater clarity on the provision of culturally competent care. It serves as a time to ask if the care was what the patient needed or desired. In our role, this feedback ensures that we are evaluating not only the care provided but also ourselves as care providers. In summary, nurse practitioners must respond to the unique and distinct needs of the diverse and ever-changing society. Attention to cultural variations as well as societal factors influencing health must be considered to care for an increasingly diverse population. Cultural awareness and sensitivity are critical to the achievement of culturally competent care.

Seminar Discussion Questions

1. Identify your own cultural beliefs and values.
2. Discuss the variety of cultures in your professional practice.
3. Reflect on your cultural journey. What do you consider as obstacles to achieving cultural competence? What strategies can be employed to overcome the barriers?
4. Describe a situation or circumstance when cultural factors influenced the care of an individual or family. Were culturally sensitive interventions/approaches implemented? If yes, please describe. If interventions/approaches were not based on the individual's or family's cultural preferences, how could the encounter have been adapted to meet the unique cultural needs?
5. What method or strategy could be implemented to evaluate the integration of cultural strategies during a patient encounter?

References

American Association of Colleges of Nursing. (1994). *The essentials of master's education for advanced practice nursing.* Retrieved from http://www.aacn.nche.edu/education-resources/MasEssentials96.pdf

American Association of Colleges of Nursing. (2006). *The essentials of doctoral education for advanced nursing practice.* Retrieved from http://www.aacn.nche.edu/publications/position/DNPEssentials.pdf

American Association of Colleges of Nursing. (2008). *The essentials of baccalaureate education for professional nursing practice.* Retrieved from http://www.aacn.nche.edu/education-resources/BaccEssentials08.pdf

American College of Physicians. (2010). *Racial and ethnic disparities in health care* (Policy paper). Philadelphia, PA: Author.

American Nurses Association. (2012). *Diversity awareness mission statement.* Retrieved from http://nursingworld.org/MainMenuCategories/ThePracticeofProfessionalNursing/Improving-Your-Practice/Diversity-Awareness/Mission-Statement.html

American Nurses Association. (2016). *Nurses rank #1 most trusted profession for 15th year in a row.* Retrieved from http://www.nursingworld.org/FunctionalMenuCategories/MediaResources/PressReleases/Nurses-Rank-1-Most-Trusted-Profession-2.pdf

Axtell, S. A., Avery, M., & Westra, B. (2010). Incorporating cultural competence content into graduate nursing curricula through community-university collaboration. *Journal of Transcultural Nursing, 21*, 183–191. doi:10.1177/1043659609357633

Baldwin, D. M. (2003). Disparities in health and health care: Focusing efforts to eliminate unequal burdens. *Online Journal of Issues in Nursing, 8*(1). Retrieved from http://www.nursingworld.org/MainMenuCategories/ANAMarketplace/ANAPeriodicals/OJIN/TableofContents/Volume82003/No1Jan2003/DisparitiesinHealthandHealthCare.aspx

Belknap, R. A., & VandeVusse, L. (2010). Listening sessions with Latinas: Documenting life contexts and creating connections. *Public Health Nursing, 27*, 337–346. doi:10.1111/j.1525-1446.2010.00864.x

Betancourt, J. R., Green, A. R., Carrillo, J. E., & Anaaeh-Firempong II, O. (2003, July-August). Defining cultural competence: A practical framework for addressing racial/ethnic disparities in health and health care. *Public Health Reports, 118*, 293–302.

Bomar, P. (2004). *Promoting health in families: Applying family research and theory to nursing practice.* Philadelphia, PA: Saunders.

Boutin-Foster, C., Foster, J., & Konopasek, L. (2008). Viewpoint: Physician, know thyself: The professional culture of medicine as a framework for teaching cultural competence. *Academic Medicine, 83*, 106–111. doi:10.1097/ACM.0b013e31815c6753

Brenick, A., Romano, K., Kegler, C., & Eaton, L. A. (2017). Understanding the influence of stigma and medical mistrust on engagement in routine healthcare among black women Who have sex with women. *LGTB, 4*(1). doi:10.1089/lgbt.2016.0083

Burks, D. J., Robbins, R., & Durtschi, J. P. (2011). American Indian gay, bisexual, and two-spirit men: A rapid assessment of HIV/AIDS risk factors, barriers to prevention, and culturally sensitive intervention. *Culture, Health & Sexuality, 13*(3), 283–298.

California Health Advocates. (2007). *Are you practicing cultural humility? The key to success in cultural competence.* Retrieved from http://www.cahealthadvocates.org/news/disparities/2007/are-you.html

Campinha-Bacote, J. (2003). Many faces: Addressing diversity in health care. *Online Journal of Issues in Nursing, 8*. Retrieved from http://www.nursingworld.org/MainMenuCategories/ANAMarketplace/ANAPeriodicals/OJIN/TableofContents/Volume82003/No1Jan2003/AddressingDiversityinHealthCare.aspx

Census Bureau. (2011). *Overview of race and Hispanic origin: 2010.* Retrieved from http://www.census.gov/prod/cen2010/briefs/c2010br-02.pdf

Corazzini, K. N., Lekan-Rutledge, D., Utley-Smith, Q., Piven, M. L., Colon-Emeric, C. S., Bailey, D., . . . Anderson, R. A. (2006, November 15). *The golden rule: Only a starting point for quality care.* Retrieved from http://www.ncbi.nlm.nih.gov/pmc/articles/PMC1636677

Davey, M. P., Waite, R., Nuñez, A., Niño, A., & Kissil, K. (2014). A snapshot of patients' perceptions of oncology providers' cultural competence. *Journal of Cancer Education, 29*(4), 657–664.

Dayer-Berenson, L. (2014). *Cultural competencies for nurses: Impact on health and illness* (2nd ed.). Burlington, MA: Jones & Bartlett.

Dodge, B., Schnarvs, P. W., Gonclaves, G., Majebranche, D., Martinez, O., Reece, M., & Fortenberry, J. D. (2012, June 1). The significance of privacy and trust in providing health-related services to behaviorally bisexual men in the United States. *AIDS Education and Prevention, 24*, 242–256.

Doorenbos, A. Z., Schim, S. M., Benkert, R., & Borse, N. N. (2005). Psychometric evaluation of the cultural competence assessment instrument among healthcare providers. *Nursing Research, 54*(5), 324–331.

Erwin, D. O., Trevino, M., Saag-Harfouche, S. G., Rodriguez, E. M., Gage, E., & Jandorf, L. (2010). Contextualizing diversity and culture within cancer control interventions for Latinas: Changing interventions, not cultures. *Social Science & Medicine, 71*, 693–701. Retrieved from http://ac.els-cdn.com.silk.library.umass.edu

Giger, J. N. (2017). *Transcultural nursing: Assessment and intervention* (7th ed.). Retrieved from https://pageburstls.elsevier.com/#/books/9780323399920/

Giger, J., Davidhizar, R., Purnell, L., Harden, J., Phillips, J., & Strickland, O. (2007). American Academy of Nursing Expert Panel Report: Developing cultural competence to eliminate health disparities in ethnic minorities and other vulnerable populations. *Journal of Transcultural Nursing, 18*(2), 95–102.

Goldbach, J. T., Thompson, S. J., & Hollaren Steiker, L. K. (2011). Special considerations for substance abuse intervention with Latino youth. *Prevention Researcher, 18*(2), 8–11.

Green, S. S., Comer, L., Elliott, L., & Neubrander, J. (2011). Exploring the value of an international service-learning experience in Honduras. *Nursing Education Perspectives, 12*, 302–307.

Ingram, M., Piper, R., Kunz, S., Navarro, C., Sander, A., & Gastelum, S. (2012). Salud sí: A case study for the use of participatory evaluation in creating effective and sustainable community-based health promotion. *Family & Community Health, 35*, 130–138. doi:10.1097/FCH.0b013e31824650ed

Institute of Medicine. (2003). *Unequal treatment: Confronting racial and ethnic disparities in health care.* Washington, DC: National Academy Press. Retrieved from http://www.nap.edu/openbook.php?record_id=12875&page=200

Issel, L. M. (2009). *Health program planning and evaluation* (2nd ed.). Sudbury, MA: Jones and Bartlett.

Johns, A., & Thompson, C. W. (2010). Developing cultural sensitivity through study abroad. *Home Health Care Management Practice, 22*, 344–348. doi:10.1177/1084822 309353153

Jones, E. D., Ivanov, L. L., Wallace, D., & VonCannon, L. (2010, August). Global service learning project influences culturally sensitive care. *Home Health Care Management Practice, 22*, 464–469. doi:10.1177/1084822310368657

Kagan, P. N. (2008). Feeling listened to: A lived experience of human becoming. *Nursing Science Quarterly, 21*(1), 59–67. doi:10.1177/0894318407310779

Kridli, S. (2011). Health beliefs and practices of Muslim women during Ramadan. *MCN, the American Journal of Maternal Child Nursing, 36*, 216–221. doi:10.1097/NMC.0b013e3182177177

Larson, K. L., Ott, M., & Miles, J. M. (2010). International cultural immersion en vivo reflections in cultural competence. *Journal of Cultural Diversity, 2*, 44–50.

LaVeist, T., Gaskin, D., & Richard, P. (2009). *The economic burden of health inequalities in the United States.* Washington, DC: Joint Center for Political and Economic Studies. Retrieved from http://www.jointcenter.org/hpi/sites/all/files/Burden_Of_Health_FINAL_0.pdf

Lee, Y., & Lin, J. L. (2011). How much does trust really matter? A study of the longitudinal effects of trust and decision-making preferences on diabetic patient outcomes. *Patient Education and Counseling, 85*, 406–412. doi:10.1016/j.pec.2010.12.005

Levin, S. J., Like, R. C., & Gottlieb, J. E. (2000). Appendix: Useful clinical interviewing mnemonics. *Patient Care: The Practical Journal for Primary Care Physicians.* Special Issue: Caring for Diverse Populations: Breaking Down Barriers, *34*(9), 189.

Luluquisen, M., Schaff, K., & Galvez, S. (n.d.). Almeda County Public Health Department Community Assessment Planning & Education Unit. *Cultural competence and cultural humility* [PowerPoint presentation]. Retrieved from http://www.acphd.org/media/133120/modii_slides_cultural_competency.pdf

Matteliano, M. A., & Street, D. (2012). Nurse practitioners' contributions to cultural competence in primary care settings. *Journal of American Academy of Nurse Practitioners, 24*, 425–435.

McFarlane, M. M., & Eipperle, M. K. (2008). Culture care theory: A proposed practice theory guide for nurse practitioners in primary care settings. *Contemporary Nurse, 28*(1/2), 46–63.

Meade, C. D., Meanard, J., Therival, C., & Riveria, M. (2009). Addressing cancer disparities through community engagement: Improving breast health among Haitian women. *Oncology Nursing Forum, 36*, 716–723. doi:10.1188/09.ONF.716-722

Nova Scotia Department of Health. (2005). *A cultural competence guide for primary health care professionals in Nova Scotia.* Halifax, Nova Scotia: Author.

Office of Disease Prevention and Health Promotion. (2010). *Healthy People 2020.* Retrieved from http://healthypeople.gov/2020/about/DisparitiesAbout.aspx

Office of Minority Health. (2011a). *About OMH.* Retrieved from http://minorityhealth.hhs.gov/templates/browse.aspx?lvl=1&lvlID=7

Office of Minority Health. (2011b). *What is cultural competency?* Retrieved from http://minorityhealth.hhs.gov/templates/browse.aspx?lvl=2&lvlID=11

Office of Minority Health. (n.d.). *National CLAS standards.* Retrieved from https://www.thinkculturalhealth.hhs.gov/Content/clas.asp#clas_standards

Office of Minority Health. (n.d.). *A physician's practical guide to culturally competent care.* Retrieved from https://cccm.thinkculturalhealth.hhs.gov

Ott, B. B., & Olson, R. M. (2011). Ethical issues of medical missions: The clinicians' view. *HEC Forum, 23*(2), 105–113. doi:10.1007/s10730-011-9154-9

Riner, M. E. (2011). Globally engaged nursing education: An academic program framework. *Nursing Outlook, 59*, 308–317. doi:10.1016/j.outlook.2011.04.005

Saha, S., Korthuis, P. T., Cohn, J. A., Sharp, V. L., Moore, R. D., & Beach, M. C. (2013). Primary care provider cultural competence and racial disparities in HIV care and outcomes. *JGIM: Journal of General Internal Medicine, 28*(5), 622–629.

Schim, S. M., Doorenbos, A., Benkert, R., & Miller, J. (2007). Culturally congruent care: Putting the puzzle together. *Journal of Transcultural Nursing, 18*, 103–110. doi:10.1177/1043659606298613

Schim, S. M., Doorenbos, A. Z., Miller, J., & Benkert, R. (2003). Development of a cultural competence assessment instrument. *Journal of Nursing Measurement, 11*(3), 29–40.

Sequist, T. D., Fitzmaurice, G. M., Marshall, R., Shaykevich, S., Marston, A., Safran, D. G., & Ayanlan, J. Z. (2010). Cultural competency training and performance reports to improve diabetes care for black patients. *Annals of Internal Medicine, 152*(4), 40–46. Retrieved from http://web.ebscohost.com.silk.library.umass.edu/ehost/pdf

Shipley, S. D. (2010). Listening: A concept analysis. *Nursing Forum, 45*(2), 125–134.

Sitzman, K., & Eichelberger, L. W. (Eds.). (2004). *Understanding the work of nurse theorists.* Sudbury, MA: Jones and Bartlett.

Stanglin, K. D. (2005). The historical connection between the Golden Rule and the second greatest love command. *Journal of Religious Ethics*, 33(2), 357–371.

Tervalon, M., & Murray-Garcia, J. (1998). Cultural humility versus cultural competence: A critical distinction in defining physician training outcomes in multicultural education. *Journal of Health Care for the Poor and Underserved, 9*(2), 117–125.

Thomas, V. J., & Cohn, T. (2006). Communication skills and cultural awareness courses for healthcare professionals who care for patients with sickle cell disease. *Issues and Innovations in Nursing Education, 53*, 480–488.

Tomey, A. M., & Alligood, M. R. (2002). *Nursing theorists and their work* (5th ed.). St Louis, MO: Mosby.

Wong, V. C. (2009). Use of complementary and alternative medicine (CAM) in autism spectrum disorder (ASD): Comparison of Chinese and Western culture. *Journal of Autism & Developmental Disorders, 39*(3), 454–463. doi:10.1007/s10803-008-0644-9

PART 3

Clinical Education for the Nurse Practitioner

CHAPTER 6

Clinical Education, Case Presentation, Consultation, and Collaboration in Primary Care

Julie G. Stewart, Susan M. DeNisco, Michelle Johnson, and Holly B. Bradley

The most exciting part of any nurse practitioner (NP) program is when the time comes to start clinical experiences. At minimum, 500 hours spent in supervised practice in the clinical setting are required for graduation and the certification examination. The American Nursing Credentialing Center (ANCC, 2013) requires 500 faculty-supervised clinical hours to take the certification exam, whereas the American Association of Colleges of Nursing (AACN, 2006) requires a total of 1,000 faculty-supervised clinical/practice hours for the nurse practitioner student graduating Doctorate of Nursing Practice (DNP). Therefore, students in a DNP program that are postmasters and are already certified as an NP still must complete 500 faculty-supervised clinical/practice hours. This chapter will first discuss traditional clinical education in a nurse practitioner program (master's NP program and post-BSN DNP program). Later, clinical education for the NP in a DNP program will be discussed.

Depending on the program track, clinical experiences could be in private medical offices, clinics, hospitals, or perhaps even national or global healthcare missions where the underserved are in great need of healthcare services. It is vital that the student, as well as the preceptor, is prepared for the experience, to avoid unnecessary frustration and possible negative outcomes. In particular, the experience needs to be focused on the goals and objectives for the clinical course, the skill level of the NP student, and the practice expectations of the preceptor. Specific goals are formulated and assessed for both the student and the preceptor throughout the clinical courses.

Each type of clinical setting has both general and site-specific planning requirements. For example, planning with the preceptor can help the student better understand how the practice functions on a daily basis, and identify the types of patients the student is able to see to meet course objectives, and in what capacity the student will see patients. Often, the first day is spent with the student observing the preceptor's interactions with patients and learning about the clinical site in general. In some practices, there may be patients who do not want to have a student do any portion of the interview or physical; however, explaining that the patient's own provider (be it an NP, MD, CNM, or PA) will always be aware of the patient's status and direct the assessment and treatment plan frequently allays any fears the patient may have. It is crucial the preceptor be aware of the role of the student NP and that the clinical should not consist of the student merely "shadowing" the provider for the entire clinical rotation. This rarely meets the expectations of the experience; preceptors (whether or not they have had a NP student in the past) need to be ready to assist the student in developing good interviewing, physical assessment, and diagnostic skills. This is especially important in the first clinical rotation, since a positive experience can give the student the confidence necessary to prevail in subsequent clinical arenas.

If the student has a clinical rotation in an outpatient clinic setting, whether it be a nurse-led clinic, community health center, federally funded health center, or an extension of a hospital-based clinic, these can be very worthwhile experiences. Although clinics tend to be very busy, and the healthcare providers often have a heavy patient load, it is a rich and rewarding opportunity for helping needy patients in addition to honing clinical skills. There may be multiple languages spoken, so the NP student must be aware of what translation services the clinic provides. In addition, there are many culturally unique approaches to care the NP student should be prepared for by reading and learning how to approach and provide culturally sensitive care. This topic is addressed in a separate chapter. Patients in clinic settings often have comorbid and complex healthcare issues in addition to psychosocial and financial difficulties. The clinical experience in this type of setting has multiple challenges as well as rewards.

An acute care site has a unique set of issues to be addressed prior to starting. The faculty and preceptor need to make sure the student is aware of the privileges awarded to the preceptor and to NPs in the setting through the credentialing process. The acute care setting may have additional policies about how much NP students are allowed to do with patients. Often, the student may be spending time shadowing the preceptor and performing portions of the history and physical together, then working collaboratively to develop a treatment plan. Faculty will need to determine if a greater scope of practice (e.g., skills or communicating with other disciplines involved in the patient's care) is needed if the scope is very narrow.

One method for gaining clinical experience is to be able to accompany faculty and other students on healthcare missions to provide care to a population needing assistance. Being prepared for the types of patients to be seen, the ability to dispense or prescribe medications, order diagnostic testing, and follow-up should be understood prior to embarking on this type of clinical immersion. Planning should be done to have local support wherever the group is going to ensure proper lodging, transportation, safety, and, importantly, to have identified specific needs of that population. It is vital that the host population dictate what the healthcare mission staff can and cannot do. Visiting mission groups are guests of the host community. NP students can learn much on these types of immersion experiences, and in particular, will discover how much they can offer patients by providing education about health and wellness, and disease management. The students may venture to a location where medications are not a viable option; therefore, diet and basic public health principles can be reviewed. It is important to remember that students may see and be exposed to infectious diseases rarely seen in the United States. This means the student must be sure to have had all appropriate travel vaccinations and bring emergency items such as Tylenol, bandages, and ointments on the trip.

Whatever the clinical site and patient population, clinical learning is a complex process for NP students. An option for the NP program and/or the individual student may consider is journaling. The ability to take the time for reflection can assist the student to process the patient interactions of the day, and help the student develop a deeper awareness of their own performance. Students can also consider concepts beyond the actual physical experience to write about such as social and cultural issues that arise in most patient encounters (Wedgeworth, Carter, & Ford, 2017). It is important for the faculty to give direction on what reflective journaling could include. Some introductory "prompting" questions are offered here (Watson, 2016):

Daily Reflective Questions:
Date/Location:

1. The images that remain with me from today are . . .
2. The best moment or part of today was . . .
3. The hardest or lowest point of today was . . .
4. Other thoughts, feelings, or learning from today:

The Role of Faculty

Nurse practitioner faculty are responsible for ensuring the NP student has adequate didactic knowledge prior to beginning clinical rotations. Nurse practitioner faculty who provide direct supervision of nurse practitioner students' clinical education should be nationally certified in the same population-focused area of practice (National Task Force on Quality Nurse Practitioner Education, 2012). Preparing students for clinical by reviewing course expectations, goals, and necessary forms, in addition to whatever the clinical site requires, needs to be accomplished prior to the start date. Leaving plenty of time for unexpected delays helps to avoid both a late start and the inability of the student to complete the necessary clinical hours for that course. Whenever possible, matching students and preceptors by the type of practice and physical location should be done. Many programs are fortunate to have clinical coordinators who are able to develop professional relationships with various practices and institutions, and they understand exactly what types of experiences will be best suited for specific student needs. The clinical coordinator is able to meet individually with students to get to know them on a more personal level, and then with the input of the responsible faculty, is apprised of the skill level of the student in order to try to match them to appropriate clinical sites.

The faculty and staff share in educating and communicating with preceptors regarding course objectives and program policies, keeping them current with expectations. Clinical advisors are either full-time faculty or adjunct faculty who are NPs that are responsible for overseeing the clinical experiences of up to six NP students. The clinical advisor is the link for the student and the preceptor, visiting the student onsite to determine that the student is progressing in a supportive learning environment, in addition to getting to know the preceptor. This role provides the student and preceptor with someone knowledgeable about the course objectives and someone who can troubleshoot any issues that may arise. One method for the clinical advisor to keep track of the types of experiences the student is getting, as well as how the student is evolving, is having the student submit nonidentifiable focused notes, with at least two per day being reasonable. The clinical advisor should also be given one to two comprehensive SOAP notes per semester, to be able to sit down with the student and give feedback and instruction in an environment outside of the clinical setting. This may also help the student to be more relaxed and able to bring up questions or comments pertinent to the role transition. At the end of the clinical rotation, the clinical advisor should be sure to obtain the student's evaluation of the clinical site and preceptor so the faculty and clinical coordinator are able to review students' evaluations of various clinical sites to maintain an up-to-date list of supportive environments.

Another option for evaluating the clinical skills of the NP student is by direct observation in a setting using actors as patients. This type of evaluation usually consists of a 20-minute direct observation assessment or "snapshot" of a trainee–patient interaction. This evaluation is based on the Mini-CEX or Objective Structured Clinical Examination (OSCE), which have been used as an evaluation of medical students or medical residents who perform the same types of patient experiences (American Board of Internal Medicine, 2012) and have become standard in most NP programs. Patient interviewing, focused physical examination, informed decision making or counseling, and clinical judgment and reasoning are evaluated by the faculty with input from the trained actors. Faculty provide timely and specific feedback to the trainee after each assessment of a trainee–patient encounter.

Another method gaining popularity among NP programs is the use of simulation. In the acute care tracks, simulation scenarios for cardiac arrest, complex procedures, and managing urgent care health problems is a safe method for allowing the student to perform these activities with no risk to an actual patient (Pittman, 2012). In addition, primary care NP tracks can use simulation or hybrid clinical scenarios for the students to evaluate abnormal heart and/or lung sounds to simulate congestive heart failure or asthma, for example. Being able to adequately assess students and provide feedback to help them learn how to improve skills in a productive manner will improve the students' abilities in real-life clinical situations.

There are approximately 1,000 simulation centers in the United States (Ross, 2012). So, in addition to students having the availability of mannequins and anatomical models, full simulation centers often include complete surgical suites, patient examination rooms fully equipped to mimic real examination rooms, and delivery rooms, in which scenarios can be played out. These simulation centers are often places where multiple disciplines can share space and work together.

The clinical instructor should also supervise students via site visits. This increases communication between the faculty and student, as well as the faculty and preceptor. Student and faculty should have open lines of communication that facilitate the student–faculty relationship. Students should be encouraged to discuss concerns, desires, and any issues that may have arisen during the clinical rotation. When visiting the clinical site, the advisor should use the opportunity to observe the student seeing a patient (with appropriate permissions). This is an excellent method for the clinical advisor, who is well aware of the level of competency the individual student should be functioning at, to assess the interaction and discuss the evaluation with the student as well as the preceptor. These site visits are also a time when not only the student performing skills can be observed, but when a face-to-face discussion related to the student's progress can be done. Brooks and Niederhauser (2010) found that preceptors expect at least two visits per semester. They further recommended that faculty be present for at least two to three patient visits and that a site visit should occur in the first 4 weeks of the clinical rotation.

The faculty should have a clear set of objectives for their site visits. Brooks and Niederhauser (2010) found that verifying that both the environment and the patients are suitable for the students to meet their learning objectives were of high priority during a site visit. In addition, answering the preceptor's questions and giving the preceptors support was imperative.

The Role of the Student

The NP student has tremendous responsibilities regarding the clinical experience. A few of the reminders may seem obvious; however, any experienced preceptor will verify that not all students adhere to these basic rules. These include being on time, being prepared, wearing appropriate dress, bringing reference materials, and coming to the clinical site with self-awareness of knowledge and skill level. The student needs to be in touch with the preceptor prior to starting the rotation to find out what time the preceptor expects the student to arrive and what time the day typically ends. Various practice sites have different policies regarding dress—some require professional attire with or without lab coats, some prefer scrubs, and so forth. Professional attire and manner is not always obvious to all students; therefore, what constitutes appropriate attire should be reviewed. Students should understand that appearing professional assists in gaining the trust of patients, as well as promoting professional communication among staff and colleagues.

Students should be aware of course goals, in order to discuss these with the preceptor, and should understand that each preceptor has a different style of teaching, as well as approach to patients. A good preceptor can teach the student through formal and informal methods. Being an engaged learner means that the student will seek out experiences that will help expand knowledge and relationship-building skills in whatever opportunities arise. It may be beneficial to expect that the first day will be spent following the preceptor as patients are being seen, to get a better feel for how the preceptor and practice setting work. As the student asks appropriate questions at the appropriate time, the preceptor will gain trust in the abilities of the student and begin to allow the student to perform the history, and then the physical examination with less and less oversight. Setting mutual goals from the beginning of the experience helps to decrease misunderstandings and avoids frustration for both the student and preceptor. Having a realistic patient load is imperative. The student must remember that the goal is not to help see as many patients as possible—it is to engage in learning how to provide safe, high-quality care with the supervision and collaboration of a competent healthcare provider. Also, one of the best ways for the student to gain clinical experience and confidence is to care for patients with diverse diagnoses with increasing acuity as time goes on.

The role transition that occurs from RN to NP is often an uncomfortable one, in particular for the expert nurse who now becomes a novice as a student NP. Numerous issues must be discussed to ease this transition. Issues include understanding the role of the NP, the expanded level of autonomy, leadership, clinical skills, and decision making (Spoelstra & Robbins, 2010). It is challenging for the student NP to fully comprehend the role of the NP, as it remains an abstract concept that is slowly coming into focus during the transition. Although numerous studies have been published on the transition from student to RN, not as many studies have investigated the transition from RN to NP. Some of these studies are discussed in the following paragraphs. They should be reviewed and discussed by student NPs in clinical seminar settings to increase awareness of the transition process and to encourage cohesion among the group.

Identity crisis and role confusion were identified in nurse practitioner students well over 30 years ago (Brown & Olshansky, 1997; Cusson & Strange, 2008; Roberts, Tabloski, & Bova, 1997). A period of resocialization was observed by Anderson, Leonard, and Yates in 1974, and was validated by NP faculty at the University of Minnesota in the late 1990s. While focusing on learning the skills of physical assessment and medical diagnosing, the NP students appeared to lose their expert nursing skills in the areas of psychosocial and developmental assessment. This return to a novice status was disconcerting and took months of guidance by the faculty to assist them in progressing through the stages of anxiety and anger to begin feeling competent and have a better understanding of the new role of nurse practitioner. Nurse practitioners' transition from novice to expert is the same as the novice RN's transition to expert as described by Benner (1984). An example of the transition process can be seen in these reflections by Bridget, a student family nurse practitioner.

IMPOSTER PHENOMENON

I had a strange dream last night. I was test riding roller coasters, one after the other. After riding a few, I was riding one along a commuter train track for a long time—seems that one of the engineers needed to be dropped off first—so we rode through the city of Philadelphia, of all places, looking at the strange scenery that can only be found in my dream. It was cloudy, grey, and foggy. There were strange-shaped buildings and structures that had very skinny foundations with elaborate buildings above them. I was waiting for the coaster to start up—it never did, but I disembarked and got onto another one. This one looked more like a hayride. I woke up before the ride began.

Could this be some strange metaphor for semester break? Perhaps the first half of the semester was more like a roller coaster, this break like a commuter train, and the latter half may be more like a hayride?

For the first time in my academic career, I had an amazing fortuitous start to the semester—half the grades are in and my average so far is a strong *A*. I cannot say that I feel any smarter than my peers; I feel lucky, if anything else, like I got lucky on the exam, for my presentation and paper, or perhaps my professor was just being kind.

In your spare time (yeah, right) check out this article:

Arena, D., & Page, N. (1992). The imposter phenomenon in the clinical nurse specialist role. *Image—The Journal of Nursing Scholarship, 24*(2), 121–125. Retrieved from MEDLINE database.

It's about imposter phenomenon, and there are many articles like this one. Basically imposter phenomenon describes people who may be successful on the outside, but they feel as if they are imposters in their chosen profession. According to the article, individuals who are experiencing the phenomenon have a deep feeling that they are fooling everyone. This describes me perfectly. I never feel as smart or accomplished as my peers; even when I do well, I tell myself that it is only because I got lucky, or that I somehow fooled my professor and peers to get the good grade, to get the kudos at work.

Essentially, the article states that to manage it, discuss your feelings with other colleagues, especially more experienced colleagues who can offer support, continue to develop your knowledge base through education and research, and seek expert assistance on topics that you are less familiar with.

I am quite certain that I don't have it mastered, but perhaps I am not unique in feeling this way.

OB/GYN CLINICAL

A few weeks ago I finished my OB/GYN rotation at a correctional institution—a women's prison in Connecticut. The good women of this correctional institution should have their sentences reduced for allowing me the privilege of performing my first gynecological assessments, Pap smears, and OB assessments on them. OB/GYN is not my strong suit, and I was definitely operating out of my comfort zone there. When I started, the thought of ever doing this independently was not on my radar.

On my final day, we had a quiet moment in the day. My preceptor went to the copy machine and left me in the clinic room. One of our patients arrived and was sitting in the hallway waiting. The least I could do was get her height, weight, and vital signs. My preceptor did not return. So I continued to get a history: She was a 27-year-old woman, there for an annual gyn exam, and she was very nice, very eager to work with a newbie like myself. I got a really long history, because my preceptor still did not return. So, she put her gown on, and I continued to make conversation with her, noting that she had a package of contraband Jolly Ranchers in her bra—I did not confiscate. My preceptor returned long before she had to "scoot to the end of the table" thank goodness, but I really felt, at that point that I could have done her exam by myself. It was a pretty good feeling that I can function in that setting—and it isn't even in my comfort area. Things just started to click.

In a grounded theory study that looked at the role transition from expert critical care nurse to advanced nurse practitioner in the critical care setting, researchers uncovered themes and categories that explained the linked processes that occur during this time frame (Fleming & Carberry, 2011). The first set of themes included the students' doubting their ability to become advanced practice nurses (APNs) after being expert critical care RNs, and issues revolving around role uncertainty and feelings of isolation and needing to fit in with other members of the healthcare team in the critical care unit (CCU). The first group of student APNs had to deal with conflict regarding boundaries between their role and the junior doctors' (residents') roles in the CCU. Peer support was identified as helpful for reducing conflict issues in a productive manner.

As the APN students started to correlate the medical knowledge to patient care their confidence improved. As their confidence rose, so did their understanding of the new role. As this new role was internalized, the student APNs began to provide a more holistic approach to patient care, using their solid nursing base to formulate a unique role as critical care APNs. The researchers identify this uniqueness, describing it as embracing both medical and nursing knowledge, which provides patients with many benefits. Researchers caution that the processes and categories/themes are not isolated points in the role transition, but that they are more complex and are interrelated. These situational, developmental, and conceptual processes are the terms used by the researchers to describe these interrelated concepts.

An ethnographical study of student NPs analyzed data from two sets of interviews; one at the beginning of the educational program and one at the conclusion of the training or education (Barton, 2007). All of the student NP participants were experienced RNs prior to attending the program. In the first phase of the training, the participants were worried about identity loss: having been expert nurses who were now novice NP students that had to disengage from their previous professional role to develop into the new role of NP. This was uncomfortable for the student NPs and was the source of much anxiety. As they moved into the transition phase, the participants remarked on the difficulty and ambiguity felt when not in the role of a nurse, nor in the role of a physician, but feeling inept in the newer role of nurse practitioner. The role boundaries that were well defined were now crossing with medical professionals in the workplace, and this increased stress levels. The students identified needing to increase group cohesion at this stressful portion of their educational program and role transition. As they progressed through their program, there was an increase in clinical skills and knowledge—called the incorporation phase. At this time, the student NPs began to look for role models from medical and nursing colleagues and to begin to merge into their new professional role identity. This also had a positive impact on the student NPs' relationships with medical staff. These social, cultural, and professional transitions were believed to closely model the rites of passage as identified by Van Gannep (1960).

Spoelstra and Robbins (2010) ran a qualitative study that sought to describe the role transition from RN to APN as it related to a role development course. This online course was based on Hamric's Model of Advanced Practice Nursing competencies (Hamric, Spross, & Hanson, 2009). These competencies are direct clinical practice, expert coaching and guidance, consultation, research, clinical/professional/systems leadership, collaboration, and ethical decision making. The overarching theme uncovered in this study was the "essence of nursing." The students integrated this theme throughout the core competencies as the basis of the APN role. The authors suggest methods to facilitate and strengthen the role transition process. Students are influenced by their preceptors, and a good preceptor and a good mentor can assist the student to enhance critical thinking skills and improve self-efficacy. Using reflective journaling is a useful tool for helping facilitate role integration.

Students must use some form of tracking method to record numbers and types of patients seen in the clinical experience, in addition to charting in the paper or electronic medical record. Keeping track of hours and procedures performed is a requirement for graduation and certification. Giving an honest evaluation of the clinical site and preceptor is also important so future students can be matched up with sites that will provide supportive learning environments.

The Role of the Preceptor

There exist many benefits of being a preceptor for an NP student. Although it may be difficult related to the need for productivity, limited physical space to accommodate students, concerns about access to electronic medical records, and cost-effectiveness related to precepting students, there are personal and professional rewards when a positive clinical experience with a student occurs (Barker & Pittman, 2010; Brooks & Niederhauser, 2010; Brykczynski, 2012; Burns, Beauchesne, Ryan-Krause, & Sawin, 2006). Motivation for becoming a preceptor varies from person to person; however, many NPs choose to precept NP students because it provides personal satisfaction, and many recall what their own student clinical experiences were like (Barker & Pittman, 2010). Qualities of a good preceptor from the students' view include the ability to be accessible, empathetic, have a good sense of humor, be flexible and fair, have enthusiasm for the role, and be consistent (Burns et al., 2006). The preceptor also needs to have a self-awareness of clinical skills and knowledge level, knowing that a recent graduate is not in the best position to be in the preceptor role. The new graduate has transitions to go through and needs time to settle into the role of a practicing NP.

It is important for the preceptor to have access to the course syllabus and thus the course objectives prior to the first face-to-face meeting with the student. The preceptor should have a contact number for both the student and the faculty for the course. In addition to having an affiliation agreement with the facility, there should be a written agreement between the preceptor, student, and faculty. The agreement should simply state what the basic expectations are of the preceptor, student, and faculty.

Once the NP has agreed to be a preceptor, the student should contact the preceptor to go over start date and essential topics that need to be covered prior to the first day of clinical. Topics for discussion during the preclinical meeting, whether face-to-face or by phone, include the expectations of the student and mutual goal setting based on the student's current knowledge level and course objectives. The student also needs to know what the appropriate dress code is, what paperwork needs to be completed, any specific requirements by employee health, how to obtain a name badge, and the typical work schedule that the student will be following.

When possible, the student and preceptor should meet 30 minutes before patients begin arriving on the first day of clinical so there is time for orienting the student to the facility (schedule, role of assistive personnel, etc.). Letting the student know the style of precepting that can be expected is beneficial for the student and helps to reduce anxiety from the unknown. Previous authors have suggested that preceptors encourage strategies that improve critical thinking skills of the student NP (Burns et al., 2006; Thompson, Kershbaumer, & Krisman-Scott, 2001). Thompson and colleagues (2001) describe the need for a comprehensive history as being a "detective," and that the student NP use reflection when considering the findings from the history and physical to develop an effective plan of care. Various approaches to teaching students have been described when working with adult learners such as graduate students. A successful approach is one where the student is given patients that are most appropriate for the individual student's previous experience and current skill level. As the student progresses, the patient load and the complexity of the patients increase. Each student may progress at varying rates, and the astute preceptor knows when to push the student to challenge his or her comfort level. Assisting the student NP with time management is necessary, particularly as the student nears graduation. Having a patient assignment reflective of what will be expected postgraduation is imperative during the final semester with close oversight to ensure the student does not forego safe and comprehensive patient care to avoid getting behind. These are often great opportunities to discuss how to manage a situation such as this when they are out in practice.

Complementary forms of clinical education can be used to help the students in addition to hours spent onsite. Some preceptors find it beneficial to assign students homework—researching a specific disease state or finding current treatment options for a patient seen during the clinical day. This is particularly beneficial when the student is rotating with a clinician who provides specialty care, such as pulmonary, cardiology, or infectious disease management. Having a student conduct this type of assignment can not only solidify his or her clinical judgment, but also assist the student in gaining new knowledge on a particular topic.

Two key components of precepting to be emphasized are discussing and using current evidence-based practice (EBP) guidelines for patient care, and, when the preceptor is an NP, role modeling. The NP preceptor has a valuable and unique opportunity to be a role model for the student. Discussing current scope of practice, legislative issues, collaborating and consulting with colleagues, and emphasizing the need to keep the nurse in nurse practitioneering is how the future NP can make a successful transition. Brykczynski (2012) investigated how student NPs are taught how to maintain the holistic approach to patient care that is the cornerstone of nursing practice. This qualitative study uncovered themes that reflected the role modeling that NP faculty perform when incorporating a mind–body–spirit approach to interviewing, listening, assessing, and devising plans of care for patients that address this holistic perspective. Brykczynski (2012) emphasized the importance of this approach, particularly when training students who do not come to NP programs with much nursing experience.

It is useful for the preceptor to be familiar with the evaluation tool used by the university and to go over each component with the student halfway through the clinical experience. Whether or not the preceptor is to complete a written evaluation should be established prior to the start of the clinical rotation. If the evaluation is complex, examples should be provided. This helps the student, as well as the preceptor, identify areas of strength and areas of weakness and then devise a plan to improve in those areas. One approach is to have the student also perform a self-evaluation at this point for comparison. The student may be reassured that certain areas are at the expected level for that point in time, or may need increased awareness that she or he needs to work harder in certain components. Pre- and postconferences can be useful in planning out goals for the day, as well as provide opportunities for the student to gain additional insight into how decision making occurs. The preceptor should discuss both what the student did well and what the student could have done differently/better, and how the student can improve. It is the preceptor's responsibility to alert the clinical advisor or faculty if there are any red flags regarding the student's performance. Keeping the lines of communication with the student and faculty open, and focusing on behaviors rather than personalities, will help to prevent potential problems from becoming serious issues leading to failure. Brooks and Niederhauser (2010) suggest a combined meeting with student, preceptor, and faculty if deficiency is observed.

Evaluation and Clinical Time Documentation

The National Task Force on Quality Nurse Practitioner Education (2012) recently published a report on criteria for evaluation of nursing programs. Criterion III.E specifically relates to NP clinical hours. Required evidence of meeting the criterion includes "documentation of the process used to verify student learning experiences and clinical hours" (p. 8). Thus, there must be a procedure in place that documents both the student's learning experience and the clinical hours he or she has obtained. Various schools use different formats; however, any clinical evaluation form needs to document the skills the student has performed and the level of proficiency to which she or he has performed. Criteria need to relate to course objectives and expected outcomes detailed in the syllabus and at the onset of the class or clinical experience.

Furthermore, evaluations should be done by the preceptor and the faculty, and there should be a method for self-evaluation by the student. In addition, there should be an evaluation of the clinical site.

Pathways to the DNP

When planning clinical experiences, one must consider the student and individual level of experience. In addition, the student's path to the DNP must also be a factor. Currently there are several paths to the DNP; these include ADN to DNP, nonnursing baccalaureate degree to DNP, BSN to DNP, postmaster's DNP, and even postdoctorate DNP. Students may enter a program with experiences ranging from little to no nursing experience, several years of nursing experience, some years of nurse practitioner experience, to several years of nurse practitioner experience. Of course, those with less experience will have quite different clinical processes than those of experienced nurse practitioners. Not everyone will be a novice, according to Benner's (1984) novice to expert theory. Ideally, the preceptor should also be a DNP-prepared nurse practitioner. For students with less experience, early on in the clinical experience it is perfectly accepted to pair them with MSN-prepared NPs so the students learn the overall role of a nurse practitioner. But, for later clinical experiences, and for more advanced students, preceptors should be doctorally prepared, assisting the students in learning the role of the doctorate-prepared nurse practitioner in a variety of roles.

Postmaster's NP Clinical Education in a DNP Program

It is essential that the curriculum of a DNP program extends beyond theory and contain structured clinical components. The AACN (2006) clearly requires a minimum of 1,000 hours of practice postbaccalaureate; however, how to achieve the additional hours for NPs who are already certified is not as clearly outlined. Thus, various programs have created varying models for students to achieve approximately 500 additional hours of clinical education. These clinical hours translate into roughly 11 credits with a ratio of 1 credit hour to 45 clinical hours.

An examination of several postmaster's DNP programs will reveal many similarities and differences. Some programs offer a "new specialty" option in which certified NPs obtain their clinical hours by becoming educated to be certified in a new area. Another option is to offer a specified subspecialty, where there would be a concentration of clinical hours in a specialty area such as cardiology or neurology, and the clinical education would be very specific to that specialty.

Many programs have an advance practice component. However, for the postmaster's student, these clinical experiences must go beyond the clinical educational experiences of their master's program. These clinical experiences must support integration of the DNP role into the complex circumstances of contemporary nursing practice.

An overarching theme that will emerge from examining varying programs is that many of the plans of study for postmaster's students will be highly individualized. Students' prior experience, program goals, individual goals, as well as final DNP project, must all be factors when determining how students will complete the remaining clinical hours.

The following are designated clinical tracks or courses that can be offered to assist students in obtaining the additional 500 clinical hours needed.

Teaching/Learning

Students with an expressed interest in teaching may choose to complete an established amount of clinical hours in a teaching capacity. These courses should include teaching/

learning theory, and clinical hours can be achieved through student teaching as well as course and curriculum development at a collegiate level.

Clinical education should not only focus on basic teaching strategies but those of educational leadership as well. Students must be exposed to the multiple facets of nursing education including management in an academic setting, regulations and industry trends, curriculum development, and leadership skills.

Community Health and Population Focus

With the ever-increasing demand for skilled care outside of the hospital setting, there is a great need for advanced nursing practice in community health, as well as population focus care. Clinical hours can be achieved through examining advanced practice nursing roles in community health and public health.

Clinical education in this area should prepare the advanced practice nurse to evaluate major health issues in populations, use various public health approaches to reduce injury and improve health, and develop and implement key strategies to maintain and improve population health and safety at all levels.

Leadership and Management

Clinical hours with a healthcare leadership or management focus will ready the doctorate-prepared NP for executive leadership in healthcare settings. The focus of the clinical education should be centered on the following competencies: leadership, business intelligence, finance, health policy, and research. Ideally, preceptors will be DNP prepared, but MSN- or PhD-prepared nurses in executive positions, such as chief nurse officer (CNO), would be a good fit for the DNP student.

Final Project

A major clinical component to all DNP nurse practitioner programs is the development, implementation, and evaluation of a final doctoral project. Although there are multiple titles for the projects, including dissertation project and capstone project, many if not all clinical hours can be achieved in this process. There are multiple ways to complete such projects. According to the AACN (2006, p. 20):

> Unlike a dissertation, the work may take a number of forms. One example of a final DNP product is a practice change initiative. This may be represented by a pilot study, a program evaluation, a quality improvement project, an evaluation of a new practice model, a consulting project, or an integrated critical literature review. Improving patient outcomes is the ultimate goal for DNP projects and should be focused on systems and/or populations (AACN, 2015). Additional examples of a DNP final product could include manuscripts submitted for publication, systematic review, research utilization project, practice topic dissemination, substantive involvement in a larger endeavor, or other practice project. The theme that links these forms of scholarly experiences is the use of evidence to improve either practice or patient outcomes.[1]

1 American Association of Colleges of Nursing, (2006). *The essentials of doctoral education for advanced nursing practice.* Washington, DC: Author.

Current Trends in NP Clinical Education

A growing trend in NP clinical education is to require institutions to pay preceptors for their services. Although providing one-on-one mentoring and direct patient care experiences for NP students by either nurse practitioners or physicians has been a time-honored tradition of service to the overall healthcare community, this is changing. With there being great competition for clinical sites, at times schools have few options and must place students at facilities where a few are required. "Some clinics are charging a minimum of $200 per week for a practicum experience. Which translates into $1,600–$2,000 for an eight to ten week session" (Brown, 2016, para 4); and, at $1,000 per credit hour, depending on the course, this could be as much as $6,000 for a 15-week course. Institutions must then find ways to either absorb the cost or pass the cost on the student, thus adding to the cost of tuition or lab fees.

Brown (2016) posed the question: Is it ethical for clinics to require payment for nursing practicums? Of course, there is no easy response. There have been requests for the Commission on Collegiate Nursing Education (CCNE), the accrediting body for many academic institutions, to regulate the guidelines for this practice (Graduate Nursing EDU, 2016).

Both the American Nurses Credentialing Center (ANCC) and the American Academy of Nurse Practitioners (AANP), through which NPs can be certified, offer precepting as a partial means to gain recertification. ANCC requires documentation of 120 hours of direct clinical supervision as one of the eligible categories, when combined with 75 hours of continuing education hours (of which 25 must be pharmacotherapeutics), the NP can gain recertification (ANCC, 2016). AANP allows 120 precepting hours to be converted to 25 nonpharmacology credits, of which 100 are required (AANP, 2017). In line with ANCC and AANP, there are states that allow precepting to be a component of renewal for state APRN licensing. North Carolina credits 30 of the required 50 contact hours for APRN license renewal for 30 hours of precepting (Nursing Center, 2017). Beginning in 2018, the state of Hawaii will allow 120 hours of precepting hours to be used as a component for renewal of APRN licensing (Department of Commerce and Consumer Affairs, 2017).

The state of Maryland has taken a unique approach to the preceptor shortage—providing an incentive, beyond that of direct pay, for nurse practitioners who serve as preceptors. In 2016 the state passed a bill that will allow a tax waiver for NP preceptors. It is called The Nurse Practitioner Preceptorship Tax Credit Fund. Preceptors are eligible for up to a $1,000 annual tax waiver subject to meeting certain requirements (Maryland Board of Nursing, 2016).

The Future of NP Clinical Education

Looking ahead, finding innovative approaches to providing effective, high-quality clinical education for NPs is challenging. Multiple issues have been identified, along with several strategies for seeking solutions (Fitzgerald, Kantrowitz-Gordon, Katz, & Hirsch, 2012). The authors identified internal challenges such as issues related to lack of diversity in the workforce, the increased workload demands on faculty, noncompetitive salaries for NP faculty, and the challenges associated with access to education for those residing in rural areas. External challenges that were identified included the difficulty of finding adequate clinical sites and preceptors, NPs whose responsibilities include teaching medical residents instead of NP students, the numerous regulatory and specialty certification requirements, and the political and control issues associated with gender relationships (p. 2).

Despite these challenges, it is possible to design innovative strategies for providing high-quality clinical education for NP students. Fitzgerald et al. (2012) suggest forming collaborative relationships with healthcare institutions as well as other educational institutions. They also suggest increasing the use of simulation and problem-based learning, distance education, interprofessional education, and international and domestic healthcare missions. It is vital to advocate for federal funding for training the future workforce of NPs in order to meet the goals of the Institute of Medicine and afford increased access to health care for the entire population.

Introduction to the Case Presentation

Preparing an oral case study presentation is an essential part of the education of nurse practitioners (NPs), but because of the burden of an overly prescribed curriculum and use of nonfaculty clinical preceptors, the art of the formal "oral presentation" is often a skill requirement that is neglected. According to the National Organization of Nurse Practitioner Faculties (NONPF), there are nine core competencies that outline specific guidelines for educational programs preparing NPs to implement the full scope of practice as licensed independent practitioners (NONPF, 2012b). Several of the practice domains state the following goals should be achieved during the education of the nurse practitioner:

- Critically analyzes data and evidence for improving advanced nursing practice
- Communicates practice knowledge effectively both orally and in writing
- Uses advanced health assessment skills to differentiate between normal, variations of normal, and abnormal findings

NONPF also purports that these competencies are acquired through mentored patient care experiences with emphasis on independent and interprofessional practice; providing evidence-based, patient-centered care across settings; and acquiring advanced knowledge of the healthcare delivery system (NONPF, 2012a). Efforts to construct frameworks to help both medical and nursing students create (and teachers evaluate) oral case presentations presume that nursing and medical educators share mutual expectations for presentations (Green, 2011).

The oral case presentation skill is at the heart of the way healthcare providers communicate. It allows the nurse practitioner to succinctly convey a clear, organized analysis of a patient's health problem(s) to another provider in order to develop an effective management plan. The case presentation also serves as a method for clinical preceptors and peers to assess the level of expertise a practitioner has regarding a particular problem and to evaluate the assessment and management portion of that patient's care. Lastly, a clearly communicated case presentation enables the nurse practitioner to get a more experienced clinician's opinion about a patient in an efficient, cost-effective manner (Coralli, 2006).

The case presentation typically presented in the SOAP (subjective, objective, assessment, and plan) format is a sequential way of arranging the facts, thereby drawing the listener down a path of critical reasoning. Building the "argument" by clearly outlining the patient's history and physical examination findings helps make linkages to define the differential diagnosis and outline a treatment plan (Hinson Brown, 2006). Much of the clinical teaching involves the nurse practitioner student interviewing and examining a patient, and then presenting the information to the clinical preceptor. This approach is common in both inpatient and outpatient primary care settings. Studies involving third-year medical students indicated that, on average, these interactions take approximately 10 minutes, and the time is divided into several different activities. Much of the time is taken up by the presentation of the patient by the learner. Additional time is spent in questioning and clarifying the content of the presentation. As a result, only about 1 minute of time is actually spent in discussion and teaching (Rollins, 2012). To do this, the nurse practitioner must learn to present in the format accepted by the medical profession and include only the most relevant information—the pertinent positives and negatives.

Physicians, over the course of their training, spend a number of years not only presenting cases to other house staff and attending physicians, but also listening to such presentations from their peers and faculty. During their residencies, it is safe to say that most house staff develop skill in case presentations. This is accomplished in three ways: (1) by repeatedly being in the position of having to present cases "off the top of the head," (2) by having their case presentations critiqued frequently, and (3) by hearing excellent case presentations from others, which they then use as models for their own presentations (Coralli, 2006). In a study of 136 internal medicine clinician teachers from five U.S. medical schools, it was found that faculty share common expectations for oral case presentation (OCP) experiences, while students often report that clinical faculty fail to share common expectations for the OCP, frustrating their attempts to use the "rules" they have learned to create an OCP (Green, 2011).

With the passage of the Affordable Care Act (ACA) and the anticipated shortage of primary care physicians, nurse practitioners will be providing medical care in a variety of interdisciplinary settings, increasing the need for excellent case presentation skills to stay on par with our physician colleagues. The nurse practitioner who presents a clear, comprehensive summary of the patient's problem to a physician or other healthcare colleague may be able to expedite that patient's care to enhance positive patient outcomes.

Organizing the Oral Case Study Presentation

Prior to the presentation, it is important for the nurse practitioner student to consider the message, the purpose, and the appropriate depth of the case in relation to the audience being addressed (Paauw, Migeon, & Burkholder, 2003). The standard outline follows the format of the written history and physical exam with several important differences. Verbal case presentations are typically 5–7 minutes in length, which makes it imperative to prioritize essential data; organizing the facts into pertinent positive findings and pertinent negative findings make for an efficient delivery of information. In addition, the review of systems that directly relate to the patient problem should be included in the history of present illness (HPI). By leaving out unnecessary information, the presenter will avoid the pitfalls of too much information that may distract the listener (Hinson Brown, 2006). It is important to note that the oral case presentation should not be a verbatim recital of the history and physical condition of the patient. Novice clinicians often have a difficult time preparing a case as they learn to distinguish how much information is enough and what is too much or nonessential information. The goal of case presentation is to establish an argument for a differential diagnosis for the patient. Important data can argue in favor of the differential diagnosis or refute the diagnosis. The nurse practitioner must recognize that leaving out relevant information can misinform the diagnosis (Paauw et al., 2003).

Components of an Effective Case Presentation

Many nurse practitioner students approach case presentations as part of their student evaluation process. As previously mentioned the main objective of the presentation is to convey the aspects of the patient's illness to the preceptor, collaborating physician, or other team members in order to participate in the patient's plan of care. The nurse practitioner student must avoid verbatim reciting of what the patient verbalized but rather deliver a critical analysis of the information gathered to develop a clear and accurate plan. Brevity, organization, eye contact, and anticipation of questions are integral to an excellent presentation. On completion of the presentation, the other clinician should understand the priority issues for the patient and what your management plan is to address those issues. **BOX 6-1** displays tips for an effective case study presentation, and **BOXES 6-2** and **6-3** represent the components of a case presentation.

Introduction or Chief Complaint

Your "opening statement" should be designed to focus the listener's attention and thinking on the patient's major concern. In general, the case study will begin with demographic information about the patient, such as age, marital status, ethnicity, sex, and occupation. The patient's chief complaint, while important to document in the medical record, should be presented as the clinician's view of the reason for the visit or patient encounter. If the reliability of the patient is in question, this should be stated early in your presentation and the reason, such as poor historian, confused, psychotic, or intoxicated.

History of the Present Illness

Following the introduction, the history of the present illness is given. It is well-known that obtaining an accurate history will provide the clinician with the differential diagnosis 90% of the time (Davenport, 2008). This is the most essential piece of your presentation, and if presented well, it should take up at least 50% of your presentation time. In this section, you will want to describe the development

BOX 6-1 Tips for an Effective Oral Case Presentation

Brevity: Do not ramble, but do not be too brief.
Organization: Present in SOAP format, and avoid jumping back and forth between different problems.
Eye contact: Engage your audience, and keep your presentation lively. Avoid reading directly from the chart.
Anticipate and expect questions: Be ready to answer any questions relevant to your patient.
Use clinical reasoning: Your listener should be able to consider a differential diagnosis.
Present the *patient* as well as the *problem*: Remember personal, family, and social factors.

BOX 6-2 Components of an Oral Case Presentation

Introduction or chief complaint
History of present illness
Physical examination
Diagnostic tests
Differential diagnosis
Management plan
Summary

BOX 6-3 Expanded Components of a Case Presentation

Chief Complaint

Mr(s) ______________ is ________ a -year-old ________ ________ who (initials) (age) (race) (sex) presented to the family health center with a chief complaint of________.

The chief complaint is a brief statement of the why the patient sought medical attention, stated in the patient's own words. No medical term or diagnosis is used.

History of Present Illness (HPI)

The HPI is a more complete description of the patient's symptoms(s). General features included in the HPI are:

- Date of onset
- Precise location
- Nature of onset, severity, and duration
- Effect of any treatment
- Degree of interference with daily activities

Past Medical History (PMH)

The PMH includes serious illness, chronic diseases, surgical procedures, and injuries the patient has experienced. Minor complaints may be omitted.

Family History (FH)

The FH includes the age and health of parents, siblings, and children. Ages and cause of death should be recorded for deceased relatives. Only include data that is pertinent to the patient case.

Social History (SH)

The SH includes not only the social characteristics of the patient, but also the environmental factors and behaviors that may contribute to the development of disease. Items included are marital status, number of children, educational background, occupation, dietary habits, and use of tobacco, alcohol, or other drugs.

Medication History (MH)

The MH should include current medications prior to office visit or admission. This includes prescription and nonprescription medications. Include name and dosing information for each.

(continues)

BOX 6-3 Expanded Components of a Case Presentation *(continued)*

Allergies

Allergies to drugs, foods, pets, and environmental factors should be included. An accurate description of the reaction that occurred should be presented.

Review of Systems and Physical Exam

In the ROS, the examiner questions the patient about the presence of symptoms that are pertinent to each body system. Only the pertinent positive and negative findings may be recorded.

The general sections for the PE are listed below. It is only necessary to list the findings that are "remarkable."

General appearance
Vital signs
Skin
HEENT
Lungs
Cardiovascular
Abdomen
Genital/rectal
Extremities
Neurological

Diagnostic Tests

The results of lab tests and diagnostic tests should be recorded. List all lab results, but comment only on those that are abnormal or pertinent to the case.

Differential Diagnosis

Based on the above information, what are the impressions, problems, or diseases? Develop a problem list according to the acuity and significance of the patient's conditions.

Management

For each problem, discuss your plan and rationale for it.
Present your plan in the following format:
Diagnostics (what tests if any will be ordered)
Therapeutics (what pharmacologic agents if any will be ordered) Patient education
Follow-up plans: Next appointment, consultation, referral

Case Summary

Provide a brief summary of the chief complaint and the treatment provided. List other problems associated with current or past treatments.

of the most important problem or "present illness" as you interpret the information the patient told you. In the outpatient setting, the typical patient will present with several issues for you to address in a limited amount of time (e.g., 15–30 minutes) depending on where you are practicing. You most likely will not have time to address each issue in a single visit and must become skilled at determining which problem is the priority for the visit and setting the goals without overlooking potentially serious problems.

The other ongoing major medical problems should reported, but you will need to condense the information about these problems and select information that is most relevant to the main issue. The seven attributes of a symptom will provide you with a framework upon which to present your information. These variables are (Bickley, 2009):

1. Timing or chronology
2. Location
3. Quality
4. Quantity or severity
5. Progression
6. Aggravating or alleviating factors
7. Associated manifestations

Do not mention any of the attributes that are not important to the diagnosis. Information from past medical history, surgical history, social history, medication, allergies, family history, and the review of other systems should be reported only if it is directly relevant to the current problem in order to keep your presentation focused and brief. Keep the report of the review of systems to pertinent positive and negative findings.

Physical Examination

As with the history, the explanation of the physical examination should be reported in a succinct format emphasizing the body systems associated with the presenting problems. A standard format for reporting the physical examination should include pertinent vital signs and the general appearance of the patient. Address all significant pertinent and abnormal findings. An accurate reporting of the pertinent physical examination should tie into your history, resulting in a critical analysis of what the differential diagnosis is for the patient. A standard format for describing the physical examination findings would be done systematically, as demonstrated in Box 6-3.

Diagnostic Studies

Presentation of diagnostic studies should follow the physical examination. Serum laboratory studies such as complete blood count and chemistries are generally presented first followed by radiologic findings such as x-rays, ultrasounds, CT scans, and MRI results, followed by electrocardiograms and other diagnostic studies. Unless directly relevant to the case, normal findings can be presented as "normal," but if important to the diagnosis the exact result should be reported. For example, in a patient with poorly controlled diabetes and chronic renal failure, although the creatinine level was "normal" it would be important to report the result of 1.2 for this case as opposed to a result of the creatinine level for a healthy 28-year-old in for a general physical examination. If the patient is presenting with a new complaint and you are considering ordering diagnostic tests, be prepared to have a rationale of the importance and reliability of the tests, as well as their risks and their cost–benefit ratio. You must present an argument to order diagnostic tests based on the facts and if they will affect management of the patient.

Differential Diagnosis

Now that the clinician has gathered all the information by asking, listening, examining, and investigating diagnostic results as applicable, it is at this point in the case presentation that you identify the differential diagnoses or the list of possibilities for the symptoms.

You must narrow to the most important one or two problems and discuss the differential diagnoses. The emphasis should be on the data that support or disprove various diagnoses and relate why the diagnosis you arrived at was made over others that were considered. Remember that the differential diagnosis should address the possible causes in the case at hand, not for the problem in general. For example, in a patient with sudden onset of fever, productive cough, rhonchi, and pulmonary infiltrate, discuss pneumonia, not the problem "cough." In your discussion, each abnormal or significant symptom or physical finding and each abnormal diagnostic study must be accounted for. If no follow-up or further study was done for some abnormal finding, provide a rationale for the decision. In addition, there is no shame in admitting that we cannot explain a particular finding or symptom. In fact, knowing what something is not has as much value as providing a specific label for a complaint or condition.

Management Plan

Lastly, the case presentation requires the nurse practitioner to discuss the management plan, being prepared to offer a strong rationale for taking proposed actions. Actions might include further diagnostics and pharmacologic or educational interventions. There are many suggested ways of developing and presenting a management plan for the clinical problem or differential diagnosis. You might find it helpful, especially if dealing with more than one or several complex clinical issues, to separate each problem into its most basic elements, with a separate plan noted for each one. By identifying the most basic components of each problem, you will be less likely to miss important issues and be better able to formulate the most complete plan possible (Coralli, 2006). Your ability to do this will obviously vary with your prior experience and knowledge base. However, this general approach applies to most clinical situations. Take, for example, a patient who presents with new dyspnea on exertion who also has known heart failure, hypertension, and hyperlipidemia. Each one of these problems is related to the patient's cardiovascular system. However, if you were to address all of them under a single "cardiovascular" heading, there is a good chance that the assessment and plan would become muddled and confusing. Describe any treatment and the patient's responses to date if known. If the patient has been followed over a period of time for the problem identified, convey some sense of the course of the illness or progression of the disease. A sample case study with management plan is presented in **BOX 6-4**.

BOX 6-4 Case Presentation Example

Chief Complaint: Blair Daniels is a 51-year-old white female administrative assistant who presents to the family health center complaining of a recent episode of rectal pain and bleeding with defecation.

HPI: The blood was bright red and was present both on the wiping paper and in the toilet bowl but was mixed with stool. The rectal pain was most severe with the passage of stool but sometimes persisted for hours after defecation. The bleeding occurred last week for 3 to 4 days and has now stopped. She reports a history of a similar but more severe episode of rectal pain and bleeding 1 year ago, which responded to dietary changes and sitz baths. A dietary inventory reveals she has been avoiding food intake to prevent bouts of pain. The patient states that she has daily loose bowel movements the past 2–3 weeks and has lost a "few pounds."

PMH:
Iron deficiency anemia secondary to heavy menses
Obesity
Irritable bowel syndrome

Surgical History:
Gallbladder surgery at 19 years old
GYN: Menarche G1 P1 AO L1, NSVD no complications age 25; history of fibroid uterus

Family History:
Mother 72 years old, irritable bowel syndrome, diverticulitis, hypertension
Father: 75 years old, type 2 diabetes, hypertension

Allergies:
Sulfa—rash

Medications:
Imodium tablets prn diarrhea

Physical Exam Findings:
Gen: Moderately obese white female, appears comfortable. BMI: 36 VS 140/92 P-76 R-12 T-101.2
Lungs: CTA. No wheeze.
CV: Normal S1 S2, no murmur, no rubs, no bruits
Abdominal exam: Hypoactive bowel sounds and diffuse RLQ tenderness. No rebound. No guarding. No organomegaly.
Rectal exam: External skin tags at the rectal verge. These are neither inflamed nor tender. A digital exam finds no masses or palpable hemorrhoids, but there is moderate tenderness at the midline inferiorly. Stool in the vault is firm, brown, and negative for occult blood.

Diagnostic Tests: No diagnostic tests available

Differential Diagnosis:
Rectal bleeding: Anal fissure, diverticulitis, colon cancer, peptic ulcer disease
Elevated blood pressure
Obesity

Management Plan:

- **Rectal bleeding**

Diagnostics: CBC, CT scan abdomen with contrast
Therapeutics: None
Patient education: Educate regards need for CT scan, refer to GI

- Elevated blood pressure:

Diagnostics: Chemistries, lipid panel, TSH
Therapeutics: Consider oral agent if BP elevated next visit in light of risk factors and family history of hypertension
Patient education: DASH diet

- **Obesity**: Deferred to next visit

Follow-up in 3 weeks following colonoscopy and GI consult

Summary: I am uncertain why she is having rectal bleeding, which warrants a complete work-up by a gastroenterologist. There may be an infectious process going on given the patient is febrile and has a history of diverticulitis. We will send the patient to the hospital for a CT scan today and have her seen by GI. We didn't address her elevated blood pressure or obesity today, but I would like to see the patient in 3 weeks to review her lab work and discuss the consultant's findings.

Summary

Whether a 1–2 minute "hallway" consult or a formal oral presentation to your preceptor or your class, conclude by summarizing the key points of the entire case in several sentences. In formal presentations, after the concluding summary, it is routine to ask if anyone has any comments or questions. Always consider the patient's personal factors that may influence his or her response to the management plan.

▸ Collaboration, Consultation, and Referral in Primary Care

According to the American Academy of Nurse Practitioners (2010), nurse practitioners (NPs) practice autonomously and in collaboration with other healthcare professionals to assess, diagnose, treat, and manage the patient's health problems and needs. Consultation, referral, and collaboration are key roles in which the primary care NP is adept at as both direct care provider and coordinator of care. Regulations vary by state dictating NPs' scope of practice and prescribing privileges. Certifying bodies and professional nursing societies have accepted certain tasks, protocols, and decisions as part of NP scope of practice, which may be in direct conflict with organizational constraints and public perceptions of NP scope of practice. NPs acknowledge that they thrive on the ability to consult with others, and that they occasionally encounter clinical circumstances outside of their scope of practice, necessitating a request for direction or guidance from a physician or other healthcare provider with additional expertise. With the predicted shortage of 91,500 primary care physicians in the United States by 2020 and the expansion of health coverage to the 32 million uninsured Americans by 2019, the American Medical Association also acknowledges the need for physicians to find ways of effectively collaborating with other healthcare professionals including NPs (Krupa, 2010). Collaboration between healthcare providers is essential to provide safe, cost-effective, high-quality healthcare services with positive patient outcomes (Maylone, Ranieri, Quinn Griffin, McNulty, & Fitzpatrick, 2011).

Defining Collaboration

Collaboration can be defined as a joint communication and decision-making process between healthcare professionals working toward a mutual goal of addressing a patient and family's medical, social, and ethical problems (O'Brien, Martin, Heyworth, & Meyer, 2009). It is essential that the collaborative relationship be vetted with mutual respect and trust for one another's unique abilities. Other elements of a collaborative team are regular and open dialogue, like-minded practice philosophies, continuing education, shared decision making, and a willingness to learn from other's clinical expertise (Makowsky, 2009). Such a relationship has the potential to improve patient care outcomes, enhance patient safety, and reduce the workload for the individual team member. Collaboration can also help to decrease burnout and enhance workplace satisfaction.

Collaboration Defined by State Statute

States define scope of practice in statutes enacted by the state legislature, or the state legislature giving the board of nursing the authority to define the scope of practice for the advanced practice nurse (Buppert, 2011). For example, according to the Connecticut General Statutes (20-87a), the term:

collaboration means a mutually agreed upon relationship between an advanced practice registered nurse and a physician who is educated, trained, or has relevant experience that is related to the work of such advanced practice registered nurse. The collaboration shall address a reasonable and appropriate level of consultation and referral, coverage for the patient in the absence of the advanced practice registered nurse, a method to review patient outcomes, and a method of disclosure of the relationship with the patient.

The above example not only defines collaboration, but subsumes the terminology of consultation and referral. Some states describe the NP's scope of practice in abbreviated formats while other states have unclear language that can be become confusing to physician colleagues as well as the consumer. There are many variables that play a role as to when a NP should collaborate with, consult with, or refer a patient to another care provider. For example, the place of employment may dictate to the NP the exact consultation process depending on whether it is a specialty site, large institution, small private practice, or the geographic location, such as an urban, suburban, or rural setting. The terms *consultation* and *referral* are often used interchangeably, but there are distinct differences.

Defining Consultation

All clinicians engage in clinical decision making and need to manage clinical uncertainty and understand the consequences of delaying an appropriate treatment plan for a patient. Nurse practitioners are faced with complex patients and need to exercise sound judgment regarding making a diagnosis, selecting an appropriate diagnostic test, observing patient care outcomes, and making a final decision on patient management. Managing clinical uncertainty is a skill that needs to be developed. Consultation can be defined as a request for direction or assistance on a diagnosis or treatment plan from another provider (Goolsby, 2002). Consultation can be either formal or informal as depicted in **BOX 6-5**.

Defining Referral

Referral can be defined as another provider accepting the ongoing treatment of a patient for a specific problem and often for a limited amount of time (Goolsby, 2002). For example, you

BOX 6-5 Mechanisms for Consultations

Informal Consultation

- Patient care rounds
- Professional meetings
- Telephone consultation
- E-mail consultation
- Video-based medical consultation

Formal Consultation

- Formal process of sending the patient to another provider for a comprehensive evaluation may refer a patient to a cardiologist to assume care for the patient's heart failure. That patient may continue to visit the cardiologist for evaluation and treatment of heart failure but will remain with her primary care provider for treatment of her other medical problems (e.g., diabetes, osteoarthritis). Consultation does not suggest continued treatment as is implied in the referral process. Although the terms are used interchangeably, there are distinct differences in regard to overall responsibility for the patient's care for specific health issues.

When Should Nurse Practitioners Seek a Consultation or Referral?

There may be multiple variables that cause the NP to initiate the consultation or referral process. The NP should consult with another healthcare provider when there is a question or uncertainty about the patient's care. The NP may have a specific question as to the treatment plan, or may need "another set of eyes" to visually assess a portion of the physical exam to confirm diagnoses. Often, in the subsequent days following the patient visit, when either laboratory results or imaging results are received and reviewed, next steps may be to include additional consultation. Under all circumstances, the nurse practitioner should clearly document the consultative discussion within the patient's medical record as well as the interventions that the NP ordered. This is important both from a legal standpoint and in an effort to provide seamless care for the patient. Another situation that should prompt a consultation or referral is when a patient expresses doubt in the NP's diagnosis and treatment plan. Patients are increasingly looking up their symptoms on the Internet, and it is common for patients to seek second opinions. The primary care NP is responsible for the coordination of care, which can become complex in particular when multiple healthcare providers are involved. Close coordination is essential to provide timely care, avoid morbidity, and decrease risk of litigation (Goolsby, 2002). The following is an example of a common patient scenario where, based on clinical experience and comfort level, the NP asks for a point-of-care consultation with her physician partner:

Miss P is a 25-year-old Caucasian female with a recent presentation of a skin lesion to her right posterior calf. She has no history of skin cancer, but has a positive family history of melanoma. The NP involved in this scenario is a recent graduate with little experience in dermatological conditions. She asks her physician colleague to visually inspect the skin lesion.

Referrals are an integral part of the NP–patient experience. It is no different from physicians who refer their patients to specialists for reasons such as exhausting treatment options or receiving abnormal test results out of the physician's scope of practice. **BOX 6-6** gives a list of common reasons to seek a consultation or referral.

BOX 6-6 Common Reasons for Consultation and Referral

- Advice on diagnosis
- Advice on treatment plan
- Advice on prognosis
- Mental health counseling
- Specialized procedure (surgical and nonsurgical)
- Patient request (second opinion)
- Insurance company guidelines
- Failure of treatment plan

Another important aspect within the referral process is the need for insurance verification and the specific procedure that needs to be followed for each carrier and plan. The patient and NP have combined ownership of the referral process and what it entails. If it has been predetermined that the insurance plan needs no formal referral, a letter of referral should be made. Also, accompanying the documentation should be any pertinent testing or ancillary information that would be helpful to the specialist/ referral provider. We can take the earlier case presentation a bit further as follows:

Miss P is a 25-year-old Caucasian female with a recent presentation of a skin lesion to her right posterior calf. She has no history of skin cancer, but has a positive family history of melanoma. The NP involved in this scenario is a recent graduate with little experience in dermatological conditions. The NP is unable to access her collaborating physician. She then makes a direct referral to dermatology for further evaluation of this lesion. The NP needs to make sure that the proper referral procedure is in place, and that this process is documented and the appointment is secured with the other provider.

The Referral and Consultation Process

There is no one set procedure or format for initiating a referral; it is often dependent upon the setting the NP works in or the institution where the referral is being generated to. Many primary care offices have ancillary staff to facilitate the acquisition of the patient's information for the specialist, understand insurance company requirements, and set up the appointment when needed. If the institution does not have a formal process or policy, the NP should write the formal referral with the relevant patient information to give the consultant a guide for approaching the patient and to avoid duplicative services. **BOX 6-7** gives an overview of the pertinent information for a formal consultation.

Tracking Referrals

Following the transmission of the patient information to the consulting physician, the patient needs to take ownership and responsibility for the overall process; very often patients do not believe they need to see the consultant and are nonadherent in attending the appointment. Giving the patient information to hand carry to the specialist may

BOX 6-7 Formal Consultation: Pertinent Information

- Demographics
- Summary of current problem
- Past medical history
- Medications
- Allergies
- Pertinent family history
- Pertinent social history
- Diagnostic test results
- Previous consultation results
- Clear outline of the problem you evaluated/treated
- Urgency of the request

increase his or her commitment to follow through with the consultation. The procedure to track referrals is dependent on the size of the practice and policies instituted, but regardless of setting all consultations should be documented appropriately within the patient's record. Some practices may have a referral book that can be referenced to make sure the appointment was booked, proper authorization was received, the patient made the appointment, and the consultant's report was received.

Consultant's Responsibilities

One of the most important areas with regards to consultations and referrals is follow-up by the NP referral originator after the patient has had the visit. A source of frustration for many primary care providers is the failure of the consulting physician to provide adequate detail and feedback regarding patient findings and treatment plans. Depending on the severity of the patient issue, the NP may hear directly back from the specialist or receive documentation electronically or via mail. That is why it is extremely important that the NP know the exact date of the specialist visit if possible; this is also another internally based tracking mechanism to ensure the patient kept the appointment as scheduled. Alerts can be instituted if using an electronic-based medical record. It is necessary to have this information in order to reduce liability or untoward patient outcomes. Maintaining referral records is a quality initiative that can be used by nursing, medical assistants, or whoever is in control of the referral procedure.

At the end of the day, the patient should be in control of his or her own health care and visits, but we as NPs need to ensure that the process in place is effective, with quality measures for further follow-up after the visit has been made. A direct patient follow-up visit should occur, if appropriate, following the specialist visit. This too would be a checkpoint to make sure proper follow-up with all parties is occurring and patient satisfaction is at a high level.

Interdisciplinary Collaboration

Interdisciplinary education is a vital component for students pursuing careers as healthcare professionals. Communication, collaboration, and cooperation across professional boundaries are essential for patients and families to receive the individualized care they deserve and need to maximize their quality of life (Haas, 2009). The shortage of nurses and other healthcare professionals is well documented, particularly in rural and urban low-income areas. The shortages are expected to worsen as the current workforce retires and the demand for health care grows. The NP is a highly skilled clinician who is in a position to collaborate with other members of the healthcare team to deliver high-quality, evidenced-based care that has the potential to improve patient care outcomes such as decreasing hospital admission rates and eliminating adverse drug reactions.

Addressing these challenges requires a transformation of our educational system and healthcare workforce. What is necessary are healthcare professionals who are better prepared and educated to care for people with multiple chronic conditions in all settings. Healthcare professionals need to be able to deliver care to the fullest extent of their education and training. Nurses represent the largest healthcare profession and are armed with the scientific knowledge and adaptive capacity to lead the changes in the healthcare system. The nursing profession as a whole must reconceptualize its roles in coaching, advocacy, chronic disease management, transitional care, prevention activities, and quality improvement.

The Institute of Medicine (IOM) in partnership with the Robert Wood Johnson Foundation (RWJF) published a landmark report on *The Future of Nursing: Leading Change, Advancing Health* (Institute of Medicine, 2010). This report is the nonpartisan work of 18 experts in nursing, medicine, economics, business, hospital administration, health policy, consumer issues, workforce policy, and health plan administration. Based on evidence from an extensive review of the research, the report outlines a blueprint for transforming the nursing profession, particularly NPs, to enhance the quality and value of U.S. health care in ways that meet the future needs of diverse populations. In launching the initiative, RWJF's president, Dr. Risa Lavizzo-Mourey, noted that "nursing is at the heart of patient care" and is therefore crucial to changing the way health care is delivered so that "patients receive better care at a cost we can afford." Echoing this sentiment, IOM president Dr. Harvey Fineberg noted that "Nurses are a linchpin for health reform and will be vital to implementing systemic changes in the delivery of care."

One of the most viewed online reports in the IOM's history, this ground-breaking report calls on the nation's leaders and stakeholders to act on its recommendations, including changes in public and institutional policies at the federal, state, and local levels. These facts spurred the need for interprofessional collaboration and diversity across the continuum of care. Studies have demonstrated how effective coordination and communication among health professionals can enhance the quality and safety of patient care. Health professionals working collaboratively as integrated teams draw on individual and collective skills and experience across disciplines. They seek input and respect the contributions of everyone involved. That allows each person to practice at a higher level. The result is inevitably better patient outcomes, including higher levels of patient satisfaction.

The passage of the Recovery and Reinvestment Act of 2009 and the Patient Protection and Affordable Care Act of 2010 has stimulated new approaches, such as the "medical home" concept, to achieving better outcomes in primary care, especially for high-risk chronically ill and other at-risk populations (Kaiser Family Foundation, 2013). Improved interprofessional teamwork and team-based care play core roles in many of the new primary care approaches.

NPs play an integral role in the foundations of the primary care model. The idea of primary care and its relationship to the broader context of health is itself being reconsidered. First, in primary care there is a focus on expanded accountability for population management of chronic diseases that links to a community context. Second, healthcare professionals and public health professionals jointly share roles and responsibilities for addressing health promotion and primary prevention needs related to behavioral change. Third, healthcare professionals and public health professionals work in collaboration with others on behalf of persons, families, and communities in maintaining healthy environments, including responding to public health emergencies.

D'Amour and Oandasan (2005) defined interprofessionality as: the process by which professionals reflect on and develop ways of practicing that provides an integrated and cohesive answer to the needs of the client/family/population. . . .[I]t involves continuous interaction and knowledge sharing between professionals, organized to solve or explore a variety of education and care issues all while seeking to optimize the patient's participation. . . . Interprofessionality requires a paradigm shift, since interprofessional practice has unique characteristics in terms of values, codes of conduct, and ways of working. These characteristics must be elucidated. (p. 9)

BOX 6-8 Core Competencies for Interprofessional Collaborative Practice

Competency 1: Values and Ethics for Interprofessional Practice
Competency 2: Roles and Responsibilities
Competency 3: Interprofessional Communication
Competency 4: Teams and Teamwork

The World Health Organization (WHO) developed a global Framework for Action on Interprofessional Education and Collaborative Practice (WHO, 2010). This illustrated the overall goal of interprofessional education as setting the stage for the preparation of a "collaborative practice-ready" workforce, which has underpinnings that are driven by the local community health needs and local community health systems designed in response and readiness for those needs.

Schmitt, Blue, Aschenbrener, and Viggiano (2011), in the *Report of Core Competencies for Interprofessional Collaborative Practice*, define four domains essential to interprofessional practice, which are discussed in the following sections (see **BOX 6-8**).

Competency Domain 1: Values and Ethics for Interprofessional Practice

Collaborative care models are based on the ability of two or more distinct and separate healthcare disciplines to respect and trust each other's clinical judgment, skills, and expertise. There is a moral obligation of all healthcare professions with respect to the care of the patient and positive, valuable outcomes.

Competency Domain 2: Roles and Responsibilities

Each profession has core competencies that define roles and responsibilities as well as scope of practice and definitive boundaries. Each member of a healthcare discipline should be able to articulate their unique role and patient care delivery methods to other members of the healthcare team. Diverse expertise builds effective teams. Through shared learning experiences, interprofessional collaboration will blossom. A diverse expertise helps build effective teams. Collaborative practice depends on maintaining this expertise through continued learning experiences and through refining, revising, and improving the roles and responsibilities of each profession involved in the collaborative effort.

Competency Domain 3: Interprofessional Communication

Effective communication is a core competency for every profession. This is especially true in the healthcare arena, where critical thinking coupled with the ability to disseminate findings in a concise manner is crucial. Transparency of information coupled with an effective communication vehicle within professions is necessary to manage any sensitive patient information.

Competency Domain 4: Teams and Teamwork

Teamwork cannot take place without a good leader. Leadership qualities are essential to building patient-centered teams where care is carefully coordinated. NPs possess the leadership skills to develop effective teams. Teamwork will enhance patient care outcomes, decrease error, and increase satisfaction among patients and team members. Understanding the functionality of the team and its influence on individual team members, daily operations, and patient care outcomes is an important part of being an effective team member.

These important steps illustrate how in the reality of practice, different disciplines can come together for the greater good of the patient, family, community, and larger health system interplay. Also, many positive benefits of effective collaboration can be shared across disciplines to illustrate a team effort to patient care. We know that the core of the NP competencies specifically set by NONPF (2012a) are acquired through mentored patient care experiences with emphasis on independent and interprofessional practice; analytic skills for evaluating and providing evidence-based, patient-centered care across settings; and advanced knowledge of the healthcare delivery system. This illustrates how NPs can be champions for their patients within the discipline of nursing as well as across disciplines in a collaborative effort approach.

Collaboration within each discipline is also a necessity for a successful treatment plan and initiatives. NPs collaborate and partner with their registered nurse workforce continuously to improve patient outcomes. This team-based approach with multiple levels of knowledge and expertise is what separates nursing from other disciplines. It really demonstrates the evolution of the care plan model that has been utilized for many years in some facilities. Each profession within health care can contribute to the care of the patient and the quality of his or her experience.

Collaborative Health Management Model

With escalating healthcare costs and an aging population with complex chronic diseases, economists, administrators, and clinicians are exploring a variety of interprofessional and team-based care models to deliver cost-effective quality care. In our current standard primary care delivery system, patients with chronic health care conditions are not receiving all recommended interventions and are failing to meet targeted treatment goals. The literature discusses six collaborative primary care models that have had a positive impact on mental health services and the management of chronic health conditions, such as end-stage renal failure, diabetes, and heart failure (Wagner, 2004). One such care model, the Collaborative Health Management Model, fosters teamwork between nurse practitioners and physicians based on an equal partnership. It serves to operationalize the call from the IOM report on the future of nursing for advanced practice registered nurses to deliver high-quality chronic disease management within their scope of practice and with a focus on team-based care and patient partnerships (Brown & Matthews, 2013). Nurse practitioners (NPs) are poised to be at the forefront of this shift in activity and to engage in the philosophy of the collaborative health management model (CHMM).

The need for a CHMM can justified by several elements: NPs have expertise in health prevention and promotion activities, which is lacking in medical education; volume-driven practices leave little time to provide comprehensive care by one clinician; and NPs are experts in facilitating effective patient self-management (Brown & Matthews, 2013). NPs in collaboration with physician partners can help streamline patient care, engage patients in the decision-making process, and provide the patients with the tools needed manage their conditions. This care model has been shown to be cost-effective as the patient receives care on a timely basis with early intervention resulting in unnecessary duplication of services and preventing medical error.

Aside from enjoying better patient outcomes, healthcare providers working in a collaborative healthcare model also experience increased job satisfaction through a structure of collegial relationships. Collaboration among healthcare providers is based on a relationship of mutual trust, shared goals and decision making, and using the collective knowledge of all the healthcare providers involved in the care of the patient. Effective CHMMs will help the patient navigate seamlessly between providers based on his or her preferences and individual healthcare needs (Naylor, 2012).

Collaborative health management models align with the educational expertise that NPs gain. The curriculum in NP education immerses graduate students in population health management with a focus on healthcare trends and communities; health promotion and preventive measures; consultation, collaboration and referral; and use of evidence-based medicine guidelines (NONPF, 2012a). The NP educational focus on patient-centered, holistic care prepares them care to care for individuals with chronic healthcare conditions, such as diabetes, hypertension, and heart failure. The educational competencies outlined by NONPF and the American Association of Colleges of Nursing, support efforts to enhance NP scope of practice, regulation, and licensure across the country.

The framework for the CHMM is designed around the following concepts (Brown & Matthews, 2013):

- Delivery system design—including goals and team member roles (families, patients, NP, MD, RN, medical assistant, pharmacist, social worker, psychologist, specialist consultants)
- Clinical information systems—including risk stratification tools, acuity tools, electronic health records, and evidenced-based practice guidelines
- Decision support—including prompts for patient preferences
- Self-management support—directed by the NP
- Organizational support—aimed at improvements and leadership at all levels of the organization
- Community resources—to assist the patient and family in using community and cultural resources to support their needs

This comprehensive framework engages all the participants in an evidenced-based, patient-focused process that will drive accountable care through meaningful patient engagement and improved relationships within the multidisciplinary team. It is based on the premise that engagement and patient empowerment is essential to driving positive health outcomes. The future success of healthcare outcomes will be determined by how NPs and their physician counterparts and other specialty providers work collaboratively to ensure the positive patient experience that demonstrates quality and cost containment.

Barriers and Benefits to Effective Interprofessional Collaboration

Barriers to implementing effective collaborative teams can be based on the individual professions' isolated evidence base, which results in a foundation of decision making and distinct communication patterns that can result in role confusion and turf battles. Each discipline perceives itself as having sole expertise, power, and leadership in one care aspect over the discipline. To adequately prepare NP students, educators must recognize a blurring of the boundaries between nursing and medicine and must acknowledge that clinical practice demands not only similar competencies but also shared language and communication. Studies show that the way to effective collaboration is through communication that results in patient-centered care.

The astute NP must be cognizant of other barriers he or she may encounter when consulting with members of the medical or allied health team. Some examples of this include scheduling/timing conflicts, in-person vs. telephone consult, and documentation and diagnostic review on a per case basis. As previously mentioned, consultation and collaboration may be site specific and directly related to the individual state statutes on scope of practice, the NP's level of experience, and access to the provider that will be providing the consultation.

Many benefits exist for effective collaboration. The creation of a bridge among professions to provide clinical and quality excellence to the patient, community, and overall population is of utmost importance. This type of collaborative experience can create major changes in how health care is perceived and provided for across local, state, and federal arenas. This allows each person to practice at a higher level. The result is inevitably better patient outcomes, including higher levels of patient satisfaction as well as professional and personal satisfaction knowing that the care provided is evidence-based best practice.

Seminar Discussion Questions

1. Reflect on your past experiences in nursing, and consider how the role change to NP may challenge your knowledge and skills.
2. What strategies for using support in the clinical experiences are available?
3. Describe a clinical experience where the assessment and plan for treatment was not according to clinical guidelines. What would you have done differently and why?
4. Use the process of reflective journaling as you progress through the NP program. During each semester, take the time to review what you have written and consider the advances made to the current time. Reflective journaling is something to consider continuing beyond the educational program.
5. Identify and discuss two patients seen this week in clinical, where one was referred for referral and one was a consultation. How will you follow up on these patients?
6. What are the different members of the healthcare team where you are doing clinical rotations? Does everyone tend to work collaboratively or do there appear to be any "turf wars"?

CASE STUDY

Joe is an NP student entering his second clinical rotation. He received positive feedback and evaluation from his first preceptor who was a physician very experienced in clinical education of NPs, PAs, and medical residents. For the current clinical experience he is at a busy federally qualified health center with a large immigrant population that are mainly Spanish-speaking. Joe does not speak Spanish but has started taking a medical Spanish course to help him communicate with these patients as well as for his future as an NP.

It has been a very different experience thus far, although it has only been 2 full clinical days. The preceptor is a fairly new NP who has only been practicing for 2 years. Her schedule is always overloaded and there are multiple issues to address with the complex patients on her panel. The first day Joe followed the preceptor and did not see any patients on his own. The second day he was directed to see a patient but to be done in 10 minutes so the preceptor could come in and go over the history and physical herself before they made a plan of care. The patient was a 62-year-old male with a history of diabetes, hypertension, and depression. He did not speak much English and so Joe had to use the translation services phone line. Joe had barely gotten the translator on the phone when the preceptor entered and was frustrated he had not completed the history and physical so she took over and saw the patient with Joe shadowing once again. The next patient he was sent to see was a 21-year-old female who was at the clinic for a discussion about contraceptive options. Joe had not covered this topic yet in didactic education so he had to go to his preceptor to inform her about this problem. The preceptor was visibly frustrated and said they would have to talk later, that this did not seem to be going well as a clinical experience for him and she was too busy to have such an "inexperienced student."

Discussion Questions

1. How could this situation have been avoided?
2. Are there steps to prepare a preceptor for what to expect with different students at different levels of experience?
3. Who should Joe reach out to?
4. Who should the preceptor reach out to? Can this clinical experience work for Joe?

References

American Academy of Nurse Practitioners. (2010). *Quality of nurse practitioner practice.* Austin, TX: Author.

American Academy of Nurse Practitioners. (2017). *Renewal requirements.* Retrieved from https://www.aanpcert.org/recert

American Association of Colleges of Nursing. (2006). *The essentials of doctoral education for advanced nursing practice.* Washington, DC: Author.

American Association of Colleges of Nursing. (2015). *The Doctoral of Nursing Practice: Current issues and clarifying recommendations.* Washington, DC: Author.

American Board of Internal Medicine. (2012). *The Mini-CEX.* Retrieved from http://www.abim.org/program-directors-administrators/assessment-tools/mini-cex.aspx#guidelines

American Nurses Credentialing Center. (2016). *ANCC 2018 certification renewal requirements.* Retrieved from http://nursecredentialing.org/RenewalRequirements

American Nursing Credentialing Center. (2013). *Family nurse practitioner certification eligibility criteria.* Retrieved from http://www.nursecredentialing.org/FamilyNP-Eligibility.aspx

Anderson, E. M., Leonard, B., & Yates, J. A. (1974). Epigenesis of the nurse practitioner role. *American Journal of Nursing, 10*(18), 12–16.

Barker, E., & Pittman, O. (2010). Becoming a super preceptor: A practical guide to preceptorship in today's clinical climate. *Journal of the American Academy of Nurse Practitioners, 22,* 144–149.

Barton, T. D. (2007). Student nurse practitioners—A rite of passage? The universality of Van Gennep's model of social transition. *Nurse Education in Practice, 7,* 338–347.

Benner, P. (1984). *From novice to expert: Excellence and power in clinical nursing practice.* Menlo Park, CA: Addison-Wesley.

Bickley, L. (2009). *Bates' guide to physical examination* (10th ed.). Philadelphia, PA: Wolters Kluwer/ Lippincott Williams & Wilkins.

Brooks, M. V., & Niederhauser, V. P. (2010). Preceptor expectations and issues with nurse practitioner clinical rotations. *Journal of the American Academy of Nurse Practitioners, 22,* 573–579.

Brown, M. A., & Matthews, S. W. (2013). APRN expertise: The collaborative health management model. *Nurse Practitioner: The American Journal of Primary Healthcare, 38*(1), 43–48.

Brown, M., & Olshansky, E. F. (1997). From limbo to legitimacy: A theoretical model of the transition to the primary care nurse practitioner role. *Nursing Research, 46*(1), 46–51.

Brown, P. (2016). A new normal: Graduate nursing students paying for clinical rotations. *Minority Nurse.* Retrieved from http://minoritynurse.com/a-new-normal-graduate-nursing-students-paying-for-clinical-rotations/

Brykczynski, K. (2012). Clarifying, affirming, and preserving the nurse in nurse practitioner education and practice. *Journal of the American Academy of Nurse Practitioners, 24,* 554–564.

Buppert, C. (2011). *Nurse practitioner's business practice and legal guide* (4th ed.). Sudbury, MA: Jones and Bartlett.

Burns, C., Beauchesne, M., Ryan-Krause, P., & Sawin, K. (2006). Mastering the preceptor role: Challenges of clinical teaching. *Journal of Pediatric Health Care, 20*(3), 172–183. doi:10.1016/j.pedhc.2005.10.012

Coralli, C. (2006). Effective case presentations—An important clinical skill. *Journal of the American Academy of Nurse Practitioners, 18,* 216–220.

Cusson, R. M., & Strange, S. N. (2008). Neonatal nurse practitioner role transition: The process of re-attaining expert status. *Journal of Perinatal and Neonatal Nursing, 22*(4), 329–337.

Department of Commerce and Consumer Affairs. (2017). *Licensing area: Nursing.* Retrieved from http://cca.hawaii.gov/pvl/boards/nursing/

D'Amour, D. O., & Oandasan, I. (2005). Interprofessionality as the field of interprofessional practice and interprofessional education: An emerging concept. *Journal of Interprofessional Care, 19*(1), 80–20.

Davenport, C. H. (2008). The 3-minute emergency medicine medical student presentation: A variation on the theme. *Society for Academic Emergency Medicine, 15*(7), 683–687.

Fitzgerald, C., Kantrowitz-Gordon, I., Katz, J., & Hirsch, A. (2012). Advanced practice nursing education: Challenges and strategies. *Nursing Research and Practice.* doi:10.1155/2012/854918

Fleming, E., & Carberry, M. (2011). Steering a course towards advanced nurse practitioner: A critical care perspective. *Nursing in Critical Care, 16*(2), 67–76.

Goolsby, M. (2002). *Nurse practitoner secrets: Questions and answers to reveal the secrets to successful NP practice.* Philadephia, PA: Hanley & Belfus.

Graduate Nursing EDU.Org. (2016). *Fee-based practicums for nursing students raise ethical concerns.* Retrieved from http://www.graduatenursingedu.org/2016/07/fee-based-practicums-for-nursing-students-raise-ethical-concerns/

Green, H. D. (2011). The oral case presentation: What internal medicine clinician–teachers expect from clinical clerks. *Teaching and Learning in Medicine, 23*(1), 58–61.

Hamric, A. B., Spross, J. A., & Hanson, C. M. (2009). *Advanced practice nursing: An integrative approach* (4th ed.). Philadelphia, PA: W. B. Saunders.

Haas, B. S.-B. (2009, October). Application of the Newell Liberal Arts Model for interdisciplinary course design and implementation. *Journal of Nursing Education, 48*(10), 579–582.

Hinson Brown, L. (2006). The case presentation as argument. *Journal of the American Academy of Nurse Practitioners, 18*(9) 395–396.

Institute of Medicine. (2010). *The future of nursing: Leading change, advancing health (consensus report).* Washington, DC: The National Academies Press. Retrieved from http://www.iom.edu/Reports/2010/The-Future-of-Nursing-Leading-Change-Advancing-Health.aspx

Kaiser Family Foundation. (2013). *Health reform source.* Retrieved from http://kff.org/health-reform

Krupa, C. (2010, October 11). Physician shortage projected to soar to more than 91,000 in a decade. *American Medical News.* Retrieved from http://www.ama-assn.org/amednews/2010/10/11/prsb1011.htm

Makowsky, M. C. (2009). Collaboration between pharmacists, physicians and nurse practitioners: A qualitative investigation of working. *Journal of Interprofessional Care, 23*(2), 169–184.

Maryland Board of Nursing. (2016). *Advanced Practice Registered Nursing: Tax benefit for nurse practitioner preceptors.* Retrieved from http://mbon.maryland.gov/Pages/advanced-practice-tax-benefit-np-preceptors.aspx

Maylone, M. M., Ranieri, L., Quinn Griffin, M. T., McNulty, R., & Fitzpatrick, J. J. (2011). Collaboration and autonomy: Perceptions among nurses. *Journal of the American Academy of Nurse Practitioners, 23*(11), 51–57.

National Task Force on Quality Nurse Practitioner Education. (2012). *Criteria for evaluation of nurse practitioner programs.* Washington, DC: National Organization of Nurse Practitioner Faculties.

Naylor, M. K. (2012). The role of nurse practitioners in reinventing primary care. *Health Affairs, 31*(11), 893–899.

National Organization of Nurse Practitioner Faculties. (2012a). *Domains and core competencies of nurse practitioner practice.* Washington, DC: Author.

National Organization of Nurse Practitioner Faculties. (2012b, October 14). *Nurse practitioner core competencies.* Retrieved from http://www.nonpf.com/associations/10789/files/NPCoreCompetenciesFinal2012.pdf

Nursing Center. (2017). *Continuing education requirements for nurses by state.* Retrieved from http://www.nursingcenter.com/ceconnection/ce-state-requirements

O'Brien, J. L., Martin, D. R., Heyworth, J. A., & Meyer, N. R. (2009). A phenomenological perspective on advanced practice. *Journal of the American Academy of Nurse Practitioners, 21*(8), 444–453.

Paauw, D., Migeon, M. B., & Burkholder, L. R. (2003). *Internal medicine clerkship guide.* St. Louis, MO: Mosby.

Pittman, O. (2012). The use of simulation with advanced practice nursing students. *Journal of the American Academy of Nurse Practitioners, 24*, 516–529. doi:10.1111/j.1745-7599.2012.00760.x

Roberts, S. J., Tabloski, P., & Bova, C. (1997). Epigenesis of the nurse practitioner role revisited. *Journal of Nursing Education, 36*, 67–73.

Robert Wood Johnson Foundation. (2013). *Reflections from the president.* Retrieved from http://www.rwjf.org/en/about-rwjf/from-the-president.html

Rollins, L. G. (2012). *The one-miniute preceptor.* University of Virgina Health System. Retrieved from http://www.med-ed.virginia.edu/courses/fm/precept/module5/m5p2.htm

Ross, K. (2012, November). Practice makes perfect: Planning considerations for medical simulation centers. *Health Facilities Management Magazine.* Retrieved from https://www.ecri.org/Documents/Reprints/Practice_Makes_Perfect_Planning_Considerations_for_Medical_Simulation_Centers%28Health_Facilities_Management%29.pdf

Schmitt, M., Blue, A., Aschenbrener, C., & Viggiano, T. (2011). Core competencies for interprofessional collaborative practice: Reforming health care by transforming health professionals' education. *Academic Medicine, 86*(11), 1351.

Spoelstra, S. L., & Robbins, L. B. (2010). A qualitative study of role transition for RN to APN. *International Journal of Nursing Education Scholarship, 7*(1), 1–14. doi:10.2202/1548-923X.2020

Suter, E., Arndt, J., Arthur, N., Parboosingh, J., Taylor, E., & Deutschlander, S. (2009). Role understanding and effective communication as core competencies for collaborative practice. *Journal of Interprofessional Care, 23*, 41–51.

Thompson, J., Kershbaumer, R., & Krisman-Scott, M. A. (2001). *Educating advanced practice nurses and midwives: From practice to teaching.* New York, NY: Springer.

Van Gannep, A. (1960). *The rites of passage.* London, England: Routledge.

Wagner, E. (2004). Effective team work and quality of care. *Medical Care, 42*(11), 1037–1039.

Watson, S. (2016). *International reflective journaling guidelines.* Unpublished paper.

Wedgeworth, M., Carter, S., & Ford, C. (2017). Clinical faculty preceptors and mental health reflections: Learning through journaling. *Journal for Nurse Practitioners, 13*(6), 411–417.

World Health Organization. (2010). *Framework for action on interprofessional education and collaborative practice.* Retrieved from http://www.who.int/hrh/resources/framework_action/en

CHAPTER 7

Evidence-Based Practice

Kerry Milner

The History of Evidence-Based Practice

The concept of evidence-based practice (EBP) originated in medicine and was first introduced to U.S. healthcare providers in the published literature in a 1992 *Journal of the American Medical Association* article (Ragan & Quincy, 2012). In this article, evidence-based medicine (EBM) was described as de-emphasizing tradition, unsystematic clinical experience, and pathology as sufficient grounds for practice decisions and it was suggested that critical examination of evidence from practice-based studies should underlie clinical decision making (Evidence-Based Medicine Working Group, 1992). The EBM movement called for physicians to learn the skills of efficient literature searching and the use of formal rules to critically evaluate evidence from the clinical literature.

In the early published definitions of EBM, the areas of foci included identifying, critically appraising, and summarizing best current evidence. However, it became clear that evidence alone was not sufficient to make clinical decisions, so in 2000 the Evidence-Based Medicine Working Group presented the second fundamental principle of EBM. This principle specified that clinical decisions, recommendations, and practice guidelines must not only focus on the best available evidence, but they also must include the values and preferences of the informed patient. Values and preferences refer not only to the patients' perspectives, beliefs, expectations, and goals for life and health, but also to the practices individuals use to consider the available options and the relative benefits, harms, costs, and inconveniences of those options (Guyatt et al., 2000).

A similar definition by Canadian medical doctor David Sackett, who is credited with pioneering EBM, emerged around the same time. His definition follows:

> *The practice of evidence-based medicine means integrating individual clinical expertise with the best available external clinical evidence from systematic research. By individual clinical expertise we mean the proficiency and judgment that individual clinicians acquire through clinical experience and clinical*

> *practice. Increased expertise is reflected in many ways, but especially in more effective and efficient diagnosis and in the more thoughtful identification and compassionate use of individual patients' predicaments, rights, and preferences in making clinical decisions about their care. (Sackett, Rosenberg, Gray, Haynes, & Richardson, 1996, p. 71)*

While EBM was being written about in U.S. scientific literature, Archie Cochrane, a British epidemiologist and physician, had been vocal about the lack of systematic reviews upon which to base medical practice, so he published a systematic review on care during pregnancy and childbirth. It was so well received that he was granted government funding for the Cochrane Center in 1992 ("Our vision, mission, and principles | Cochrane," n.d.). The central mission of the Cochrane Collaboration is to promote healthcare decision making throughout the world that is informed by high-quality, timely research evidence. Today the Cochrane Collaboration is an international network of nearly 30,000 people from over 100 countries helping healthcare providers, policy makers, patients, their advocates, and caregivers make well-informed decisions about health care by preparing, updating, and promoting the accessibility of systematic reviews.

While the United States, Canada, and England were implementing EBM, in Australia, in response to the growing trend of evidence-based health care, the Joanna Briggs Institute was created at the Royal Adelaide Hospital in 1996 to facilitate evidence-based health care globally (Jordan, Donnelly, & Piper, 2006). The institute's original focus was on nursing, and later it changed to incorporating medicine and allied health practitioners. The institute's definition of evidence-based health care is consistent with early definitions of EBM, stating that clinical decisions should be based on best available scientific evidence while recognizing patient preferences, the context of health care, and the judgment of the clinician (Jordan, Munn, Aromataris, & Lockwood, 2015).

Nursing and EBP

Concern about overlooking the patient's values and preferences in the early definition of EBM by Evidence-Based Medicine Working Group (1992) prompted nursing to adopt a definition similar to those written by Sackett et al. (1996) and the Joanna Briggs Institute. In 2000, Ingersoll articulated the following definition of EBP for nursing:

> *Evidence-based nursing practice is the conscientious, explicit, and judicious use of theory-derived, research-based information in making decisions about care delivery to individuals or groups of patients and in consideration of individual needs and preferences. (Ingersoll, 2000, p. 154)*

Unique to this EBP definition was the inclusion of the use of theory as well as evidence when making clinical practice decisions. Leaders in nursing believed that theory and clinical research should be the basis for evidence-based nursing instead of ritual, isolated, and unsystematic clinical experiences, ungrounded opinion, and tradition (Fain, 2014; Ingersoll, 2000). The goal of EBP is to promote effective nursing practice, efficient care, and improved outcomes for patients, and to provide the best available evidence for clinical, administrative, and educational decision making (Newhouse, Dearholt, Poe, Pugh, & White, 2007). Key assumptions of EBP in nursing practice include:

1. Nursing is both a science and an applied profession.
2. Knowledge is important to professional practice, and there are limits to knowledge that must be identified.
3. Not all evidence is created equal, and there is a need to use the best available evidence.
4. Evidence-based practice contributes to improved outcomes.

Two nurse practitioners (NP), who are educators and researchers in nursing, (Melnyk & Fineout-Overholt, 2014), define EBP using Sackett's definition as a platform and identify seven steps in the EBP process. The EBP process, per this definition, starts with an organizational culture that supports EBP and encourages nurses at all levels to wonder are we doing the best thing. Nurses turn a clinical question into a searchable format using an established method (e.g. PICO) and use this focused question to search for the most relevant evidence. Step 3 involves critically appraising the evidence found in step 2, summarizing the strength and quality of the best relevant evidence, and formulating recommendations. The evidence is integrated with a nurses' clinical expertise and patients' values and goals when making a decision or practice change. The next step is to evaluate the outcomes of the EBP decision or practice change. The last step is to disseminate the outcomes of the decision or change locally (e.g. grand rounds) or through traditional methods (e.g. poster or podium presentation, publishable manuscript).

Evidence-based practice for nursing is not EBM, because it is imperative that many sources of evidence are critically appraised when making practice decisions. While randomized controlled trials or systematic reviews may provide the most rigorous scientific evidence for EBM, that evidence may not be applicable to nursing and patient care, which requires a holistic approach and a broad range of methodologies as the basis for care (Houser & Oman, 2010). No one research design is better than another when evaluating evidence on effective nursing practices, and appropriate clinical decision making can only be achieved by using several sources of evidence (DiCenso, Cullum, & Ciliska, 1998; Rycroft-Malone et al., 2004).

Non-research evidence is useful for answering some types of clinical questions. For example, practice-based evidence includes "evidence concerning the contexts, experiences, and practices of healthcare providers working in real-world practice settings" (Leeman & Sandelowski, 2012, p. 171), and the use of qualitative methodologies play an essential role in creating more practice-based evidence in the evidence base for nursing practice used for problem solving and clinical decision making.

Missing from the earlier definitions of EBM and EBP is clinical decision making related to available resources. The reality is that there is a limited amount of healthcare dollars. Therefore, when making evidence-based clinical decisions, nurses and other healthcare professionals must also weigh the cost of benefit, cost of harm, and cost to the system when providing evidence-based care (Hopp & Rittenmeyer, 2012).

NPs are actively championing the advancement of EBP in health care and academia. The Center for Transdisciplinary Evidence-based Practice (CTEP) is a world-renowned center, based at The Ohio State University, that serves as a leader and resource to health professionals, healthcare systems, and academic institutions for implementing best practices through an EBP approach to decision making and sustaining a culture of EBP for the ultimate purpose of improving quality of health care and outcomes for all ("Overview | CTEP," n.d.). The founders are NURSE PRACTITIONERS whose mission is to:

- Improve EBP knowledge, skills, and attitudes in clinicians from all disciplines
- Facilitate EBP across the care continuum and healthcare systems
- Assist with creating sustainable EBP culture in healthcare systems
- Synthesize and disseminate evidence to advance evidence-based care
- Influence health policy by advocating for EBP
- Assist clinicians and healthcare organizations with expediting the process of translation of evidence into practice
- Disseminate findings of EBP implementation and research
- Conduct ongoing research on many aspects of EBP

It is clear from the inception of EBM and evidence-based nursing that all healthcare disciplines should be making decisions based on the best available evidence, clinical expertise, patient values and preferences, and available resources. Moreover, leaders in nursing are calling for EBP to be the foundation for everything healthcare providers do ("Overview | CTEP," n.d.).

Why Should NPs use EBP?

If you were diagnosed with breast cancer and were faced with the decision of whether to have a lumpectomy versus mastectomy and chemotherapy versus radiation, would you want your NP to give you the best and latest information on treatment options and the risks and benefits associated with each treatment from systematic reviews or randomized control trials (RCT) including patients with the same diagnosis and similar personal characteristics? Would you want to know about how others with your type of cancer coped with the treatment based on evidence from well-designed descriptive or qualitative studies?

There are many reasons why NPs should base their practice on the EBP process. First and foremost is, care that is not evidence based is likely unethical and incompetent (Vincent, Hastings-Tolsma, Gephart, & Alfonzo, 2015). Thus, as the basis of patient care, NP should integrate research evidence with clinical evidence and patient values while considering available resources in order to provide the best care. NPs should use the EBP paradigm to promote optimal patient outcomes, stimulate innovation in clinical practice, and promote the value of the nursing profession in the healthcare system (Melnyk, 2014). In today's complex and dynamic patient-care environment, nursing practice informed by the best evidence is vital to realizing healthcare improvements and cost savings (Dearholt & Dang, 2012). The role of the NP has expanded over the years to include a wider scope of practice in many states, thus prompting the need for all NPs to acquire EBP skills and use best current evidence for clinical decision making (Facchiano & Snyder, 2012a). NPs need to practice using the EBP process because studies have shown that patient care outcomes are substantially improved when health care is based on well-designed studies rather than relying on tradition and clinical expertise alone (Houser & Oman, 2010; Melnyk, 2016a).

Existing practices based on tradition or clinical expertise may be harming patients. It is unethical to continue using untested interventions. NPs need to use and understand the EBP process so they can take a lead role in facilitating the evaluation of evidence to develop EBP guidelines, form EBP teams, identify practices and systems that need study, and collaborate with nurse scientists to initiate research (Melnyk, 2016b).

Evidence-Based Competencies for Advanced Practice Nurses

The Doctor of Nursing Practice (DNP) is a practice-focused doctorate that prepares advanced practices nurses for clinical, faculty, and leadership roles; to improve practice and patient outcomes; and to strengthen practice and health care delivery ("AACN Position Statement on the Practice Doctorate in Nursing," 2004). The AACN and the DNP essentials are clear that DNP prepared nurses are the leaders and experts in EBP (Melnyk, 2016b). The following EBP competencies have been developed for NP nurses working in health systems and should be a part of NP performance evaluations (Melnyk, Gallagher-Ford, Long, & Fineout-Overholt, 2014).

1. Questions clinical practice in order to improve healthcare outcomes.
2. Uses internal evidence (e.g., data from clinical setting) to describe clinical problems.
3. Develops clinical questions in a searchable format (e.g., PICO = Patient population; Intervention; Comparison intervention; Outcome).
4. Conducts systematic, exhaustive searches for external evidence (e.g., evidence from research studies) to answer clinical questions in PICO format.
5. Critically appraises all different evidence types (e.g., clinical practice guidelines, systematic reviews, research studies, evidence reviews; manufacture guidelines).
6. Synthesizes a body of evidence to determine its strength and worth to clinical practice.
7. Collects data from practice (e.g., patient, system, or quality/performance improvement data) to inform clinical decision making.
8. Plans and implements evidence-based practice changes using internal and external evidence, clinical expertise, and patient preferences to improve healthcare processes and outcomes.
9. Evaluates evidence-based decisions and practice changes for individuals, populations, and systems to determine best practices.
10. Develops evidence-based policies and procedures.
11. Participates in research studies with other healthcare professionals.
12. Is an EBP mentor.
13. Disseminates evidence-based best practices that improve healthcare outcomes.
14. Implements strategies to sustain an EBP culture.
15. Shares best evidence with individuals, colleagues, and policy makers.[1]

Incorporating these competencies into the standards of practice for NPs working in health systems should facilitate higher quality, efficient care, and improved healthcare outcomes (Melnyk et al., 2014).

---

1 Reproduced from Melnyk, B. M., Gallagher-Ford, L., Long, L. E., & Fineout-Overholt, E. (2014). The Establishment of Evidence-Based Practice Competencies for Practicing Registered Nurses and Advanced Practice Nurses in Real-World Clinical Settings: Proficiencies to Improve Healthcare Quality, Reliability, Patient Outcomes, and Costs. *Worldviews on Evidence-Based Nursing, 11*(1), 5-15. Used with permission from John Wiley.

How to Translate EBP into Practice

Many EBP models exist that help to guide healthcare systems and their clinicians with implementing EBP policies, protocols, and guidelines. It is important for organizations or healthcare systems to have EBP models that assist clinicians with translating research evidence into the practice setting. A central goal of these EBP models is to speed up the transfer of new knowledge into practice, because in the past this has taken years. Use of a model provides an organized approach to EBP implementation and can maximize use of nursing time and resources (Gawlinski & Rutledge, 2008). There are several EBP models that help with translating research into practice. Common aspects of these models include the EBP process that identifies problems and practice questions and reviews latest evidence, existing clinical practices and practice guidelines, and other data specific to quality indicators in that setting. No one model of EBP exists that meets the needs of all nursing environments. For the purposes of this chapter, some of the more popular models are described in **TABLE 7-1**.

The ACE Star model, ARCC, PARIHS, EBP Model for Change, and Trinity EBP model are all models or frameworks for systematically putting the EBP process into operation within a healthcare system. The Johns Hopkins Nursing EBP Model and the

TABLE 7-1 Evidence-Based Practice Models

Model	Description	Processes
ACE Star (Stevens, 2004)	EBP framework for systematically putting EBP processes into operation	1. Knowledge discovery 2. Evidence summary 3. Translation into practice recommendations 4. Integration into practice 5. Evaluation
Advancing Research and Clinical Practice through Close Collaboration Model (ARCC Model) (Melnyk & Fineout-Overholt, 2014)	Provides healthcare systems with a guide for implementation and sustainability of EBP to achieve quality outcomes	1. Assessment of organizational culture and readiness for EBP 2. Identification of strengths and major barriers 3. Development and use of EBP mentors 4. EBP implementation
Johns Hopkins Nursing Evidence-Based Practice Model (Dearholt & Dang, 2012)	Assists nurses at the bedside in translating evidence to clinical, administrative, and educational practice	1. Practice question 2. Evidence 3. Translation

TABLE 7-1 Evidence-Based Practice Models *(continued)*

Model	Description	Processes
Iowa Model of Evidence-Based Practice to Promote Quality Care (Titler et al., 2001)	A guide for nurses and clinicians in making decisions about day-to-day practices that affect patient outcomes	1. Identify type of organizational trigger: problem or knowledge focused 2. Form a team 3. Gather and critically appraise evidence 4. Assess if sufficient evidence 5. Pilot practice change or conduct research 6. Evaluate pilot practice change 7. Institute practice change
Promoting Action on Research Implementation in Health Services Framework (PARIHS framework) (Kitson, Harvey, & McCormack, 1998)	Provides healthcare systems a framework for how research findings can be successfully implemented into practice with equal recognition of level of evidence, the context into which the evidence is being implemented, and the method of facilitating the change	1. Critical appraisal of evidence 2. Gain understanding of practice area where change will happen 3. Create a strategic plan for practice change 4. Successful implementation is a function of evidence, context, and facilitation
Model for EBP Change (Rosswurm & Larabee, 1999)	Model for translating EBP into healthcare organization	1. Assess the need for change in practice 2. Locate the best evidence 3. Critically analyze the evidence 4. Design practice change 5. Implement and evaluate change in practice 6. Integrate and maintain change in practice
Transdisciplinary Model of EBP (Newhouse & Spring, 2010)	Interdisciplinary EBP model to accelerate the translation of EBP across disciplines	1. Primary researcher 2. Systematic reviewer 3. Practitioner
Trinity Evidence-Based Practice Model (Vratney & Shriver, 2007)	A conceptual model for EBP that addresses how to overcome barriers to implementation; a guide for growing EBP in your organization while weeding out barriers	1. Breaking ground 2. Planting seeds 3. Sprouting up 4. Showering of education 5. Heating things up 6. Branching out 7. Bearing fruit

Iowa Model of Evidence-Based Practice to Promote Quality Care are geared toward clinical decision making at the bedside. The goal of the Transdisciplinary Model of EBP is to accelerate the translation of the EBP process across disciplines within an organization. In summary, there are many models and frameworks that nurse leaders can choose to help guide and integrate EBP into their healthcare system.

Searching for Evidence

Before you can find the best current evidence for clinical decision making, you must identify a clinical problem and translate it into a searchable, answerable question. The PICOT method is a widely accepted format for creating clinical questions. Melnyk and Fineout-Overholt (2014) have developed question templates for asking PICOT questions in nursing based on the type of clinical problem (e.g., intervention/therapy, prevention, diagnosis) (see **FIGURE 7-1**). Examples of intervention and prognosis/prediction PICOT questions are displayed in **FIGURE 7-2**.

The definition of PICOT is as follows:

P: Population/disease (age, gender, ethnicity, with a certain disorder)
I: Intervention or variable of interest (therapy, exposure to a disease, risk behavior, prognostic factor)
C: Comparison: (alternate therapy, placebo or usual practice, absence of risk factor)
O: Outcome: (risk of disease, accuracy of a diagnosis, rate of occurrence of adverse outcome)
T: Time: The time it takes to demonstrate an outcome (time it takes for the intervention to achieve an outcome or time populations are observed for outcome)

The templates for PICOT questions based on the type of clinical problem are as follows:

Intervention/therapy query:
In __________(P), how does __________(I) compare to __________(C) affect __________(O) within __________(T)?

Prevention query:
For __________ (P), does the use of __________ (I) reduce the future risk of __________ (O) compared with __________ (C)?

Prognosis/prediction query:
In __________(P), how does __________(I) compare to __________(C) influence/predict __________(O) over __________(T)?

Diagnosis or diagnostic test query:
In __________(P), are/is __________(I) compared with __________(C) more accurate in diagnosing __________(O)?

Etiology query:
Are __________(P) who have __________(I), compared with those without __________ (C), at __________risk for/of __________(O) over __________(T)?

Meaning query:
How do __________(P) with __________(I) perceive __________(O) during __________(T)?

FIGURE 7-1 PICOT Definitions and Questions

Reproduced from Melnyk, B., & Fineout-Overholt, E. (2010). *Evidence-based practice in nursing & healthcare*. New York, NY: Lippincott Williams & Wilkins, p. 26. Reprinted by permission of Lippincott Williams & Wilkins.

PICOT QUESTION USING INTERVENTION TEMPLATE

Clinical scenario: You are an extremely busy NP in the primary care division of a Veterans Administration Health System. It has been challenging to meet the complex care needs of veterans with diabetes in the traditional 20-minute clinic visit. You wonder what other care delivery models (e.g., shared medical appointment) may lead to improved clinical outcomes, patient satisfaction, and provider efficiency.

Population: Veterans with diabetes
Intervention: Shared medical appointments
Comparison: Routine clinic visit
Outcome: Improved clinical outcomes
Time: 1-year period

In veterans with diabetes, how does shared medical appointment compared to standard care (routine clinic visit) improve clinical outcomes over 1 year?

PICOT QUESTION USING PROGNOSIS/PREDICTION TEMPLATE

Clinical scenario: A 65-year-old male comes to the cardiology clinic for his regularly scheduled physical examination. He shares that he has seen advertisements for anticoagulant medicine that does not require frequent laboratory testing. He is apprehensive about switching to one of these newer anticoagulant medicines (e.g., dabigatran etexilate) because he has also seen news reports for increased complications related to these newer medicines. The PICOT question would be: Are adult patients who have dabigatran etexilate prescribed compared to warfarin at increased risk for complications? In this scenario you do not need "T."

FIGURE 7-2 Examples of Intervention and Prognosis/Prediction PICOT Questions

Searching Databases for Best Current Evidence

Successful searching for the best current evidence after developing a PICOT question is the next step in the EBP process. Melnyk and Fineout-Overholt (2014) identified eight steps for an efficient search:

1. Begin with a PICOT question and the P, I, C, O, T should be used as the key words (e.g., P = veteran with diabetes, I = shared medical appointment, C = routine office visit, O = clinical outcomes, T = 1 year) that will be used for the search.
2. Establish inclusion and exclusion criteria before searching (e.g., studies published in last 5 years).
3. Use controlled vocabulary headings when available (e.g., MeSH).
4. Expand search using explode option.
5. Use tools to limit the search so the topic of interest is the main point of article.
6. Combine searches generated from PICOT key words.
7. Limit final search results with meaningful limits, such as year, type of study, age, gender, and language.

8. Organize studies in a meaningful way using evidence summary tools (e.g., Johns Hopkins Nursing Evidence Based Practice [JHNEBP] Individual Evidence Summary Tool).

Bibliographic databases commonly used for searches by NPs include the Cochrane Library, Cumulative Index to Nursing and Allied Health Literature (CINAHL), Medical Literature Online (MEDLINE), PubMed, National Guideline Clearinghouse, and Embase. Several of these databases require a subscription fee. **TABLE 7-2** includes a variety of sources for finding evidence to aid clinical decision making; a description of the evidence for each source; the website addresses; and if a fee is needed to access. In the following paragraphs, some of the more popular databases are described in more detail.

TABLE 7-2 Sources of Evidence

Name of Source	Type of Evidence	Access	Fee
ACP PIER (American College of Physicians—Physicians Information & Education Resource)	Includes guidelines and recommendations based on all levels of medical evidence including RCTs, cohort and observational studies, case reports, and expert opinions	https://www.acponline.org/clinical-information	ACP member/fee
Agency for Healthcare Research and Quality (AHRQ)	Clinical Information Effectiveness: ■ Evidence-based practice ■ Outcomes and effectiveness ■ Technology assessments ■ Guidelines: ■ Preventive services ■ Clinical practice guidelines ■ National Guideline Clearinghouse	http://www.ahrq.gov	Free
Campbell Collaboration	Systematic reviews and other evidence synthesis for evidence-based social policy and practice Emphasis on reviews of research evidence on the effectiveness of social and behavioral interventions	https://www.campbellcollaboration.org/	Free

TABLE 7-2 Sources of Evidence *(continued)*

Name of Source	Type of Evidence	Access	Fee
Center for Evidence-Based Medicine (Oxford)	Conferences, workshops, and EBM tools for how to access, appraise, and use evidence	http://www.cebm.net	Some free, some fee to access
Clinical Evidence	Database of best available evidence on common clinical interventions	http://clinicalevidence.bmj.com	Subscription
CINAHL Plus with Full Text	Comprehensive nursing and allied health research database, providing full text for more than 770 journals Evidence-based care sheets	http://www.ebscohost.com/academic/cinahl-plus-with-full-text	Subscription
Cochrane Collaboration	Cochrane Reviews	http://www.cochrane.org	Free abstract Subscription for full text
DARE: Database of Abstract Reviews of Effects	Contains 15,000 abstracts of systematic reviews	http://site.ovid.com/products/ovidguide/daredb.htm	Subscription
EBN Online, Evidence-Based Nursing	Electronic journal providing EBN	http://ebn.bmj.com	Subscription
Joanna Briggs Institute	Reliable evidence for health professionals to use to inform their clinical decision making; tools for how to access, appraise, and use evidence	http://joannabriggs.org/	Subscription
National Guidelines Clearinghouse	A comprehensive free database of evidence-based clinical practice guidelines and related documents, an initiative of the Agency for Healthcare Research and Quality (AHRQ); browse the database by condition or treatment/intervention	http://www.guideline.gov	Free

(continues)

TABLE 7-2 Sources of Evidence *(continued)*

Name of Source	Type of Evidence	Access	Fee
NICE: National Institutes of Health and Clinical Excellence	NICE develops evidence-based clinical guidelines on the most effective ways to diagnose, treat, and prevent disease and ill health; also have patient-friendly versions of guidelines to help educate and empower patients, caregivers, and the public to take an active role in managing their conditions	http://www.nice.org.uk	Free
Prospero	Protocol details for systematic reviews relevant to health and social care, welfare, public health, education, crime, justice, and international development, where there is a health-related outcome	https://www.crd.york.ac.uk/PROSPERO	Free
PubMed/ MEDLINE/ NLM	Provides free access to Medline and the NLM database of indexed citations and original abstracts in medicine, nursing, and health care; search tutorials; evidence-based medical reviews (EBMR)	http://www.ncbi.nlm.nih.gov/pubmed	Free abstracts Some free articles Subscription for full text
RePort	Access to reports, data, and analyses of NIH research activities and the results of NIH-supported research	http://report.nih.gov	Free
Turning Research into Practice Database (TRIP) Database: For Evidence Based Medicine	Meta-search engine for evidence-based healthcare topics; searches hundreds of EBM and EBN websites that contain synopses, clinical answers, textbook information, clinical calculators, systematic reviews, and guidelines	http://www.tripdatabase.com	Free
UpToDate	Clinical decision support system that combines the most recent evidence with the experience of expert clinicians	http://www.uptodate.com	Subscription

The Cochrane Library is a collection of seven databases that may be used to find best current evidence in health care. The most popular database is the Cochrane Database of Systematic Reviews. This database contains systematic reviews of primary research in human health care and health policy. This database is maintained by the Cochrane Working Group, and their reviews are held to the highest scientific standards. Abstracts of reviews are available free of charge from the Cochrane website; however, full reviews are available by subscription. The Cochrane Database of Systematic Reviews is found online at http://www.cochrane.org/cochrane-reviews.

The CINAHL database produced by EBSCO Information Systems has more than 2.6 million records and provides indexing to more than 3,000 journals from nursing and allied health fields. In addition to journals, this database has publications from the National League for Nursing, American Nurses Association, references to healthcare books, nursing dissertations, legal cases, clinical innovations, critical paths, drug records, evidence-based care sheets, research instruments, and clinical trials. To access this database, you need a subscription.

The MEDLINE database is provided by the National Library of Medicine and is widely known as the premier source for bibliographic and abstract coverage of biomedical literature. It has indices that reference more than 5,000 journals, and includes at least 300 journals specific to nursing. PubMed is the National Library of Medicine's Web interface, through which MEDLINE can be accessed for free. PubMed has free tutorials on how to conduct searches. Abstracts are free as well as some full text articles; otherwise, a fee is charged to retrieve full text articles. A guide of MEDLINE and PubMed resources can be found at http://www.nlm.nih.gov/bsd/pmresources.html.

The Joanna Briggs Institute is an international collaboration involving nursing, medical, and allied health researchers, clinicians, academics, and quality managers across 40 countries in every continent. The Joanna Briggs Institute connects healthcare professionals with the best available international evidence at the point of care. They offer systematic reviews, best practice information sheets, and critical appraisal tools. Some information is free but most information is accessed by paying a fee.

The National Guideline Clearinghouse is a search engine for finding clinical practice guidelines. This database is available free of charge from the Agency for Healthcare Research and Quality (AHRQ) and is a mechanism for obtaining objective, detailed information on clinical practice guidelines from all over the world. Guidelines can be searched using medical subject headings (MeSH) or by disease/condition, treatment/intervention, or health services administration. You can also sign up for email alerts based on a topic of interest.

Embase is a subscription-based international biomedical and pharmaceutical database that includes over 24 million indexed records and 7,600 peer-reviewed journals. All MEDLINE records produced by the National Library of Medicine are included, as well as over 5 million records not covered on MEDLINE. Embase has in-depth indexing of the drug-related and clinical literature, with a particular focus on comprehensive indexing of adverse drug reactions, systematic reviews, and development and use of medical devices.

Busy NPs with limited resources or limited time should start their search in PubMed because it is a free database that can be accessed via the Internet from any mobile device (Facchiano & Snyder, 2012b). Natural language or key words can be used for the search by typing in words from your PICOT question (e.g., diabetes). Searches may also be done using controlled vocabulary called medical subject headings (MeSH).

In PubMed, when you type in key words or natural language you will automatically get MeSH and you can click on these words and continue the search with these words. You can use built-in filters within PubMed to further refine the search. One example is the clinical queries filter that extracts evidence based on the best study design to answer that PICOT question. Boolean operators include *AND*, *OR*, and *NOT*. They can link key words and further define the search, such as *diabetes care and veterans*. Searches can be further defined using the limit feature. This feature includes many categories such as age, gender, English language, year of publication, and humans or animals. It is important to become familiar with how to do searches efficiently. PubMed offers free tutorials on how to search their database and can be accessed via the homepage.

NPs should investigate gaining access to a health science librarian to aid with searches for evidence. Librarian-provided services have been shown to be effective in saving time for health professionals and providing relevant information for decision making (Perrier et al., 2014). Moreover, studies demonstrated decreased patient length of stay when clinicians requested literature searches related to a patient's case.

▸ What Counts as Evidence?

NPs use a variety of sources of evidence to make clinical decisions regarding diagnoses, treatments, and interventions on a daily basis. Evidence can come from external sources such as published research studies or internal sources such as quality improvement (QI) data or clinical data. What is important to remember is that not all evidence is equally rigorous or applicable to your practice setting or the patient populations that you manage. Evidence from a textbook, colleague, or single journal article is not the same as evidence from a systematic review of randomized controlled trials that answers a particular research question. Moreover, the evidence must match the type of clinical question in PICOT format being asked. For example, a synthesis of cohort or case control studies is the highest level of evidence for answering prediction/prognostics questions. Lastly, NP must be adept at assessing the level, quality, and strength of evidence in order to make a judgment about whether or not to translate that evidence into practice.

Evidence hierarchies exist to help healthcare providers assess the level of evidence that is based on type of research design (quantitative or qualitative), summaries of research (e.g., systematic review of quantitative, qualitative, or both), and types of non-research evidence (e.g., clinical practice guideline). In most evidence hierarchies, the strongest evidence is from rigorous scientific research or systematic reviews with or without meta-analysis of single randomized control trials and the weakest evidence is manufacture recommendations. Evidence hierarchies that contain other evidence types in addition to research studies are most useful to the practicing nurse because many nursing care problems cannot be investigated using research designs such as RCT (Jones, 2010). In this section, select evidence hierarchies from different organizations in nursing and medicine are described.

The American Association of Critical Care Nurses (AACN) created their own evidence-leveling system for all their publications outlined in **TABLE 7-3** (Armola et al., 2009). The AACN's system is unique in that it includes meta-analysis of multiple controlled trials or meta-synthesis of qualitative studies in the highest level of evidence and manufacturer's recommendations in the lowest level of evidence. All AACN resources include the evidence-leveling system so practitioners have a reliable guide to assist in determining the strength of evidence.

TABLE 7-3 AACN Evidence-Leveling System

Level	Evidence Type
A	Meta-analysis of multiple controlled studies or meta-synthesis of qualitative studies with results that consistently support specific action, intervention, or treatment.
B	Well-designed controlled studies, both randomized and nonrandomized, with results that consistently support a specific action, intervention, or treatment
C	Qualitative studies, descriptive or correlational studies, integrative reviews, systematic reviews, or randomized controlled trials with inconsistent results
D	Peer-reviewed professional organizational standards, with clinical studies to support recommendations
E	Theory-based evidence from expert opinion or multiple case reports
M	Manufacturers' recommendations only

Reproduced from Armola, R. R., Bourgault, A. M., Halm, M. A., Board, R. M., Bucher, L., Harrington, L., . . . Medina, J. (2009). AACN levels of evidence: What's new? *Critical Care Nurse 2009, 29*(4), 70–73. © AACN. Reprinted by permission.

The Oxford Centre for Evidence-Based Medicine 2011 Levels of Evidence is a hierarchy of evidences described in **TABLE 7-4**. The OCEBM hierarchy of evidences was designed to help busy clinicians, researchers, or patients find the best evidence for a particular type of clinical question (e.g., intervention/diagnosis, prognosis/prediction or etiology, meaning). A clinician who needs to find the best evidence for a treatment clinical query should look for systematic reviews of randomized trials first because they usually provide the most reliable answers. If no evidence is found, the search should continue with individual randomized trials, and so on down the OCEBM Levels of Evidence table.

An important concept raised early in this section that the OCEBM Levels of Evidence table highlights, is that different types of evidence are appropriate for answering different clinical questions. For example, an NP working in obstetrics may ask the health sciences librarian to do a literature search to answer the question: How do pregnant women (P) with gestational diabetes (I) perceive reporting their blood sugar results (O) to their healthcare providers during pregnancy and 6 weeks postpartum (T)? Because this is a meaning PICOT question the highest level of evidence appropriate for answering this question would be meta-synthesis of qualitative or descriptive studies. Conversely, an NP working in labor and delivery has seen a 3-month spike in postpartum hemorrhage after a practice change from an oxytocin infusion dosage of 80 mg/500 mL to 10 mg/500 mL. The NP should use the PICOT intervention question template to develop a searchable clinical question; and systematic reviews with meta-analysis of RCTs would be the appropriate highest level of evidence to answer the question.

TABLE 7-4 OCEBM Levels of Evidence

Type of Question	Level of Evidence
Diagnostic or diagnostic test	1. Systematic review/meta-analysis of RCTs 2. RCTs 3. Nonrandomized controlled trials 4. Cohort study or case-control studies 5. Meta-synthesis of qualitative or descriptive studies 6. Qualitative or descriptive single studies 7. Expert opinion
Prognosis/prediction or etiology	1. Synthesis of cohort study or case-control studies 2. Single cohort study or case-control studies 3. Meta-synthesis of qualitative or descriptive studies 4. Single qualitative or descriptive studies 5. Expert opinion
Meaning	1. Meta-synthesis of qualitative or descriptive studies 2. Single qualitative studies 3. Synthesis of descriptive studies 4. Expert opinion

Reproduced from OCEBM Levels of Evidence Working Group*. (2011). The Oxford Levels of Evidence 2. Oxford Centre for Evidence-Based Medicine. Retrieved from http://www.cebm.net/index.aspx?o=5653. Reprinted by permission.
** OCEBM Levels of Evidence Working Group = Jeremy Howick, Iain Chalmers (James Lind Library), Paul Glasziou, Trish Greenhalgh, Carl Heneghan, Alessandro Liberati, Ivan Moschetti, Bob Phillips, Hazel Thornton, Olive Goddard, and Mary Hodgkinson.*

Multiple evidence hierarchies can be overwhelming so this author created a single general level of evidence hierarchy based on evidence type for the busy NP to refer to when rating level of evidence (**TABLE 7-5**). The type of PICOT question each evidence type answers is included.

In practice there is often a lack of clarity among the terms, level of evidence, quality of evidence, and strength of evidence (Jones, 2010). In this section, level of evidence was described and examples of different hierarchies of evidence that can help the NP to rate level of evidence provided. Rating the level of evidence is the first in a three-step process for assessing evidence for translation into practice outlined by Jones (2010). The additional steps of assessing quality of evidence and strength of evidence are described in the next section.

Critical Appraisal of Evidence

Critical appraisal of evidence is an important step in the EBP process that comes after the search for best current evidence. Publication of research studies and other types of evidence do not guarantee quality, value, or applicability to clinical practice. Thus, NPs must have strong research and statistical literacy to critically appraise all types of evidence sources and determine their worth to practice.

TABLE 7-5 General Levels of Evidence Hierarchy Based on Evidence Type

Evidence Type	Type of PICOT Question Answered	Level
Systematic review with or without meta-analysis of single randomized control trials	Intervention, Diagnostic	1
Single randomized control trial	Intervention, Diagnostic	2
Systematic review with or without meta-analysis of mixed experimental study designs (RCT or quasi-experimental)	Intervention, Diagnostic	3
Nonrandomized control trial or systematic review of mixed experimental and nonexperimental study designs	Intervention, Diagnostic, Prognosis/prediction, Etiology	4
Observational studies (cohort, case-control)	Intervention, Diagnostic, Prognosis/prediction, Etiology	5
Meta-synthesis or single qualitative or descriptive studies	Prognosis/prediction, Etiology, Meaning	6
Peer-reviewed professional and organizational standards with clinical studies to support recommendations	Intervention, Diagnostic, Prognosis/prediction, Etiology	7
Expert opinion or literature review or peer-reviewed professional and organizational standards without clinical studies to support recommendations	Meaning	8
Manufacturer recommendations	Meaning	9

There are many types of critical appraisal tools that NPs can use to assess the quality of research and non-research evidence (**TABLE 7-6**). These tools are designed to help the user systematically examine and critique evidence to determine its validity, clinical significance, and applicability to practice. Critical appraisal tools include specific questions based on a particular methodology or research design; therefore, it is important to pick the correct tool based on the type of evidence you are critically appraising.

Johns Hopkins Nursing (Dearholt & Dang, 2012), Melnyk and Fineout-Overholt (2014), Oxford England Centre for Evidence-Based Medicine, and United Kingdom Critical Appraisal Skills Programme (CASP) have created critical appraisal tools for

TABLE 7-6 Critical Appraisal Tools for Different Sources of Evidence

Author	Tools	Research Method	Access
Critical Appraisal Tools by Research Method			
Johns Hopkins Nursing Evidence-Based Practice Research Evidence Appraisal	Research appraisal questions organized by research design	RCTs Meta-analysis of RCTs Quasi-experimental Nonexperimental Qualitative Meta-synthesis of qualitative studies	Dearholt, S., & Dang, D. (2012). Johns Hopkins Nursing Evidence-based Practice: Models and Guidelines. Sigma Theta Tau.
Melnyk & Fineout-Overholt	Rapid Critical Appraisal (RCA) Checklist; method specific	Case-control Cohort RCTs Systematic reviews Qualitative	Melnyk, B. M., & Fineout-Overholt, E. (2014). Evidence-based practice in nursing and health care: A guide to best practice (3rd ed.). Philadelphia, PA: Lippincott Williams & Wilkins.
Centre for Evidence-Based Medicine	Critical Appraisal Sheets	Systematic Prognostic Diagnostic RCT Educational Prescription	http://www.cebm.net/critical-appraisal/
United Kingdom Critical Appraisal Skills Programme (CASP)	CASP critical appraisal checklists	Systematic reviews RCTs Qualitative research Economic evaluation studies Cohort studies Case-control studies Diagnostic studies Clinical prediction rule	http://www.casp-uk.net
Craig Hospital, Englewood, CO	Appraisal support tool in the form of a bookmark	All types of research methods	

TABLE 7-6 Critical Appraisal Tools for Different Sources of Evidence *(continued)*

Author	Tools	Research Method	Access
Critical Appraisal Tools for Clinical Guidelines			
The Agree Collaboration	AGREE II Instrument and My AGREE Plus Software	Clinical practice guideline	http://www.agreetrust.org
Melnyk & Fineout-Overholt	RCA for Evidence-Based Guidelines	Clinical practice guideline	Melnyk, B. M., & Fineout-Overholt, E. (2014). Evidence-based practice in nursing and health care: A guide to best practice (3rd ed.). Philadelphia, PA: Lippincott, Williams & Wilkins.

specific research designs and non-research evidence. Craig Hospital in Colorado created a pocket-sized general critical appraisal tool for their nurses to carry and use as a quick guide when reading research (**FIGURE 7-3**).

Strength of the evidence is determined by synthesizing the information on the level of evidence (hierarchy of evidence) and quality of evidence (critical appraisal tool) (Jones, 2010). This process begins by organizing the important pieces of information from the completed critical appraisal tools for each evidence source in a meaningful way, and this can be done by using a summary of evidence table. Using Word or Excel software you may create your own table or use **TABLE 7-7**. If your evidence is solely from experimental studies, you may want to use **TABLE 7-8**, which is an example of an evidence summary table for RCT/non-RCT created by Facchiano and Snyder (2013). The underlying concept is to choose a table format that will help you organize evidence from multiple studies or sources in the most efficient manner that answers your PICOT question. The summary table should provide a succinct, stand-alone account of the important study/article details that is understandable to anyone viewing the table. The summary of evidence table will form the basis for creating an evidence synthesis table and recommendations described in the next section.

Evidence Synthesis and Recommendations

Evidence synthesis is the next step after organizing the evidence in a meaningful way. This can be done using the evidence synthesis table (**TABLE 7-9**). This table is organized by number of evidence sources for each level of evidence, and overall summary

<table>
<tr>
<td>

Credibility:
- Authors credentials
- Credibility of publication
- No evidence of conflict of interest

Validity:
- Research question has PICO elements (below)
- Clear design matches the question
- Extraneous variables controlled
- Instrument reliability and validity (> 0.7)
- Sampling procedure (key: randomness)
- Sample size/power (> 80%)
- Results reported clearly
- Evidence of significance (P < .05)

Generalizability:
- Sample represents similar patients
- Setting is similar

Elements of research question:
P: Population
I: Intervention or trait of interest
C: Comparison group or time
O: Outcome of interest

Evaluating a research opportunity:
F: Feasible
I: Interesting
N: Novel
E: Ethical
R: Relevant

Linking evidence to practice:
Level I: Required
Level II: Recommended
Level III: Recommended
Level IV: Optional

</td>
<td>

Level I evidence:
Multiple studies reported as meta-analysis, systematic review, or integrative review, or an evidence-based practice guideline

Well-designed studies with large sample sizes or large effect sizes

Level II evidence:
Evidence from at least one well-designed randomized trial

Single randomized trials with small samples

Single studies with small to moderate effect sizes

Level III evidence:

IIIA:
Evidence from well-designed trials without randomization

IIIB:
Evidence from studies of intact groups
Ex post facto and causal-comparative studies
Case/control or cohort studies

IIIC:
Evidence obtained from time series with and without an intervention

Single experimental or quasi-experimental studies with dramatic effect sizes

Level IV evidence:
Evidence from expert panels
Systematic reviews of descriptive studies
Case series and uncontrolled studies

</td>
</tr>
</table>

FIGURE 7-3 Craig Hospital Critical Appraisal Tool

Journal Club Critique Book Mark. Research/EBP/Quality Committee, Craig Hospital, Englewood, CO. Used with permission.

of evidence source results and overall rating of quality of evidence sources. Strength of evidence is determined from the evidence synthesis table.

Strength of a body of evidence has been defined in terms of quality, quantity, and consistency for intervention studies (Manchikanti, Abdi, & Lucas, 2005). Quality is the extent to which relevant studies for a given topic minimized bias. Quantity includes number of studies that have evaluated the given topic, intervention effect size, and overall sample size across all studies. Consistency reflects the extent to which similar findings are reported from work on a given topic using similar and different study designs.

The JHNEBP Model includes a broadly defined quality of evidence rating scale for research and non-research evidence sources (Dearholt & Dang, 2012) that has characteristics of the domains (quality, quantity, and consistency) for rating overall

TABLE 7-7 Summary of Evidence Table

Clinical question in PICOT Format						
					Evidence Rating	
Citation	Evidence Type	Sample, Sample Size, Setting	Findings that help to answer clinical question	Limitations	Level/Quality	
Author, year, first few words of title	Type of evidence being critically appraised (e.g., systematic review with meta-analysis, RCT, QI study, meta-synthesis clinical practice guideline, expert opinion)	If applicable (e.g., single study) describe the sample, sample size, setting	Describe findings that answer clinical question	Describe limitations that should be considered when assessing the quality of evidence and worth to practice	Identify the level of evidence and with the first entry, state the evidence hierarchy used	Identify the quality rating of evidence and with the first entry state the quality rating system used

Modified from JHNEBP Tools

TABLE 7-8 Evidence Summary Table for Randomized or Nonrandomized Trials

Clinical Question in PICOT Format							
Citation	**Funding Source**	**Level of Evidence**	**Purpose/ Research Design**	**Intervention/ Comparison Group**	**Results**	**Strengths/ Weaknesses**	**Worth to Practice**
Authors and title	*Funding agency, note any conflicts*	*Use level of evidence table from this chapter*	*Trial's purpose/ number of subjects invited to participate, attrition rate, trial length*	*Describe intervention group and comparison group*	*Include results that answer clinical question*	*Critically appraise study using appropriate critical appraisal tool*	*Clinical significance*
Study 1							
Study 2 etc.							

TABLE 7-9 Evidence Synthesis

Level of Evidence (LOE)	Total Number of Evidence Sources for LOE	Overall Summary of Evidence Source Results	Overall Rating for Quality of Evidence Sources
Level 1			
Level 2			
Level 3			
Etc.			

strength of a body of evidence by Manchikanti et al. (2005). For research evidence, a rating of high is defined as "consistent, generalizable results; sufficient sample size for study design; adequate control; definitive conclusions; consistent recommendations based on comprehensive literature review that includes thorough reference to scientific evidence" (p. 108). A rating of good is defined as "reasonably consistent results; sufficient sample size for the study design; some control; fairly definitive conclusions; reasonably consistent recommendations based on fairly comprehensive literature review that include some reference to scientific evidence" (p. 108). A rating of low or major flaw is considered "little evidence with inconsistent results; insufficient sample size for the study design; conclusions cannot be drawn" (p. 108).

The JHNEBP Model has a *Quality Rating System for Organizational Experience* that can be used to rate the quality of evidence sources from QI, financial evaluation, or program evaluation (Dearholt & Dang, 2012). A high quality rating has "clear aims and objectives; consistent results across multiple settings; formal quality improvement or financial evaluation methods used; definitive conclusions; consistent recommendations with thorough reference to scientific evidence" (p. 244). Good quality is defined as "clear aims and objectives; formal quality improvement or financial evaluation methods used; consistent results in single setting; reasonably consistent recommendations with some reference to scientific evidence" (p. 244). Evidence rated as low quality or major flaws is "unclear or missing aims and objectives; poor defined quality improvement/financial analysis method; recommendations cannot be made" (p. 244).

Judgments about a body of evidence are used to support recommendations. For example, the strength of evidence (level of evidence + quality of rating of evidence) may be very strong with consistent, high quality evidence to support a practice change. Conversely there may be very little strong, consistent, quality evidence so original research is needed. It is also possible to find good evidence but conflicting results and a practice change is not recommended until more consistent research evidence becomes available. A pilot of the practice change may be in order if there is good evidence with consistent results from lower level of evidence sources and quality ratings.

In the next two sections, critical appraisal skills for single intervention study and clinical practice guidelines are described.

Critical Appraisal of a Single Intervention Study

It is probable as an NP that you will hear about results from a single RCT and ask, "Should I incorporate these findings into my practice?" To answer this question, you should follow the EBP process from the critical appraisal step. Step one is to assess level of evidence and based on the evidence hierarchy in Table 7-5, a single RCT is level 2 evidence. Next, read the study abstract to assess if the study is relevant to your practice and patients in your practice. If the clinical problem is one you encounter frequently then you should read the whole article to determine if the treatment is feasible given the resources in your practice (Vincent et al., 2015). Step two involves an assessment of the quality of evidence and you could use any of the tools for RCTs listed in Table 7-6 under *Critical Appraisal Tools by Research Method*. The next step is to determine the clinical significance. This can be done by looking at number needed to treat (NNT) and absolute relative risk, otherwise known as the effect size. The absolute risk reduction (ARR) compares the event rate in the treatment group to the event rate in the control group. If a study found 80% of patients in the treatment group improved and 20% of patients in the control group improved, the ARR would be 80% − 20% = 60%. The NNT is calculated by dividing 100 by the ARR: 100/60 = 1.6; so for every two patients exposed to the treatment one will benefit. After validating the findings from the study, the last step is to determine if patients in your practice mirror the patients described in the study. If this were a real-life example and your patients' values and preferences were open to the treatment, costs were low, and the treatment could be easily adopted into your setting, then you would adopt this new treatment.

Critical Appraisal of a Clinical Practice Guidelines

NPs should be able to rapidly appraise the strength of clinical practice guidelines and the quality of evidence used to create the guidelines. Guidelines should be critically appraised in terms of validity, usefulness, when last updated, and clinical context, including environment and patient values and preferences. Rapid critical appraisal checklists for clinical practice guidelines have been developed by the AGREE Collaboration and Melnyk and Fineout-Overholt (2014). At the bottom of Table 7-6 there is a listing of the tools for appraising clinical guidelines and where they can be accessed.

The AGREE II tool is a free, valid, and reliable 23-item tool that is organized into the domains of scope and purpose, stakeholder involvement, rigor of development, clarity of presentation, applicability, and editorial independence. Each of the 23 items focuses on an area of the clinical practice guideline quality. The AGREE II tool also includes two overall guideline assessment items where the appraiser rates the overall quality of the practice guideline and makes a determination of whether or not to use the practice guideline (see **BOX 7-1**).

A new feature is My AGREE PLUS that allows users to complete individual AGREE II Appraisals, contribute to and coordinate group AGREE II appraisals, save appraisals to a personal library, and share appraisals with colleagues. The AGREE II website http://www.agreetrust.org/agree-ii/ has excellent tutorials on how to use the tool and the software.

Grading recommendation systems have been created to assist the clinician with evaluating the strength of recommendations and quality of underlying evidence that the clinical guideline is based upon. The strength of a recommendation reflects the extent to which the clinician can be confident that the clinical guideline has the desired effect

BOX 7-1 AGREE II Instrument

Scope and Purpose

The overall objective(s) of the guideline is (are) specifically described.
The health question(s) covered by the guideline is (are) specifically described.
The population (patients, public, etc.) to whom the guideline is meant to apply is specifically described.

Stakeholder Involvement

The guideline development group includes individuals from all relevant professional groups.
The views and preferences of the target population (patients, public, etc.) have been sought.
The target users of the guideline are clearly defined.

Rigor of Development

Systematic methods were used to search for evidence.
The criteria for selecting the evidence are clearly described.
The strengths and limitations of the body of evidence are clearly described.
The methods for formulating the recommendations are clearly described.
The health benefits, side effects, and risks have been considered in formulating the recommendations.
There is an explicit link between the recommendations and the supporting evidence.
The guideline has been externally reviewed by experts prior to its publication.
A procedure for updating the guideline is provided.

Clarity of Presentation

The recommendations are specific and unambiguous.
The different options for management of the condition or health issue are clearly presented.
Key recommendations are easily identifiable.

Applicability

The guideline describes facilitators and barriers to its application.
The guideline provides advice and/or tools on how the recommendations can be put into practice.
The potential resource implications of applying the recommendations have been considered.
The guideline presents monitoring and/or auditing criteria.

Editorial Independence

The views of the funding body have not influenced the content of the guideline.
Competing interests of guideline development group members have been recorded and addressed.

Overall Guideline Assessment

Rate overall quality of guideline.
I would recommend this guideline for use.

rather than the undesired effect (Guyatt et al., 2008). A systematic approach in the grading of recommendations is important, to cut down on bias and aid in the interpretation of clinical guidelines developed by experts. Two examples of grading systems are the United States Preventative Services Task Force (USPSTF) and the Grading of Recommendations, Assessment, Development and Evaluations (GRADE) approach that is used by clinical decision-making systems like UpToDate and Cochrane Collaboration.

The USPSTF grading system is displayed in **TABLE 7-10**. In this system, Grade A is the strongest recommendation, and clinicians should offer this service to

TABLE 7-10 USPSTF Task Force Recommendation Grades and Suggestions

Grade	Grade Definitions	Suggestions for Practice
A	The USPSTF recommends the service. There is high certainty that the net benefit is substantial.	Offer or provide this service.
B	The USPSTF recommends the service. There is high certainty that the net benefit is moderate or there is moderate certainty that the net benefit is moderate to substantial.	Offer or provide this service.
C	The USPSTF recommends selectively offering or providing this service to individual patients based on professional judgment and patient preferences. There is at least moderate certainty that the net benefit is small.	Offer or provide this service only if other considerations support offering or providing the service in an individual patient.
D	The USPSTF recommends against the service. There is moderate or high certainty that the service has no net benefit or that the harms outweigh the benefits	Discourage the use of this service.
I Statement	The USPSTF concludes that the current evidence is insufficient to assess the balance of benefits and harms of the service. Evidence is lacking, of poor quality, or conflicting, and the balance of benefits and harms cannot be determined.	Read the clinical considerations section of USPSTF Recommendation Statement. If the service is offered, patients should understand the uncertainty about the balance of benefits and harms.

Reproduced from USPSTF. (2017). Grade definitions. Retrieved from https://www.uspreventiveservicestaskforce.org/Page/Name/grade-definitions

their patients. Grade D is the weakest recommendation, and clinicians should not provide this service to patients. There is an additional recommendation of Grade I, which means clinicians should proceed with caution, and patients who want the service need to be aware of the uncertainty of the benefits and harms. Clinicians can visit the website and access free clinical guidelines for many clinical categories (e.g., cancer, heart and vascular diseases, mental health conditions). The guidelines are created by rigorously evaluating clinical research and assessing the merits of preventive measures, including screening tests, counseling, immunizations, and preventive medications. The USPSTF provides a grade for each clinical guideline.

The GRADE is a method of linking evidence-quality evaluations to clinical recommendations that begin in 2000 (Guyatt et al., 2008). In the GRADE approach, recommendations are classified as strong or weak, according to the balance between desirable effects (health benefits, less burden, cost savings) versus undesirable effects (harms, more burdens, costs). A strong recommendation means that the most informed patients would choose the recommended management, and clinicians can recommend the intervention to patients. Weak recommendations mean the intervention has too many undesirable consequences (Guyatt et al., 2008). The GRADE approach also includes quality of evidence and patient preferences. UpToDate, a clinical decision system, uses the GRADE approach (see **TABLE 7-11**). In this system, a grade of 1A means a strong recommendation to use this intervention and the guideline has high-quality evidence backing it. Conversely, a grade of 2C means a weak recommendation with low-quality evidence, and other options should be explored. Both the GRADE Working Group and UpToDate have GRADE resources and tutorials that are free and can be accessed at http://www.gradeworkinggroup.org/ and http://www.uptodate.com/home/grading-tutorial, respectively.

▸ Outcomes of the EBP Process

The EBP process should be the core foundation from which all NPs practice. NPs should routinely question practice, describe practice problems using internal evidence (e.g., QI data), formulate clinical questions to answer practice problems in PICOT format, systematically search for external evidence, critically appraise evidence, synthesize evidence, and make recommendations. Outcomes of the EBP process can take the form of research, EBP, QI, and program evaluation. Therefore, a comparison of these outcomes with an example of each is displayed in **TABLE 7-12**.

▸ Shared Decision Making: An Important Often Missed Part of EBP

Despite the varied definitions of shared decisions making (SDM) in the literature (Makoul & Clayman, 2006), Charles, Gafni, and Whelan (1997) first described this collaborative process between patient and provider where information is exchanged, deliberated, and treatment decisions are made. Healthcare reform, including the passage of the Affordable Care Act and subsequent regulations, has spurred healthcare delivery systems to engage patients and families in SDM (Friedberg, Van Busum,

TABLE 7-11 UpToDate Grading System for Clinical Practice Recommendations

Grade of Recommendation	Clarity of Risk/Benefit	Quality of Supporting Evidence	Implications
1A Strong recommendation, high-quality evidence	Benefits clearly outweigh risks and burdens, or vice versa.	Consistent evidence from well-performed randomized, controlled trials or overwhelming evidence of some other form. Further research is unlikely to change our confidence in the estimate of benefit and risk.	Strong recommendation, can apply to most patients in most circumstances without reservation. Clinicians should follow a strong recommendation unless a clear and compelling rationale for an alternative approach is present.
1B Strong recommendation, moderate-quality evidence	Benefits clearly outweigh risks and burdens, or vice versa.	Evidence from randomized, controlled trials with important limitations (inconsistent results, methodologic flaws, indirect or imprecise), or very strong evidence of some other research design. Further research (if performed) is likely to have an impact on our confidence in the estimate of benefit and risk and may change the estimate.	Strong recommendation and applies to most patients. Clinicians should follow a strong recommendation unless a clear and compelling rationale for an alternative approach is present.
1C Strong recommendation, low-quality evidence	Benefits appear to outweigh risks and burdens, or vice versa.	Evidence from observational studies, unsystematic clinical experience, or from randomized, controlled trials with serious flaws. Any estimate of effect is uncertain.	Strong recommendation, and applies to most patients. Some of the evidence base supporting the recommendation is, however, of low quality.

TABLE 7-11 UpToDate Grading System for Clinical Practice Recommendations *(continued)*

Grade of Recommendation	Clarity of Risk/Benefit	Quality of Supporting Evidence	Implications
2A Weak recommendation, high-quality evidence	Benefits closely balanced with risks and burdens	Consistent evidence from well-performed randomized, controlled trials or overwhelming evidence of some other form. Further research is unlikely to change our confidence in the estimate of benefit and risk.	Weak recommendation, best action may differ depending on circumstances or patients or societal values.
2B Weak recommendation, moderate-quality evidence	Benefits closely balanced with risks and burdens, some uncertainty in the estimates of benefits, risks, and burdens.	Evidence from randomized, controlled trials with important limitations (inconsistent results, methodologic flaws, indirect or imprecise), or very strong evidence of some other research design. Further research (if performed) is likely to have an impact on our confidence in the estimate of benefit and risk and may change the estimate.	Weak recommendation, alternative approaches likely to be better for some patients under some circumstances.
2C Weak recommendation, low-quality evidence	Uncertainty in the estimates of benefits, risks, and burdens; benefits may be closely balanced with risks and burdens.	Evidence from observational studies, unsystematic clinical experience, or from randomized, controlled trials with serious flaws. Any estimate of effect is uncertain.	Very weak recommendation; other alternatives may be equally reasonable.

Reproduced with permission from UpToDate and GRADE. Grading Guide. In: UpToDate and GRADE. (2013). Grading guide. In UpToDate, D.S. Basow (Ed). UpToDate, Waltham, MA, 02013. For more information visit www.uptodate.com and http://www.gradeworkinggroup.org.

TABLE 7-12 Comparison of Research, EBP, QI, and Program Evaluation Characteristics

	Research	EBP	QI	Program Evaluation
Definition	Prescribed, methodical, meticulous technique of investigation	A problem-solving process that integrates existing evidence (research, QI), nursing expertise and patient preferences to guide care decisions	Appraise the efficiency of clinical interventions and provide guidance for achieving quality outcomes, productivity, cost containment	Evaluate a specific program using a well-defined conceptual framework to judge success or failure
Prompted by	Gap in knowledge	New evidence from research	Process breakdown or system failure	Ineffectiveness, inefficiency, new guidelines
Purpose	Generate new knowledge	Integrate best evidence, clinician's expertise, and patient values and preferences to improve health outcomes	Improve system and process of healthcare delivery; real-life experience and data on application of best practices	Provide timely information/data for decision making for particular programs
The Questions	What is the best thing to do?	Are we doing the best thing?	Are we doing the best thing right, all of the time?	Is the thing we are doing successful?
IRB approval	Yes, unless analysis of public data	No, but health systems may require a review to protect their data	No, but health systems may require a review to protect their data	No, but health systems may require a review to protect their data
Sample	Subset of population	Patient population	Unit, service line, institution wide or health system	Specific programs
Method	Quantitative or qualitative	Level of evidence matches question asked; assess strength and quality of evidence; make recommendations based on evidence; translate evidence into practice using translation strategies	PDSA Lean Thinking Six Sigma Structure, process, outcome	Quantitative or qualitative

TABLE 7-12 Comparison of Research, EBP, QI, and Program Evaluation Characteristics *(continued)*

	Research	EBP	QI	Program Evaluation
Rigor/ Control	Maximum rigor/ control	More rigor than QI but not as rigorous as research	Least rigorous	Can be as rigorous as research
Data collection	Follow specific procedures and don't deviate	Research and non-research evidence sources and critically appraise evidence	Pre-data and evaluation, data can come from patient record or surveys	Formative and summative evaluation
Results	Generalizable to population	Recommendation for practice change, clinical research study, or no change	Applicable to the patients studied	Direct, persuasive, or conceptual utilization
Dissemination	Presentation or publish	Presentation or publish	Presentation or publish	Presentation or publication
Example	Emergency department weekend presentation and mortality in patients with acute myocardial infarction (de Cordova, Johansen, Martinez, & Cimiotti, 2017)	Alternate light sources in sexual assault examinations: An evidence-based practice project (Eldredge, Huggins, & Pugh, 2012)	Large-scale implementation of the I-PASS handover system at an academic medical centre (Shahian, McEachern, Rossi, Chisari, & Mort, 2017)	Using the program logic model to evaluate ¡cuídate!: A sexual health program for Latino adolescents in a school-based health center (Serowoky, George, & Yarandi, 2015)

Wexler, Bowen, & Schneider, 2013). Existing evidence suggests that SDM benefits patients of all ages and educational levels (Wexler et al., 2015).

Both patient-centered care and evidence-based practices are foundational to the SDM process between providers and patients. Although SDM is the preferred model for engaging patients in the process of decisions about care when more than one reasonable option is available, no option has a clear advantage, or the options have benefits and harms that the patient may value differently (Stacey et al., 2014; Stiggelbout, Pieterse, & De Haes, 2015), use of this model in practice by clinicians is lacking (Couët et al., 2015; Légaré et al., 2008).

The SHARE Approach is a model for SDM developed by AHRQ (AHRQ, 2016). It is a five-step process that includes exploration and comparison of the benefits, harms, and risks of care options using meaningful provider–patient dialogue. Step 1 is seeking the patient's participation. Step 2 is helping the patient explore and compare treatment options. Step 3 is assessing the patient's values and preferences. Step 4 involves reaching a decision with your patient. Step 5 is to evaluate the patient's decision. In situations where the patient cannot make decisions the family may participant in each step.

Decision aids (DA) are effective tools to facilitate the SDM discourse between the patient and the provider (Stacey & Légaré, 2015). These tools can be used to prepare the patient to make informed, value-based decisions with their provider. High-quality evidence exists that DA improve patients' knowledge of options and facilitate informed, clear decisions based on preferences (Stacey & Légaré, 2015). Moderate quality evidence suggests that patients participate more in decision making when using DA. Despite the availability of hundreds of free DA through AHRQ and the Ottawa Hospital Research Institute (OHRI), translation of these tools into practice is slow. NPs must be the leaders in implementing SDM and DA in the practice setting as part of the EBP process.

Barriers to EBP

If EBP is as much about removing harmful or ineffective practices as it is about implementing robust evidence into practice (Vincent et al., 2015) and it is unethical to practice using evidence-less care (Jones, 2010), why do barriers to EBP continue to exist? Houser and Oman (2010) identified three categories associated with barriers to using evidence in clinical practice that continue to be relevant today (Warren et al., 2016). The first category includes limitations in EBP systems caused by an overwhelming amount of evidence and sometimes contradictory findings in the research. The second category is human factors that create barriers. These factors include lack of knowledge about EBP and skills needed to conduct EBP, nurses' negative attitudes toward research and evidence-based care, nurses' perception that research is only for medicine and is a cookbook approach, and patient expectations. The last category identifies the lack of organizational systems or infrastructure to support clinicians using EBP. Causes for barriers in this category include lack of authority for clinicians to make changes in practice, peer emphasis on practicing the way they always have practiced, lack of time during the workday, lack of administrative support or incentives, and conflicting priorities between unit work and research.

The barriers described above may seem overwhelming; however, all healthcare-related disciplines are becoming evidence based, and professional organizations, accrediting bodies, insurers, and third-party payers are requiring nurses to use evidence to support clinical practices and decision making. Therefore, organizations need to address these barriers and put systems in place to support EBP (Warren et al., 2016). Moreover, NP with Doctor of Nursing Practice degrees must be EBP leaders who mentor others and promote the EBP process as the foundation upon which practice is built.

Chapter Summary Points

Evidence-based nursing practice is the conscientious, explicit, and judicious use of theory-derived, research-based information in making decisions about care delivery to individuals or groups of patients and considers individual needs and preferences. It is vital to a practice-based profession like nursing to use the best current evidence from many sources when making clinical decisions. EBP competencies have been described for the NP and should be part of performance evaluation criteria.

There are several steps in the EBP process beginning with fostering a spirit of inquiry, asking the right clinical question in a PICOT format, finding the best current evidence, critically appraising the evidence, and integrating the synthesis of evidence with patient values and preferences.

Best current research evidence can be found in many web-based electronic databases, such as the Cochrane Database of Systematic Reviews. There are databases for clinical practice guidelines such as the National Guidelines Clearinghouse. There are quantitative, qualitative, and non-research tools specific to study design or evidence type to assist clinicians with rapid systematic appraisal of evidence.

Strength of the evidence is determined by synthesizing the information on the level of evidence (hierarchy of evidence) and quality of evidence (critical appraisal tool). An evidence summary table provides a succinct, stand-alone account of the important study/article details and the critical appraisal results. An evidence synthesis table incorporates data from the evidence summary table to make recommendations that are based on the strength of the evidence.

Existing EBP models can be used to implement and sustain a culture of EBP. These models may aid with translation of evidence into practice. Outcomes of EBP can take the form of NP collaborating on original research, QI studies, or program evaluation.

Shared decision making and the AHRQ SHARE Approach can be used by NPs to facilitate the incorporation of patient values, preferences, and goals when making care decisions. Existing decision aids for many health conditions or treatments are available for free. NP should be leaders in adopting this practice.

Health systems continue to face the same barriers to implementing and sustaining EBP. NPs need to take an active role in breaking down these barriers, being EBP mentors, and promoting the EBP process as the foundation from which all practice is built.

Seminar Discussion Questions

1. Explain the steps of the EBP process.
2. Write a clinical question in PICOT format for each template type for common practice problems encountered by NPs. Swap answers with a peer and provide feedback.
3. Sign up for clinical practice alerts from the TRIP database in your specialty area.

4. Think about a patient problem you have had in the clinical setting and answer the following:
   a. What formal structures were in place to help you address the problem?
   b. How did you use evidence to investigate the problem?
   c. Did you have time to search for evidence? If no, what were the barriers?
   d. What databases did you access for evidence and why?
   e. Did you use a health sciences librarian to help with your search? Explain why or why not.
5. Go to http://www.guideline.gov and search for chronic pain management clinical practice guidelines. Compare and contrast two guidelines.
6. Find a clinical practice guideline from National Guideline Clearinghouse. Use the AGREE II Plus software to critically appraise the guideline with two or more peers.
7. Find a recent randomized control trial on a topic of interest. Critically appraise the study using a tool from this chapter. Using an evidence hierarchy from this chapter identify the level of evidence. Enter the relevant data into an evidence summary table. Rate the quality of evidence using the JHNEBP quality rating. Summarize clinical significance using NNT and effective size.
8. Using the databases described in this chapter find two or more of the following evidence types (research study, QI study, EBP project, or program evaluation). Describe the search process used. After reading the articles, compare and contrast the different methodologies. Did the authors provide support for the selected methodology? Give examples to support your answer.
9. Identify areas where SDM can be used in your practice. Go to https://decisionaid.ohri.ca/ and browse the decision aids by topic. Select a decision aid and write a plan for how it can be incorporated into your practice setting.

References

AACN Position Statement on the Practice Doctorate in Nursing. (2004). Retrieved from http://www.aacn.nche.edu/publications/position/DNPpositionstatement.pdf

AHRQ. (2016). *The SHARE approach: A model for shared decision making.* Retrieved from https://www.ahrq.gov/sites/default/files/publications/files/share-approach_factsheet.pdf

Armola, R. R., Bourgault, A. M., Halm, M. A., Board, R. M., Bucher, L., Harrington, L., . . . Medina, J. (2009). AACN levels of evidence: What's new? *Critical Care Nurse, 29*(4), 70–73. Retrieved from https://doi.org/10.4037/ccn2009969

Brouwers, M. C., Kho, M. E., Browman, G. P., Burgers, J. S., Cluzeau, F., Feder, G., . . . Littlejohns, P. (2010). AGREE II: Advancing guideline development, reporting and evaluation in health care. *Canadian Medical Association Journal, 182*(18), E839–E842. doi:10.1503/cmaj.090449

Charles, C., Gafni, A., & Whelan, T. (1997). Shared decision-making in the medical encounter: What does it mean? (or it takes at least two to tango). *Social Science & Medicine, 44*(5), 681–692. Retrieved from http://www.ncbi.nlm.nih.gov/pubmed/9032835

Couët, N., Desroches, S., Robitaille, H., Vaillancourt, H., Leblanc, A., Turcotte, S., . . . Légaré, F. (2015). Assessments of the extent to which health-care providers involve patients in decision making: A systematic review of studies using the OPTION instrument. *Health Expectations, 18*(4), 542–561. Retrieved from https://doi.org/10.1111/hex.12054

de Cordova, P. B., Johansen, M. L., Martinez, M. E., & Cimiotti, J. P. (2017). Emergency department weekend presentation and mortality in patients with acute myocardial infarction. *Nursing Research, 66*(1), 20–27. Retrieved from https://doi.org/10.1097/NNR.0000000000000196

Dearholt, S., & Dang, D. (2012). *Johns Hopkins nursing evidence-based practice: Models and guidelines.* Sigma Theta Tau.

DiCenso, A., Cullum, N., & Ciliska, D. (1998). Implementing evidence-based nursing: Some misconceptions. *Evidence Based Nursing, 1*(2), 38–39.

Eldredge, K., Huggins, E., & Pugh, L. C. (2012). Alternate light sources in sexual assault examinations: An evidence-based practice project. *Journal of Forensic Nursing, 8*(1), 39–44. Retrieved from https://doi.org/10.1111/j.1939-3938.2011.01128.x

Evidence-Based Medicine Working Group. (1992). Evidence-based medicine. A new approach to teaching the practice of medicine. *JAMA, 268*(17), 2420–2425.

Facchiano, L., & Snyder, C. H. (2012a). Evidence-based practice for the busy nurse practitioner: Part one: Relevance to clinical practice and clinical inquiry process. *Journal of the American Academy of Nurse Practitioners, 24*(10), 579–586. Retrieved from https://doi.org/10.1111/j.1745-7599.2012.00748.x

Facchiano, L., & Snyder, C. H. (2012b). Evidence-based practice for the busy nurse practitioner: Part two: Searching for the best evidence to clinical inquiries. *Journal of the American Academy of Nurse Practitioners, 24*(11), 640–648. Retrieved from https://doi.org/10.1111/j.1745-7599.2012.00749.x

Facchiano, L., & Snyder, C. H. (2013). Evidence-based practice for the busy nurse practitioner: Part four: Putting it all together. *Journal of the American Academy of Nurse Practitioners, 25*(1), 24–31. Retrieved from https://doi.org/10.1111/j.1745-7599.2012.00751.x

Fain, J. (2014). *Reading, understanding, and applying nursing research* (4th ed.). Philadelphia, PA: F.A. Davis.

Friedberg, M. W., Van Busum, K., Wexler, R., Bowen, M., & Schneider, E. C. (2013). A demonstration of shared decision making in primary care highlights barriers to adoption and potential remedies. *Health Affairs, 32*(2), 268–275. Retrieved from https://doi.org/10.1377/hlthaff.2012.1084

Gawlinski, A., & Rutledge, D. (2008). Selecting a model for evidence-based practice changes: A practical approach. *AACN Advanced Critical Care, 19*(3), 291–300. Retrieved from https://doi.org/10.1097/01.AACN.0000330380.41766.63

Guyatt, G. H., Haynes, R. B., Jaeschke, R. Z., Cook, D. J., Green, L., Naylor, C. D., . . . Richardson, W. S. (2000). Users' guides to the medical literature: XXV. Evidence-based medicine: principles for applying the users' guides to patient care. Evidence-Based Medicine Working Group. *JAMA, 284*(10), 1290–1296.

Guyatt, G. H., Oxman, A. D., Vist, G. E., Kunz, R., Falck-Ytter, Y., Alonso-Coello, P., . . . GRADE Working Group. (2008). GRADE: An emerging consensus on rating quality of evidence and strength of recommendations. *BMJ* (Clinical Research Ed.), *336*(7650), 924–926. Retrieved from https://doi.org/10.1136/bmj.39489.470347.AD

Hopp, L., & Rittenmeyer, L. (2012). *Introduction to evidence-based practice: A practical guide for nursing.* Philadelphia, PA: F.A. Davis.

Houser, J., & Oman, K. (2010). *Evidence-based practice: An implementation guide for healthcare organizations.* Burlington, MA: Jones & Bartlett.

Ingersoll, G. L. (2000). Evidence-based nursing: What it is and what it isn't. *Nursing Outlook, 48*(4), 151–152. Retrieved from https://doi.org/10.1067/mno.2000.107690

Jones, K. R. (2010). Rating the level, quality, and strength of the research evidence. *Journal of Nursing Care Quality, 25*(4), 304–312.

Jordan, Z., Donnelly, P., & Piper, R. (2006). *A short history of a BIG idea: The Joanna Briggs Institute 1996-2006.* Retrieved from https://hekyll.services.adelaide.edu.au/dspace/handle/2440/35988

Jordan, Z., Munn, Z., Aromataris, E., & Lockwood, C. (2015). Now that we're here, where are we? The JBI approach to evidence-based healthcare 20 years on. *International Journal of Evidence-Based Healthcare, 13*(3), 117–120. Retrieved from https://doi.org/10.1097/XEB.0000000000000053

Kitson, A., Harvey, G., & McCormack, B. (1998). Enabling the implementation of evidence based practice: A conceptual framework. *Quality in Health Care, 7*(3), 149–158.

Leeman, J., & Sandelowski, M. (2012). Practice-based evidence and qualitative inquiry. *Journal of Nursing Scholarship: An Official Publication of Sigma Theta Tau International Honor Society of Nursing, 44*(2), 171–179. Retrieved from https://doi.org/10.1111/j.1547-5069.2012.01449.x

Légaré, F., Elwyn, G., Fishbein, M., Frémont, P., Frosch, D., Gagnon, M.-P., . . . van der Weijden, T. (2008). Translating shared decision-making into health care clinical practices: Proof of concepts. *Implementation Science: IS, 3*, 2. Retrieved from https://doi.org/10.1186/1748-5908-3-2

Makoul, G., & Clayman, M. L. (2006). An integrative model of shared decision making in medical encounters. *Patient Education and Counseling, 60*(3), 301–312. Retrieved from https://doi.org/10.1016/j.pec.2005.06.010

Manchikanti, L., Abdi, S., & Lucas, L. F. (2005). Evidence synthesis and development of guidelines in interventional pain management. *Pain Physician, 8*(1), 73–86.

Melnyk, B. M. (2014). Building cultures and environments that facilitate clinician behavior change to evidence-based practice: What works? *Worldviews on Evidence-Based Nursing, 11*(2), 79–80. Retrieved from https://doi.org/10.1111/wvn.12032

Melnyk, B. M. (2016a). An urgent call to action for nurse leaders to establish sustainable evidence-based practice cultures and implement evidence-based interventions to improve healthcare quality. *Worldviews on Evidence-Based Nursing, 13*(1), 3–5. Retrieved from https://doi.org/10.1111/wvn.12150

Melnyk, B. M. (2016b). The doctor of nursing practice degree = evidence-based practice expert. *Worldviews on Evidence-Based Nursing, 13*(3), 183–184. Retrieved from https://doi.org/10.1111/wvn.12164

Melnyk, B. M., & Fineout-Overholt, E. (2014). *Evidence-based practice in nursing & healthcare* (3rd ed.). New York, NY: Lippincott Williams & Wilkins.

Melnyk, B. M., Gallagher-Ford, L., Long, L. E., & Fineout-Overholt, E. (2014). The establishment of evidence-based practice competencies for practicing registered nurses and advanced practice nurses in real-world clinical settings: Proficiencies to improve healthcare quality, reliability, patient cutcomes, and costs. *Worldviews on Evidence-Based Nursing, 11*(1), 5–15. Retrieved from https://doi.org/10.1111/wvn.12021

Newhouse, R. P., Dearholt, S., Poe, S., Pugh, L. C., & White, K. M. (2007). Organizational change strategies for evidence-based practice. *Journal of Nursing Administration, 37*(12), 552–557. Retrieved from https://doi.org/10.1097/01.NNA.0000302384.91366.8f

Newhouse R. P., & Spring B. (2010). Interdisciplinary evidence-based practice: Moving from silos to synergy. *Nursing Outlook, 58*(6), 309–317.

Our vision, mission, and principles | Cochrane. (n.d.). Retrieved from http://www.cochrane.org/about-us/our-vision-mission-and-principles

Overview | CTEP. (n.d.). Retrieved from https://ctep-ebp.com/about-overview

Perrier, L., Farrell, A., Ayala, A. P., Lightfoot, D., Kenny, T., Aaronson, E., . . . Weiss, A. (2014). Effects of librarian-provided services in healthcare settings: A systematic review. *Journal of the American Medical Informatics Association: JAMIA, 21*(6), 1118–1124. Retrieved from https://doi.org/10.1136/amiajnl-2014-002825

Ragan, P., & Quincy, B. (2012). Evidence-based medicine: Its roots and its fruits. *Journal of Physician Assistant Education: The Official Journal of the Physician Assistant Education Association, 23*(1), 35–38.

Rosswurm, M. A., & Larrabee, J. H. (1999). A model for change to evidence-based practice. *Sigma Theta Tau International, 31*(4), 317–322.

Rycroft-Malone, J., Seers, K., Titchen, A., Harvey, G., Kitson, A., & McCormack, B. (2004). What counts as evidence in evidence-based practice? *Journal of Advanced Nursing, 47*(1), 81–90. Retrieved from https://doi.org/10.1111/j.1365-2648.2004.03068.x

Sackett, D. L., Rosenberg, W. M., Gray, J. A., Haynes, R. B., & Richardson, W. S. (1996). Evidence based medicine: What it is and what it isn't. *BMJ* (Clinical Research Ed.), *312*(7023), 71–72.

Serowoky, M. L., George, N., & Yarandi, H. (2015). Using the program logic model to evaluate ¡cuídate!: A sexual health program for Latino adolescents in a school-based health center. *Worldviews on Evidence-Based Nursing, 12*(5), 297–305. Retrieved from https://doi.org/10.1111/wvn.12110

Shahian, D. M., McEachern, K., Rossi, L., Chisari, R. G., & Mort, E. (2017). Large-scale implementation of the I-PASS handover system at an academic medical centre. *BMJ Quality & Safety*, bmjqs-2016-006195. Retrieved from https://doi.org/10.1136/bmjqs-2016-006195

Stacey, D., & Légaré, F. (2015). Engaging patients using an interprofessional approach to shared decision making. *Canadian Oncology Nursing Journal = Revue Canadienne de Nursing Oncologique, 25*(4), 455–469.

Stacey, D., Légaré, F., Col, N. F., Bennett, C. L., Barry, M. J., Eden, K. B., . . . Wu, J. H. C. (2014). Decision aids for people facing health treatment or screening decisions. *The Cochrane Database of Systematic Reviews, 1*, CD001431. Retrieved from https://doi.org/10.1002/14651858.CD001431.pub4

Stevens, K. R. (2004). *ACE star model of EBP: Knowledge transformation*. San Antonio, TX: Academic Center for Evidence-Based Practice. Retrieved from http://www.acestar.uthscsa.edu

Stiggelbout, A. M., Pieterse, A. H., & De Haes, J. C. J. M. (2015). Shared decision making: Concepts, evidence, and practice. *Patient Education and Counseling, 98*(10), 1172–1179. Retrieved from https://doi.org/10.1016/j.pec.2015.06.022

Titler, M. G., Kleiber, C., Steelman, V. J., Rakel, B. A., Budreau, G., Everett L. Q., . . . Goode, C. J. (2001). The Iowa model of evidence-based practice to promote quality care. *Critical Care Nursing Clinics North America, 13*, 497–509.

UptoDate (2013). Grading Guide. Retrieved from: https://www.uptodate.com/home/grading-guide

Vincent, D., Hastings-Tolsma, M., Gephart, S., & Alfonzo, P. M. (2015). Nurse practitioner clinical decision-making and evidence-based practice. *Nurse Practitioner, 40*(5), 47–54. Retrieved from https://doi.org/10.1097/01.NPR.0000463783.42721.ef

Vratny, A., & Shriver, D. (2007). A conceptual mode for growing evidence-based practice. *Nursing Administration Quarterly, 31*(2), 162–170.

Warren, J. I., McLaughlin, M., Bardsley, J., Eich, J., Esche, C. A., Kropkowski, L., & Risch, S. (2016). The strengths and challenges of implementing EBP in healthcare systems. *Worldviews on Evidence-Based Nursing, 13*(1), 15–24. Retrieved from https://doi.org/10.1111/wvn.12149

Wexler, R., Gerstein, B. S., Brackett, C., Fagnan, L. J., Fairfield, K. M., Frosch, D. L., . . . Fowler, F. J. (2015). Decision aids in the United States: The patient response. *International Journal of Person Centered Medicine, 5*(3).

CHAPTER 8

Clinical Prevention/ Community and Population Health

Julie G. Stewart

For almost 50 years, nurse practitioners have been providing primary care to a large variety of patient populations. Traditionally, nurses have been the backbone of health prevention and health promotion (Sullivan-Marx, McGivern, Fairman, & Greenberg, 2010). Lillian Wald coined the term *public health nursing* in 1893 and stated that the focus of public health nursing was the prevention of disease. Indeed, nurses have done an excellent job of initiating and managing nurse-managed health centers (NMHCs), providing health care to the multitudes of underserved and vulnerable populations in the United States. Nurses have also been contributing to the providing of health care to populations in need across the globe (Sullivan-Marx et al., 2010). A recent report from the Institute of Medicine (IOM) emphasized finding ways to link primary care and public health to improve population health (IOM, 2012). Nurse practitioners are in the perfect position to take advantage of this mandate. NPs learn about the intersection of social determinants of health, and the need to do thorough physical, psychosocial, and lifestyle assessments to incorporate appropriate prevention strategies, screenings, immunizations, and lifestyle changes. Cawley (2012) suggests that future curricular offerings include more depth in the areas of health education, nutrition, and culturally sensitive outreach services. Healthcare providers in community health centers, as well as public health departments and services, need to know how to perform data analysis and apply it to the principles of population health.

▸ Clinical Prevention and Population Health

In most DNP programs there are specific courses that focus solely on these important topics in response to DNP essential VII: clinical prevention and population health for improving the nation's health.

> *Clinical prevention* is defined as health promotion and risk reduction/illness prevention for individuals and families. *Population health* is defined to include aggregate, community, environmental/occupational, and cultural/socioeconomic dimensions of health. Aggregates are groups of individuals defined by a shared characteristic such as gender, diagnosis, or age. These framing definitions are endorsed by representatives of multiple disciplines including nursing. (AACN, 2006, p. 15)

Courses typically introduce students to methods used by epidemiologists to assess factors associated with the distribution and determinants of health and disease in populations and to read, interpret, and apply literature using epidemiological and statistical methods. Understanding the historical background as well as the practical applications of epidemiology, methods for identifying and evaluating sources of health information, calculation of key epidemiological measures and investigation techniques, and an evaluation of the strengths and weaknesses of different study designs are key elements for NPs. Current concepts of public health, health promotion, evidence-based recommendations, determinants of health, environmental and occupational health, and cultural diversity and sensitivity are interrelated concepts that provide the foundation for "nurse practitionering" in a local to global worldview. Specifics should be included for examining methods for describing disease rates and other vital statistics; cohort, case control, and cross-sectional studies; odds ratios, relative risks, their confidence intervals, and tests of significance; and concepts of confounding, effect modification, and bias.

Epidemiology is derived from the Greek words *epi*, meaning "on"; *demos*, meaning "the people"; and *logos*, "the study of." According to the World Health Organization (WHO, 2012), "epidemiology is the study of the distribution and determinants of health-related states or events (including disease), and the application of this study to the control of diseases and other health problems." From the memorable work of Jenner in developing the smallpox vaccination in 1798, to the landmark work of Snow uncovering the transmission of cholera in the Soho area of London in 1854, the world of epidemiology is fascinating. In the 19th century, it was believed that the cause of most illnesses was related to infectious diseases. Today, we have insight into the myriad of factors that contribute to illness and disease—which include infectious agents, elements within the environment, our nutrition, and effects from trauma—and surveillance and research continue to uncover emerging factors.

One example of a disease that has plagued public health and direct healthcare providers for hundreds of years is tuberculosis. Today, despite medications to treat and cure tuberculosis, it is a disease that causes approximately 1 million deaths per year worldwide (Keshavjee & Farmer, 2012). Experts in the topic attribute the inability to contain this epidemic to numerous factors, including the fact that the associated social determinants are most often "extreme poverty, severe malnutrition, and overcrowded living conditions" (p. 932). The countries who continue to suffer most from tuberculosis are the countries where incomes are low. Despite multifaceted efforts by global agencies such as the World Bank and the WHO to control tuberculosis, we now face multidrug-resistant strains of tuberculosis that have been fueled by HIV and inadequate funding to properly treat tuberculosis. Succinctly summarized, Keshavjee and Farmer (2012) stated,

> The contours of global efforts against tuberculosis have always been mediated by both biologic and social determinants, and the reasons for the divergence in the rates of tuberculosis and drug resistance between rich and poor countries are biosocial. (p. 934)

Efforts to curtail the AIDS epidemic are worthwhile and have made substantial impact; healthcare practitioners must work on similar concentrated, multifaceted efforts to curtail tuberculosis. As NPs, we need to stay informed regarding global and national trends in all diseases; be on the lookout for patients with any forms of infectious diseases; appropriately assess, treat, and report patients who need treatment; and with our ability to develop trusted patient–NP relationships, see our patients finish appropriate treatment regimens and reduce infectivity within our own communities.

Terminology in Epidemiology

Understanding terminology in the domain of public health and research is important for the NP. Common demographic and social data include age and gender distribution, socioeconomic status, family structure (marital, single parent, etc.), as well as racial, ethnic, and religious composition. Variables that describe the community infrastructure include availability of social and health services (hospitals, ER), the quality of housing (lead, asbestos), social stability, safety and community policing, and employment opportunities. Examples of health-related outcomes that are commonly monitored are interpersonal violence (including homicide and suicide rates), infant mortality rate, mortality from selected conditions, prevalence of chronic and infectious diseases, alcohol and substance abuse rates, teenage pregnancy rates, the occurrence of sexually transmitted diseases (STDs), and the birth rate. Important variables related to the environment include air pollution from stationary and mobile sources, access to parks and recreation, availability of clean water, availability of markets that supply healthy groceries, number of liquor stores and fast-food restaurants, nutritional quality of foods and beverages at school, and radon and lead levels in the soil. The importance of health statistics has been demonstrated by such projects as the Framingham Heart Study, community intervention trials of fluoride supplementation in water, the surgeon general's report on smoking and health, and a study that 238,000 of us participated in—the Nurses' Health Study. Although the main focus of the Nurses' Health Study (2012) has been on cancer prevention, much of the data collected has shown the effects that diet, exercise, and lifestyle have on maintaining health and disease prevention.

Morbidity and *mortality* should be familiar terms. As a quick reminder, morbidity rates indicate how fast a disease is occurring in a population, the proportion is what fraction of the population is affected by the disease, and the incidence rate is the number of new cases of the disease in a specific time period (Fos, 2011). **BOX 8-1** provides a mathematical method to calculate an incidence rate per 1,000 people.

Understanding illness and disease requires the NP to be aware first of the natural history of disease and the *epidemiological triangle*. When considering the course of

BOX 8-1 Incidence Rate per 1,000

$$\frac{\text{\# of new cases of a disease occuring in the population during a specific time period}}{\text{\# of persons who are at risk of developing the disease during that time period}} \times 1{,}000$$

Mortality rates can be used for the overall population or be cause or age specific. Typically, mortality rates are going to increase as age increases, unless reviewing suicide and homicide rates (Fos, 2011). For example, to calculate a mortality (death) rate, one would use the following:

$$\frac{\text{\# of deaths in the population during a specified time period}}{\text{\# of persons in the population during the specified time period}}$$

infectious diseases, this triad posits that infections result from the interaction of agent, host, and environment. Transmission occurs when the agent leaves its reservoir or host through a portal of exit, is conveyed by some mode of transmission, and enters through an appropriate portal of entry to infect a susceptible host (Centers for Disease Control, 2012). **FIGURE 8-1** is a graphic depiction of the chain of infection.

Using an example to apply to this triad approach, we can consider the agent anthrax as a single-celled bacillus bacterium called *Bacillus anthracis*. The bacterium most often causes illness in host animals such as cows and sheep; however, it can infect humans. Transmission most commonly occurs through the skin, when spores get into the body via a scrape, but spores can also be inhaled or ingested by eating tainted meat. Anthrax has been used as a biological weapon, but typically those most at risk are veterinarians and farm, wool, and tannery workers.

Other important terms are *epidemic*, *pandemic*, and *endemic*. An epidemic is when there is an outbreak that is limited in time and locations. An example of an epidemic is when in 2003, the severe acute respiratory syndrome (SARS) epidemic took the lives of nearly 800 people worldwide. A *pandemic* is an epidemic extending to an entire country or a large part of the world. HIV/AIDS is an example of a global pandemic disease. Multiple times we have experienced influenza pandemics: Spanish influenza killed 40–50 million people in 1918, the Asian influenza killed 2 million people in 1957, and the Hong Kong influenza killed 1 million people in 1968. Current epidemics, such as Zika virus and Ebola virus, have the potential to become pandemic if efforts to curtail the diseases are ineffective. A disease is said to be endemic if it remains present in an area for a long period of time. For example, malaria is endemic in tropical climates, and hepatitis B (HBV) is endemic in China and many Asian countries. Vietnam is hyperendemic for HBV, meaning it is found in excessively high rates within a host population.

The natural history of a disease refers to the progression of that disease if there were no intervention or treatment to alter the disease process. For instance, from researching history, and unfortunately from data obtained through the Tuskegee study, much information has been obtained about the natural history of an infectious disease that has likely been around for over a thousand years—syphilis. According to the National Center for HIV/AIDS, Viral Hepatitis, STD, and TB Prevention (2011), "In 1932 the Public Health Service, working with the Tuskegee Institute, began a study

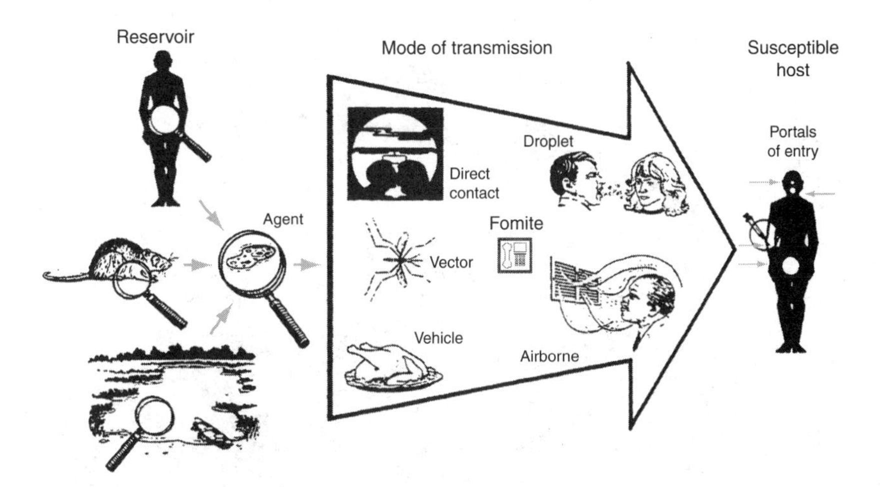

FIGURE 8-1 Chain of Infection

Reproduced from CDC. (1992). *Principles of epidemiology* (2nd ed.). Atlanta, GA: Author.

to record the natural history of syphilis in hopes of justifying treatment programs for blacks" (para. 1). The tragedy of following the natural history of syphilis in this case included many facets: misleading the participants about the real purpose of the study, not offering treatment when it became available, nor offering the option to stop being a participant in the study. Today we know that syphilis is easily cured in its early stages, and treatment can be given in the secondary and tertiary stages.

The natural history of HIV infection includes various stages, as shown in **FIGURE 8-2**.

Acquisition of the virus is through a portal for transmission, which includes ingesting infected breastmilk, blood exposure (e.g., by sharing infected needles), or exposure to HIV-infected seminal or vaginal fluids during unprotected sex. HIV may also be perinatally transmitted in utero or during the birth process.

The course of the primary infection begins with an acute retroviral syndrome that occurs early in the new HIV infection. Approximately 50%–70% of infected people will experience an influenza-like illness with fever, rash, pharyngitis, lymphadenopathy, and myalgia. About 3 to 6 weeks after acquiring an HIV infection, the CD4 cell count in the peripheral blood drops dramatically as the virus replicates rapidly and is widely disseminated throughout the body, where it is predominantly trapped in lymph nodes. During this time, which can last from 2–3 months, the amount of virus in the serum (viral load) is very high and can be detected by measuring viral copies in the serum; however, the HIV antibody test may be negative at this time.

The seroconversion period is the time it takes an infected person's body to make antibodies to HIV. This can take 3 months (more common) to 6 months (less common) after infection.

The asymptomatic period of HIV infection can last from a few months to many years (up to 15 years). This varies from person to person, and it is usually associated with the level of HIV viral load; typically, those with higher viral loads deteriorate faster than those with lower viral loads. During this time, the CD4 cells typically decline at an average rate of approximately 50 cells/μL/year. Over time the body cannot keep up, and as CD4 cells decline, opportunistic infections and diseases will cause symptoms.

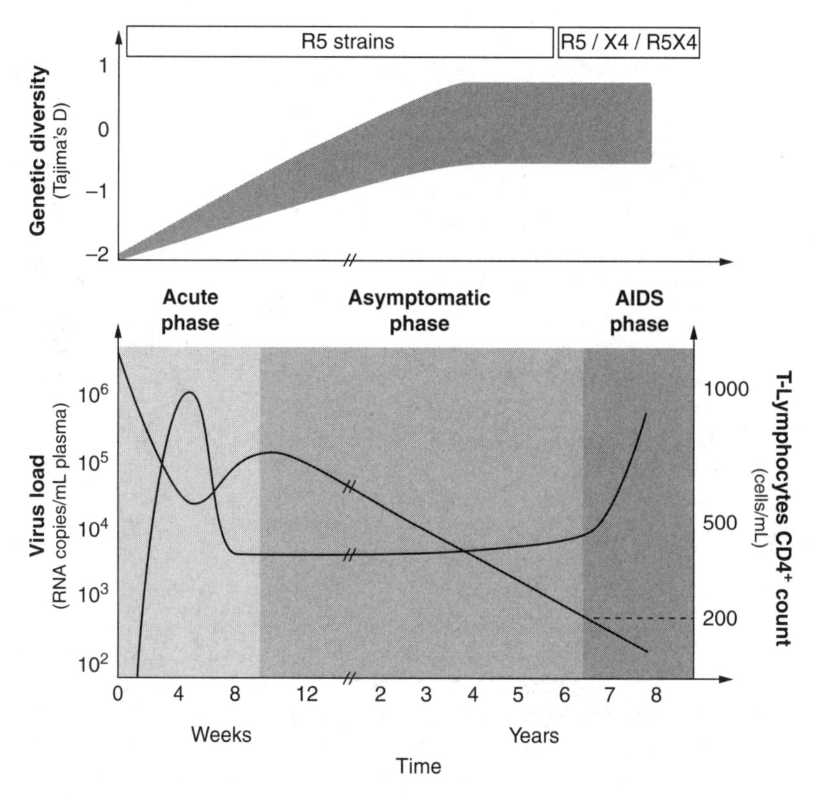

FIGURE 8-2 Typical Course of HIV Infection

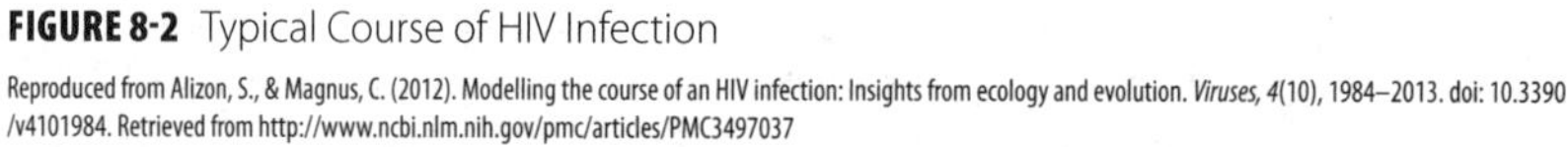
Reproduced from Alizon, S., & Magnus, C. (2012). Modelling the course of an HIV infection: Insights from ecology and evolution. *Viruses, 4*(10), 1984–2013. doi: 10.3390/v4101984. Retrieved from http://www.ncbi.nlm.nih.gov/pmc/articles/PMC3497037

If left untreated, the HIV infection develops into AIDS. The rapid replication of HIV eventually depletes the immune system in most people to such an extent that the patient loses critical body defenses and succumbs to infections, cancers, and ultimately death.

Population Health

Most, if not all, textbooks describing population health ascribe public health professionals with expertise in epidemiology and biostatistics to that larger domain. The health of an individual is then posited to be the focus of the clinician. However, the NP, and in particular the NP/DNP, is charged with being educated on the health of communities, and indeed, even reaching to make a difference in global health initiatives.

What constitutes a population? A population consists of a group of people who have some common characteristics (Fos, 2011; Friis & Sellers, 2004). It can be large (an entire nation) or small (a neighborhood). Characteristics are not solely related to physical boundaries of where one may reside (Fries & Stewart, 2012). A community may include members who share interpersonal and intrapersonal connections, known as a *phenomenological community* (Maurer & Smith, 2009). The types of characteristics held in common for a population subset or community can include age, gender, health behaviors, exposure to a virus, among others.

The concept of vulnerability as it relates to healthy and unhealthy communities must be noted. Promoting healthy communities as part of population-based nursing curricula is emphasized in the book *Caring for the Vulnerable: Perspectives in Nursing Theory, Practice, and Research, Third Edition* (de Chesnay & Anderson, 2016). One method for identifying an unhealthy community is by determining the lack of support for vulnerable populations that exists within the community. Including all members of the community in addressing poverty and providing adequate housing, healthy food, job opportunities, and proper air, water, and sanitation for all of its community members is vital to the health and development of resilience of the population. One method to build a healthy community is to focus on the strengths within the community and its vulnerable populations. This is quite different than the typical approach, which is to first seek to find and identify problems within a community.

Nurse practitioners provide health care to certain populations as part of their professional practice site. Therefore, it is imperative that the NP remain current in what issues are contributing to health issues and be actively engaged in health promotion and disease prevention efforts. Having a concrete knowledge base from which to intertwine concepts of epidemiology with clinical prevention and population health is vital to be a successful NP or DNP.

Prevention Levels

There exist three levels of prevention: (1) avoiding disease altogether, (2) early diagnosis of disease, and (3) measures taken to prevent or limit disease progression.

Primary Prevention

Primary prevention includes a cadre of activities that are aimed at preventing disease. This step is the most important of all the prevention levels when you consider that half of all deaths that occur are preventable. Lifestyle management, proper nutrition, school health, immunizations, and proper waste disposal are all forms of primary prevention. For instance, it is estimated that smoking causes more than $96 billion in health-related costs and over 400,000 premature deaths per year (Curley & Vitale, 2012). Smoking is the leading cause of preventable morbidity and mortality. It is obvious that there is a huge potential for health and cost savings by preventing the use of tobacco.

As we all learned in nursing school, perhaps even in nursery school, hand-washing is the most important activity we can encourage to prevent the spread of infectious diseases. In 1900, pneumonia, tuberculosis, and diarrheal diseases were the top three causes of death in the United States (CDC, 2009). Because of efforts to reduce morbidity and mortality from infectious diseases, they are no longer the leading causes of death in the United States (CDC, 2016). See **BOX 8-2** and **TABLE 8-1**.

Methods to avoid illness are part of primary prevention. Vaccinations to prevent pneumococcal pneumonia, influenza, tetanus, varicella, human papilloma virus, and so on should be part of the NP's routine health management for each patient. Not all practice sites have electronic health records to help the healthcare provider with tracking vaccinations, so it is imperative to review the chart to keep the patient up to date. See **FIGURE 8-3A** for a sample vaccine administration record for adults, and **FIGURE 8-3B** for a screening questionnaire for adult immunizations.

BOX 8-2 Leading Causes of Death in the United States, 2011

1. Diseases of the heart
2. Malignant neoplasms
3. Chronic lower respiratory diseases
4. Cerebrovascular diseases
5. Accidents (unintentional injuries)
6. Alzheimer's disease
7. Diabetes mellitus
8. Influenza and pneumonia
9. Nephritis, nephrotic syndrome, and nephrosis
10. Intentional self-harm (suicide)
11. Septicemia
12. Chronic liver disease and cirrhosis
13. Essential hypertension and hypertensive renal disease
14. Parkinson's disease
15. Pneumonitis due to solids and liquids

Data from CDC. (2017). Leading causes of death. Retrieved from https://www.cdc.gov/nchs/fastats/leading-causes-of-death.htm

TABLE 8-1 World Health Organization Leading Causes of Death Worldwide, 2008

World	Deaths in Millions	% of Deaths
Ischemic heart disease	7.25	12.8
Stroke and other cerebrovascular disease	6.15	10.8
Lower respiratory infections	3.46	6.1
Chronic obstructive pulmonary disease	3.28	5.8
Diarrheal diseases	2.46	4.3
HIV/AIDS	1.78	3.1
Trachea, bronchus, and lung cancers	1.39	2.4
Tuberculosis	1.34	2.4
Diabetes mellitus	1.26	2.2
Road traffic accidents	1.21	2.1

Data from World Health Organization. (2012). *Epidemiology*. Retrieved from http://www.who.int/topics/epidemiology/en

PAGE 1 OF 2

Vaccine Administration Record for Adults

Patient name ______

Birthdate ______ Chart number ______

PRACTICE NAME AND ADDRESS

Before administering any vaccines, give the patient copies of all pertinent Vaccine Information Statements (VISs) and make sure he/she understands the risks and benefits of the vaccine(s). Always provide or update the patient's personal record card.

Vaccine	Type of Vaccine[1]	Date vaccine given (mo/day/yr)	Funding Source (F,S,P)[2]	Route[3] and Site[3]	Vaccine		Vaccine Information Statement (VIS)		Vaccinator[5] (signature or initials and title)
					Lot #	Mfr.	Date on VIS[4]	Date given[4]	
Tetanus, Diphtheria, Pertussis (e.g., Tdap, Td) Give IM.[3]									
Hepatitis A[6] (e.g., HepA, HepA-HepB) Give IM.[3]									
Hepatitis B[6] (e.g., HepB, HepA-HepB) Give IM.[3]									
Human papillomavirus (HPV2, HPV4, HPV9) Give IM.[3]									
Measles, Mumps, Rubella (MMR) Give Subcut.[3]									
Varicella (VAR) Give Subcut.[3]									
Meningococcal ACWY (e.g., MenACWY [MCV4], MPSV4) Give MenACWY IM.[7] Give MPSV4 Subcut.[7]									
Meningococcal B (e.g., MenB) Give MenB IM.[7]									

▶ **See page 2** to record influenza, pneumococcal, zoster, Hib, and other vaccines (e.g., travel vaccines).

How to Complete this Record

1. Record the generic abbreviation (e.g., Tdap) or the trade name for each vaccine (see table at right).
2. Record the funding source of the vaccine given as either F (federal), S (state), or P (private).
3. Record the route by which the vaccine was given as either intramuscular (IM), subcutaneous (Subcut), intradermal (ID), intranasal (NAS), or oral (PO) and also the site where it was administered as either RA (right arm), LA (left arm), RT (right thigh), or LT (left thigh).
4. Record the publication date of each VIS as well as the date the VIS is given to the patient.
5. To meet the space constraints of this form and federal requirements for documentation, a healthcare setting may want to keep a reference list of vaccinators that includes their initials and titles.
6. For combination vaccines, fill in a row for each antigen in the combination.

Abbreviation	Trade Name and Manufacturer
Tdap	Adacel (Sanofi Pasteur); Boostrix (GlaxoSmithKline [GSK])
Td	Decavac, Tenivac (Sanofi Pasteur); generic Td (MA Biological Labs)
HepA	Havrix (GSK); Vaqta (Merck)
HepB	Engerix-B (GSK); Recombivax HB (Merck)
HepA-HepB	Twinrix (GSK)
HPV2	Cervarix (GSK)
HPV4, HPV5	Gardasil, Gardasil 9 (Merck)
MMR	MMRII (Merck)
VAR	Varivax (Merck)
MenACWY	Menactra (Sanofi Pasteur); Menveo (GSK)
MPSV4	Menomune (Sanofi Pasteur)
MenB	Bexsero (GSK); Trumenba (Pfizer)

Technical content reviewed by the Centers for Disease Control and Prevention

IMMUNIZATION ACTION COALITION Saint Paul, Minnesota • 651-647-9009 • www.immunize.org • www.vaccineinformation.org

www.immunize.org/catg.d/p2023.pdf • Item #P2023 (4/16)

FIGURE 8-3A Vaccine Administration Record for Adults

Reproduced from Immunization Action Council. (n.d.). Vaccine administration record for adults. Retrieved from http://www.immunize.org/catg.d/p2023.pdf

Vaccine Administration Record for Adults (continued)

Patient name____________________

Birthdate____________ Chart number____________

PRACTICE NAME AND ADDRESS

Before administering any vaccines, give the patient copies of all pertinent Vaccine Information Statements (VISs) and make sure he/she understands the risks and benefits of the vaccine(s). Always provide or update the patient's personal record card.

Vaccine	Type of Vaccine[1]	Date vaccine given (mo/day/yr)	Funding Source (F,S,P)[2]	Route[3] and Site[3]	Vaccine		Vaccine Information Statement (VIS)		Vaccinator[5] (signature or initials and title)
					Lot #	Mfr.	Date on VIS[4]	Date given[4]	
Influenza (e.g., IIV3, IIV4, ccIIV3, RIV3, LAIV4) Give IIV3, IIV4, ccIIV3, and RIV3 IM.[3] Give LAIV4 NAS.[3]									
Pneumococcal conjugate (e.g., PCV13) Give PCV13 IM.[3]									
Pneumococcal polysaccharide (e.g., PPSV23) Give PPSV23 IM or Subcut.[3]									
Zoster (HZV) Give Subcut.[3]									
Hib Give IM.[3]									
Other									

▶ **See page 1** to record Tdap/Td, hepatitis A, hepatitis B, HPV, MMR, varicella, MenACWY, and MenB vaccines.

How to Complete this Record

1. Record the generic abbreviation (e.g., Tdap) or the trade name for each vaccine (see table at right).
2. Record the funding source of the vaccine given as either F (federal), S (state), or P (private).
3. Record the route by which the vaccine was given as either intramuscular (IM), subcutaneous (Subcut), intradermal (ID), intranasal (NAS), or oral (PO) and also the site where it was administered as either RA (right arm), LA (left arm), RT (right thigh), or LT (left thigh).
4. Record the publication date of each VIS as well as the date the VIS is given to the patient.
5. To meet the space constraints of this form and federal requirements for documentation, a healthcare setting may want to keep a reference list of vaccinators that includes their initials and titles.

Abbreviation	Trade Name and Manufacturer
IIV3 (inactivated influenza vaccine, trivalent); IIV4 (inactivated influenza vaccine, quadrivalent); ccIIV3 (cell culture-based inactivated influenza vaccine, trivalent); RIV3 (inactivated recombinant influenza vaccine, trivalent)	Fluarix (GSK); Flublok (Protein Sciences Corp.); Afluria, Fluad, Flucelvax, Fluvirin (Seqirus); FluLaval (GSK); Fluzone, Fluzone Intradermal, Fluzone High-Dose (Sanofi Pasteur)
LAIV (live attenuated influenza vaccine, quadrivalent]	FluMist (MedImmune)
PCV13	Prevnar 13 (Pfizer)
PPSV23	Pneumovax 23 (Merck)
HZV (shingles)	Zostavax (Merck)
Hib	ActHIB (Sanofi Pasteur); Hiberix (GSK); PedvaxHib (Merck)

Immunization Action Coalition • Saint Paul, Minnesota • 651-647-9009 • www.immunize.org • www.vaccineinformation.org

www.immunize.org/catg.d/p2023.pdf • Item #P2023 – page 2 (4/16)

FIGURE 8-3A Continued

Vaccine Administration Record for Adults

Patient name *Mahamud Omar*

Birthdate *5/31/1971* Chart number

Before administering any vaccines, give the patient copies of all pertinent Vaccine Information Statements (VISs) and make sure he/she understands the risks and benefits of the vaccine(s). Always provide or update the patient's personal record card.

PRACTICE NAME AND ADDRESS

Small Rural Clinic
135 County Road D
Small Town, CD 46902

Vaccine	Type of Vaccine[1]	Date vaccine given (mo/day/yr)	Funding Source (F,S,P)[2]	Route[3] and Site[3]	Vaccine		Vaccine Information Statement (VIS)		Vaccinator[5] (signature or initials and title)
					Lot #	M[illegible]	Date on VIS[4]	Date given[4]	
Tetanus, Diphtheria, Pertussis (e.g., Tdap, Td) Give IM.[3]	Td	8/1/2002	P	IM/LA	U0376AA	A[illegible]	6/[illegible]0/1994	8/1/2002	JTA
	Td	9/1/2002	P	IM/LA	U0376AA	[illegible]VP	6/10/1994	9/1/2002	RVO
	Td	3/1/2003	P	IM/LA	U0376[illegible]A	A[illegible]P	6/10/1994	3/1/2003	TAA
	Tdap	3/1/2015	P	IM/LA	AC52B[illegible]AA	GSK	2/24/2015	3/1/2015	JA
Hepatitis A[6] (e.g., HepA, HepA-HepB) Give IM.[3]									
Hepatitis B[6] (e.g., HepB, HepA-HepB) Give IM.[3]									
Human papillomavirus (HPV2, HPV4, HPV9) Give IM.[3]									
Measles, Mumps, Rubella (MMR) Give Subcut.[3]	MMR	8/1/2002	P	Subcut/RA	0025L	MSD	6/13/2002	8/1/2002	JTA
	MMR	11/1/2002	P	Subcut/RA	0025L	MSD	6/13/2002	11/1/2002	TAA
Varicella (VAR) Give Subcut.[3]	VAR	8/1/2002	P	Subcut/LA	0799M	MSD	12/16/1998	8/1/2002	JTA
	VAR	11/1/2002	P	Subcut/LA	0689M	MSD	12/16/1998	11/1/2002	TAA
Meningococcal ACWY (e.g., MenACWY [MCV4], MPSV4) Give MenACWY IM.[7] Give MPSV4 Subcut.[7]	MenACWY	7/12/2011	P	IM/RA	M28011	NOV	1/2/2008	7/12/2011	LTB
	Menveo	7/15/2016	P	IM/LA	M12115	NOV	3/31/16	7/15/2016	RVO
Meningococcal B (e.g., MenB) Give MenB IM.[7]	MenB	1/14/2016	P	IM/LA	J296203	PFR	8/14/2015	1/14/2016	RVO
	Trumenba	3/15/2016	P	IM/LA	J296203	PFR	8/14/2015	3/15/2016	RVO
	Trumenba	7/15/2016	P	IM/RA	J296203	PFR	8/14/2015	7/15/2016	RVO

▶ **See page 2** to record influenza, pneumococcal, zoster, Hib, and other vaccines (e.g., travel vaccines).

How to Complete this Record

1. Record the generic abbreviation (e.g., Tdap) or the trade name for each vaccine (see table at right).
2. Record the funding source of the vaccine given as either F (federal), S (state), or P (private).
3. Record the route by which the vaccine was given as either intramuscular (IM), subcutaneous (Subcut), intradermal (ID), intranasal (NAS), or oral (PO) and also the site where it was administered as either RA (right arm), LA (left arm), RT (right thigh), or LT (left thigh).
4. Record the publication date of each VIS as well as the date the VIS is given to the patient.
5. To meet the space constraints of this form and federal requirements for documentation, a healthcare setting may want to keep a reference list of vaccinators that includes their initials and titles.
6. For combination vaccines, fill in a row for each antigen in the combination.

Abbreviation	Trade Name and Manufacturer
Tdap	Adacel (Sanofi Pasteur); Boostrix (GlaxoSmithKline [GSK])
Td	Decavac, Tenivac (Sanofi Pasteur); generic Td (MA Biological Labs)
HepA	Havrix (GSK); Vaqta (Merck)
HepB	Engerix-B (GSK); Recombivax HB (Merck)
HepA-HepB	Twinrix (GSK)
HPV2	Cervarix (GSK)
HPV4, HPV5	Gardasil, Gardasil 9 (Merck)
MMR	MMRII (Merck)
VAR	Varivax (Merck)
MenACWY	Menactra (Sanofi Pasteur); Menveo (GSK)
MPSV4	Menomune (Sanofi Pasteur)
MenB	Bexsero (GSK); Trumenba (Pfizer)

Technical content reviewed by the Centers for Disease Control and Prevention

IMMUNIZATION ACTION COALITION Saint Paul, Minnesota • 651-647-9009 • www.immunize.org • www.vaccineinformation.org

www.immunize.org/catg.d/p2023.pdf • Item #P2023 (4/16)

FIGURE 8-3A Continued

Vaccine Administration Record for Adults (continued)

Patient name *Mahamud Omar*

Birthdate *5/31/1971* Chart number

PRACTICE NAME AND ADDRESS
Small Rural Clinic
135 County Road D
Small Town, CD 46902

Before administering any vaccines, give the patient copies of all pertinent Vaccine Information Statements (VISs) and make sure he/she understands the risks and benefits of the vaccine(s). Always provide or update the patient's personal record card.

Vaccine	Type of Vaccine[1]	Date vaccine given (mo/day/yr)	Funding Source (F,S,P)[2]	Route[3] and Site[3]	Vaccine Lot #	Vaccine Mfr.	VIS Date on VIS[4]	VIS Date given[4]	Vaccinator[5] (signature or initials and title)
Influenza (e.g., IIV3, IIV4, ccIIV3, RIV3, LAIV4) Give IIV3, IIV4, ccIIV3, and RIV3 IM.[3] Give LAIV4 NAS.[3]	Flulaval	10/2/2009	F	IM/RA	2F600411	GSK	8/11/09	10/2/09	PWS
	H1N1	12/7/2009	P	IM/RA	10092224P	NOV	10/2/09	12/7/09	DLW
	Afluria	9/12/2010	P	IM/RA	06949111A	CSL	8/10/10	9/12/10	TAA
	Flulaval	10/1/2011	P	IM/LA	2F600411	GSK	8/10/11	10/1/11	JTA
	IIV3	9/5/2012	P	IM/RA	M50907	CSL	7/2/12	9/5/12	KKC
	RIV3	12/2/2013	P	IM/RA	350603F	PSC	7/26/13	12/2/13	DCP
	IIV4	10/5/2014	P	IM/RA	UI196AA	PMC	8/19/14	10/5/14	JTA
	IIV4	11/2/2015	P	IM/LA	111773P	NOV	8/7/15	11/2/15	DCP
Pneumococcal conjugate (e.g., PCV13) Give PCV13 IM.[3]	PCV13	11/1/2012	P	[illegible]	7-5096-06A	WYE	4/16/10	11/1/12	CJP
Pneumococcal polysaccharide (e.g., PPSV23) Give PPSV23 IM or Subcut.[3]	PPSV23	9/10/2011	P	[illegible]	663012/1163X	MSD	10/6/09	9/10/11	DLW
	PPSV23	9/15/2015	[illegible]	[illegible]	663860/1626X	MSD	4/24/15	9/15/15	TAA
Zoster (HZV) Give Subcut.[3]									
Hib Give IM.[3]	ActHIB	11/1/201[illegible]	P	IM/RA	D05561	PMC	2/4/14	11/1/14	MAT
Other									

▶ **See page 1** to record Tdap/Td, hepatitis A, hepatitis B, HPV, MMR, varicella, MenACWY, and MenB vaccines.

How to Complete this Record

1. Record the generic abbreviation (e.g., Tdap) or the trade name for each vaccine (see table at right).
2. Record the funding source of the vaccine given as either F (federal), S (state), or P (private).
3. Record the route by which the vaccine was given as either intramuscular (IM), subcutaneous (Subcut), intradermal (ID), intranasal (NAS), or oral (PO) and also the site where it was administered as either RA (right arm), LA (left arm), RT (right thigh), or LT (left thigh).
4. Record the publication date of each VIS as well as the date the VIS is given to the patient.
5. To meet the space constraints of this form and federal requirements for documentation, a healthcare setting may want to keep a reference list of vaccinators that includes their initials and titles.

Abbreviation	Trade Name and Manufacturer
IIV3 (inactivated influenza vaccine, trivalent); IIV4 (inactivated influenza vaccine, quadrivalent); ccIIV3 (cell culture-based inactivated influenza vaccine, trivalent); RIV3 (inactivated recombinant influenza vaccine, trivalent)	Fluarix (GSK); Flublok (Protein Sciences Corp.); Afluria, Fluad, Flucelvax, Fluvirin (Seqirus); FluLaval (GSK); Fluzone, Fluzone Intradermal, Fluzone High-Dose (Sanofi Pasteur)
LAIV (live attenuated influenza vaccine, quadrivalent)	FluMist (MedImmune)
PCV13	Prevnar 13 (Pfizer)
PPSV23	Pneumovax 23 (Merck)
HZV (shingles)	Zostavax (Merck)
Hib	ActHIB (Sanofi Pasteur); Hiberix (GSK); PedvaxHib (Merck)

Immunization Action Coalition • Saint Paul, Minnesota • 651-647-9009 • www.immunize.org • www.vaccineinformation.org

www.immunize.org/catg.d/p2023.pdf • Item #P2023 – page 2 (4/16)

FIGURE 8-3A Continued

Screening Checklist for Contraindications to Vaccines for Adults

PATIENT NAME ______________________

DATE OF BIRTH ____ / ____ / ____ (month / day / year)

For patients: The following questions will help us determine which vaccines you may be given today. If you answer "yes" to any question, it does not necessarily mean you should not be vaccinated. It just means additional questions must be asked. If a question is not clear, please ask your healthcare provider to explain it.

	yes	no	don't know
1. Are you sick today?	☐	☐	☐
2. Do you have allergies to medications, food, a vaccine component, or latex?	☐	☐	☐
3. Have you ever had a serious reaction after receiving a vaccination?	☐	☐	☐
4. Do you have a long-term health problem with heart disease, lung disease, asthma, kidney disease, metabolic disease (e.g., diabetes), anemia, or other blood disorder?	☐	☐	☐
5. Do you have cancer, leukemia, HIV/AIDS, or any other immune system problem?	☐	☐	☐
6. In the past 3 months, have you taken medications that affect your immune system, such as prednisone, other steroids, or anticancer drugs; drugs for the treatment of rheumatoid arthritis, Crohn's disease, or psoriasis; or have you had radiation treatments?	☐	☐	☐
7. Have you had a seizure or a brain or other nervous system problem?	☐	☐	☐
8. During the past year, have you received a transfusion of blood or blood products, or been given immune (gamma) globulin or an antiviral drug?	☐	☐	☐
9. For women: Are you pregnant or is there a chance you could become pregnant during the next month?	☐	☐	☐
10. Have you received any vaccinations in the past 4 weeks?	☐	☐	☐

FORM COMPLETED BY ______________________ DATE ________

FORM REVIEWED BY ______________________ DATE ________

Did you bring your immunization record card with you? yes ☐ no ☐

It is important for you to have a personal record of your vaccinations. If you don't have a personal record, ask your healthcare provider to give you one. Keep this record in a safe place and bring it with you every time you seek medical care. Make sure your healthcare provider records all your vaccinations on it.

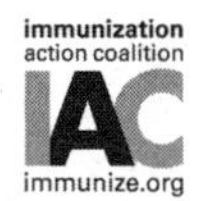

Technical content reviewed by the Centers for Disease Control and Prevention

Saint Paul, Minnesota • 651-647-9009 • www.immunize.org • www.vaccineinformation.org

www.immunize.org/catg.d/p4065.pdf • Item #P4065 (8/17)

FIGURE 8-3B Screening Questionnaire for Adult Immunization

Reproduced from Immunization Action Council. (n.d.). Screening checklist for contraindications to vaccines for adults. Retrieved from http://www.immunize.org/catg.d/p4065.pdf

Information for Healthcare Professionals about the Screening Checklist for Contraindications to Vaccines for Adults

Are you interested in knowing why we included a certain question on the screening checklist? If so, read the information below. If you want to find out even more, consult the references listed at the end.

1. Are you sick today? *[all vaccines]*

There is no evidence that acute illness reduces vaccine efficacy or increases vaccine adverse events.[1] However, as a precaution with moderate or severe acute illness, all vaccines should be delayed until the illness has improved. Mild illnesses (such as upper respiratory infections or diarrhea) are NOT contraindications to vaccination. Do not withhold vaccination if a person is taking antibiotics.

2. Do you have allergies to medications, food, a vaccine component, or latex? *[all vaccines]*

An anaphylactic reaction to latex is a contraindication to vaccines that contain latex as a component or as part of the packaging (e.g., vial stoppers, prefilled syringe plungers, prefilled syringe caps). If a person has anaphylaxis after eating gelatin, do not administer vaccines containing gelatin. A local reaction to a prior vaccine dose or vaccine component, including latex, is not a contraindication to a subsequent dose or vaccine containing that component. For information on vaccines supplied in vials or syringes containing latex, see reference 2; for an extensive list of vaccine components, see reference 3.

People with egg allergy of any severity can receive any recommended influenza vaccine (i.e., any IIV or RIV) that is otherwise appropriate for the patient's age. For people with a history of severe allergic reaction to egg involving any symptom other than hives (e.g., angioedema, respiratory distress), or who required epinephrine or another emergency medical intervention, the vaccine should be administered in a medical setting, such as a clinic, health department, or physician office. Vaccine administration should be supervised by a healthcare provider who is able to recognize and manage severe allergic conditions.[4]

3. Have you ever had a serious reaction after receiving a vaccination? *[all vaccines]*

History of anaphylactic reaction (see question 2) to a previous dose of vaccine or vaccine component is a contraindication for subsequent doses.[1] Under normal circumstances, vaccines are deferred when a precaution is present. However, situations may arise when the benefit outweighs the risk (e.g., during a community pertussis outbreak).

4. Do you have a long-term health problem with heart disease, lung disease, asthma, kidney disease, metabolic disease (e.g., diabetes), anemia, or other blood disorder? *[MMR, LAIV]*

A history of thrombocytopenia or thrombcytompenic purpura is a precaution to MMR vaccine. The safety of intranasal live attenuated influenza vaccine (LAIV) in people with these conditions has not been established. These conditions, including asthma in adults, should be considered precautions for the use of LAIV.

5. Do you have cancer, leukemia, HIV/AIDS, or any other immune system problem? *[LAIV, MMR, VAR, ZOS]*

Live virus vaccines (e.g., LAIV, measles-mumps-rubella [MMR], varicella [VAR], zoster [ZOS]) are usually contraindicated in immunocompromised people. However, there are exceptions. For example, MMR vaccine is recommended and varicella vaccine should be considered for adults with CD4+ T-lymphocyte counts of greater than or equal to 200 cells/μL. Immunosuppressed people should not receive LAIV. For details, consult the ACIP recommendations.[4,5,6]

6. In the past 3 months, have you taken medications that affect your immune system, such as cortisone, prednisone, other steroids, or anticancer drugs; drugs for the treatment of rheumatoid arthritis, Crohn's disease, or psoriasis; or have you had radiation treatments? *[LAIV, MMR, VAR, ZOS]*

Live virus vaccines (e.g., LAIV, MMR, VAR, ZOS) should be postponed until after chemotherapy or long-term high-dose steroid therapy has ended. For details and length of time to postpone, consult the ACIP statement.[1,5] Some immune mediator and immune modulator drugs (especially the antitumor-necrosis factor agents adalimumab, infliximab, and etanercept) may be immunosuppressive. The use of live vaccines should be avoided in persons taking these drugs (*MMWR* 2011;60 [RR-2]:23). To find specific vaccination schedules for stem cell transplant (bone marrow transplant) patients, see reference 7. LAIV can be given only to healthy non-pregnant people ages 2 through 49 years.

> **NOTE: Live attenuated influenza vaccine (LAIV4; FluMist), is not recommended by CDC's Advisory Committee on Immunization Practices for use in the U.S. during the 2017–18 influenza season.**

7. Have you had a seizure or a brain or other nervous system problem? *[influenza, Td/Tdap]*

Tdap is contraindicated in people who have a history of encephalopathy within 7 days following DTP/DTaP given before age 7 years. An unstable progressive neurologic problem is a precaution to the use of Tdap. For people with stable neurologic disorders (including seizures) unrelated to vaccination, or for people with a family history of seizure, vaccinate as usual. A history of Guillain-Barré syndrome (GBS) is a consideration with the following: 1) Td/Tdap: if GBS has occurred within 6 weeks of a tetanus-containing vaccine and decision is made to continue vaccination, give Tdap instead of Td if no history of prior Tdap; 2) Influenza vaccine (IIV/LAIV): if GBS has occurred within 6 weeks of a prior influenza vaccine, vaccinate with IIV if at increased risk for severe influenza complications.

8. During the past year, have you received a transfusion of blood or blood products, or been given immune (gamma) globulin or an antiviral drug? *[LAIV, MMR, VAR, ZOS]*

Certain live virus vaccines (e.g., LAIV, MMR, VAR, ZOS) may need to be deferred, depending on several variables. Consult the most current ACIP recommendations for current information on intervals between antiviral drugs, immune globulin or blood product administration and live virus vaccines.[1]

9. For women: Are you pregnant or is there a chance you could become pregnant during the next month? *[HPV, IPV, MMR, LAIV, VAR, ZOS]*

Live virus vaccines (e.g., MMR, VAR, ZOS, LAIV) are contraindicated one month before and during pregnancy because of the theoretical risk of virus transmission to the fetus. Sexually active women in their childbearing years who receive live virus vaccines should be instructed to practice careful contraception for one month following receipt of the vaccine. On theoretical grounds, inactivated poliovirus vaccine should not be given during pregnancy; however, it may be given if risk of exposure is imminent and immediate protection is needed (e.g., travel to endemic areas). Inactivated influenza vaccine and Tdap are both recommended during pregnancy. Both vaccines may be given at any time during pregnancy but the preferred time for Tdap administration is at 27–36 weeks' gestation. HPV vaccine is not recommended during pregnancy.[1,4,5,6,8,9]

10. Have you received any vaccinations in the past 4 weeks? *[LAIV, MMR, VAR, yellow fever, ZOS]*

People who were given either LAIV or an injectable live virus vaccine (e.g., MMR, VAR, ZOS, yellow fever) should wait 28 days before receiving another vaccination of this type. Inactivated vaccines may be given at any spacing interval if they are not administered simultaneously.

REFERENCES

1. CDC. General best practice guidelines for immunization. Best Practices Guidance of the Advisory Committee on Immunization Practices (ACIP) at www.cdc.gov/vaccines/hcp/acip-recs/downloads/general-recs.pdf.
2. Latex in Vaccine Packaging: www.cdc.gov/vaccines/pubs/pinkbook/downloads/appendices/B/latex-table.pdf.
3. Table of Vaccine Components: www.cdc.gov/vaccines/pubs/pinkbook/downloads/appendices/B/excipient-table-2.pdf.
4. CDC. Prevention and control of seasonal influenza with vaccines: Recommendations of the Advisory Committee on Immunization Practices – United States, 2017–18 Influenza Season at www.cdc.gov/mmwr/volumes/66/rr/pdfs/rr6602.pdf.
5. CDC. Measles, mumps, and rubella – vaccine use and strategies for elimination of measles, rubella, and congenital rubella syndrome and control of mumps. *MMWR* 1998; 47 (RR-8).
6. CDC. Prevention of varicella: Recommendations of the Advisory Committee on Immunization Practices. *MMWR* 2007; 56 (RR-4).
7. Tomblyn M, Einsele H, et al. Guidelines for preventing infectious complications among hematopoietic stem cell transplant recipients: a global perspective. Biol Blood Marrow Transplant 15:1143–1238; 2009 at www.cdc.gov/vaccines/pubs/hemato-cell-transplts.htm.
8. CDC. Notice to readers: Revised ACIP recommendation for avoiding pregnancy after receiving a rubella-containing vaccine. *MMWR* 2001; 50 (49).
9. CDC. Updated recommendations for use of tetanus toxoid, reduced diphtheria toxoid, and acellular pertussis vaccine (Tdap) in pregnant women: Recommendations of the ACIP. *MMWR* 2012; 62 (7):131–4.

Immunization Action Coalition • Saint Paul, Minnesota • 651-647-9009 • www.immunize.org • www.vaccineinformation.org

www.immunize.org/catg.d/p4065.pdf • Item #P4065 – page 2 (8/17)

FIGURE 8-3B Continued

When we look at the top leading causes of death worldwide, the picture has been changing. Ischemic heart disease tops this list as well, and HIV/AIDS has made it off this list. Diarrheal diseases and tuberculosis are in the top 10 causes of death globally but cancer is only on the U.S. list. It is important to think globally when caring for recent immigrants to the United States in order to not miss accurately diagnosing and treating infectious diseases.

Secondary Prevention

Secondary prevention includes actions that lead to early identification, diagnosis, and treatment of disease. Health screenings and various detection activities are used in secondary prevention efforts. Collection and analysis of clinical data give us a starting point for identifying, selecting, and implementing interventions that target specific populations at risk.

The United States Preventive Services Task Force (USPSTF) is a source of evidence-based information for NPs to use in improving population health. The USPSTF offers expert advice on preventive services that focus on primary prevention. The task force performs a rigorous review of research on specific health topics prior to making recommendations on the merits of preventive measures. This includes screening tests, counseling, immunizations, and medications given for prevention of diseases. Topics include type 2 diabetes mellitus, lipids, breast and colorectal cancer, depression, tobacco use, and many more. Nurse practitioners are encouraged to visit the CDC website for selective preventative screening recommendations at http://www.cdc.gov/nccdphp/dnpao/hwi/resources/preventative_screening.htm to review information on your topic of interest.

Tertiary Prevention

Actions that promote activities of daily living to limit progression and complications of disease are what constitute tertiary prevention. Probably the most important factor affecting tertiary prevention is that the population is aging. The expectation is that there will be a 60% increase in people over the age of 65 years by the year 2030 (He, Goodkind, & Kowal, 2016). Many factors have played a part in this phenomenon. One of the reasons is the increase in lifespan related to medical advancements; other factors include public health efforts to improve sanitation and the availability of clean water, as well as the impact of prevention efforts aimed at reducing risk factors for cardiovascular disease (Van Leuven, 2012). This change in population demographics has an enormous impact on nurse practitioners. Health services will be focused on chronic comorbid diseases including cardiovascular disease, diabetes, cancer, dementia, depression, osteoarthritis, and lung disease (Van Leuven, 2012).

HIV and Prevention Levels

One example of a comprehensive approach to primary, secondary, and tertiary prevention is the worldwide effort to reduce HIV infection. As noted in Chapter 3, *Vulnerable Populations*, HIV/AIDS continues to be a global issue. Clearly, this is an area that needs collaborative efforts to reduce transmission, screening to identify and treat those already infected, and tertiary measures to avoid death due to complications from AIDS.

In 2006 the CDC issued recommendations for HIV testing in healthcare settings (Branson et al., 2006). Routine voluntary testing for patients ages 13 to 64 years in healthcare settings was encouraged, and testing was not to be based solely on patient risk for acquiring HIV as in the past. Opt-out testing includes no separate consent for HIV and pretest counseling not being required. Patients can decline testing, but the test would be performed unless the patient specifically refuses to have it done. The CDC's goal was threefold:

1. To get "late testers," or patients who were diagnosed with AIDS within 12 months of a diagnosis of HIV, representing about 40% of all HIV diagnoses, into care sooner, thereby extending their lives.
2. To curtail unsafe practices that spread HIV by having people who are HIV positive know their status and take measures to reduce transmission.
3. To have HIV testing be part of routine medical screenings for everyone, which would help to reduce the stigma associated with being offered an HIV test.

You can see the levels of prevention addressed by screening for HIV in the above goals. The goal of primary HIV prevention is to reduce the incidence of transmission, whereas secondary HIV prevention aims to reduce the prevalence and severity of the disease through early detection and prompt treatment.

Primary HIV prevention efforts include the following:

- Community and peer-based prevention and intervention programs
- School-based skills education and prevention
- The use of needleless technologies in healthcare settings to reduce injury and risk of blood-borne virus transmission
- Post-exposure prophylaxis, including nonoccupational post-exposure prophylaxis
- Pre-exposure prophylaxis

One of the advancements in primary prevention of HIV was approved by the Centers for Disease Control and Prevention in 2014. Pre-exposure prophylaxis (PrEP) using Truvada (tenofovir/emtricitabine) has shown to reduce sexual transmission of HIV by 90% and transmission by injection drug use by 70% (CDC, 2017). Primary care providers must do a thorough history of each patient and identify those who may be at high risk for acquiring HIV and offer PrEP. This includes anyone in a relationship with a partner who is HIV positive, or has unprotected sex with partners of unknown HIV status, and/or injection drug users who share needles or drug paraphernalia. Baseline laboratory assessment and education about adherence to taking the once-daily medication is critical to avoid adverse events including HIV infection.

Secondary HIV prevention includes removing barriers to HIV testing and detection by removing the requirement for pretest counseling and permission forms. Secondary prevention also includes increasing healthcare providers' knowledge about HIV and testing, the signs of acute antiretroviral infection, and what to do when a patient tests positive for HIV. According to research done on the topic of HIV testing and barriers (Burke et al., 2007), barriers in clinical settings included insufficient time, a burdensome consent process, lack of knowledge or training, lack of patient acceptance, pretest counseling requirements, competing priorities, and inadequate reimbursement. In the emergency department, barriers also included the need to inform an HIV-positive patient, institutional costs, unavailability of testing, administrative barriers, and the feeling that testing should be done at the patient's request. Other identified barriers included a lack of trust with the patient, gender differences between the provider and patient, differences in sexual orientation, the concept that HIV and sexually transmitted diseases were not an issue in the community, and a lack of institutional policies for testing. There are many areas for improvement regarding HIV testing related to the barriers identified.

The goal of tertiary prevention is to reduce disability and complications from HIV infection. Much work is done in this area, and guidelines are frequently updated. In addition to the CDC's recommendations for HIV testing, there are standard guidelines for the treatment of HIV infection, as well as guidelines for preventing and treating opportunistic infections in children, adolescents, and adults (CDC, 2016a; CDC, 2016b; 2017; U.S. Department of Health and Human Services [DHHS], 2017). For example, the standard of care in the United States for preventing *Pneumocystis jirovecii* pneumonia (PCP) is to put any patient on a medication such as trimethroprim-sulfamethoxazole (TMP-SMX), dapsone, or atovaquone when the absolute CD4 count falls below 200 cells/μL. The guidelines are evidence based and help all HIV care providers offer the most current high-quality care to their patients.

Population Health and *Healthy People 2020*

In 1979, the DHHS launched an initiative aimed at improving the health of the U.S. population. This effort was titled *Healthy People 2000,* which was followed by *Healthy People 2010*, and the current edition is now *Healthy People 2020.* The DHHS amassed baseline data and then set goals on the prioritized health targets (Koh, 2010). *Healthy People 2020* keeps the previous overarching goals of *Healthy People 2010* to increase the quality of life, increase the lifespan, and decrease health disparities. *Healthy People 2020* has supplemented those goals with: "promoting quality of life, healthy development, and healthy behaviors across life stages; and creating social and physical environments that promote good health" (Koh, 2012, p. 1656). These goals are tailor-made for nurse practitioners and their ability to have an enormous impact on the health of the nation. **BOX 8-3** outlines the leading health indicators as defined by the DHHS.

BOX 8-3 Healthy People 2020 Leading Health Indicators

Physical activity
Tobacco use
Responsible sexual behavior
Injury and violence
Immunization
Overweight and obesity
Substance abuse
Mental health
Environmental quality
Access to health care
Focus areas
Access to quality health services
Cancer
Diabetes
Educational and community-based programs

(continues)

BOX 8-3 Healthy People 2020 Leading Health Indicators *(continued)*

Family planning
Health communication
Human immunodeficiency virus
Injury and violence prevention
Medical product safety
Nutrition and overweight
Oral health
Public health infrastructure
Sexually transmitted diseases
Tobacco use
Arthritis, osteoporosis, and chronic back conditions
Chronic kidney disease
Disability and secondary conditions
Environmental health
Food safety
Heart disease and stroke
Immunization and infectious diseases
Maternal, infant, and child health
Mental health and mental disorders
Occupational safety and health
Physical activity and fitness
Respiratory diseases
Substance abuse
Vision and hearing

The Clinical Prevention and Population Health (CPPH) Curriculum Framework was developed by the Healthy People Curriculum Task Force, which includes representatives from eight health professional education associations, including allopathic and osteopathic medicine, nursing and nurse practitioners, allied health, dentistry, pharmacy, and physician assistants (Association for Prevention Teaching and Research [APTR], 2009). The CPPH Curriculum Framework was developed to assist educators in teaching about health promotion to meet the goals identified by *Healthy People* initiatives. The framework comprises four components that include evidence-based practice (EBP), clinical preventive services and health promotion, health systems and health policy, and population health and community aspects.

The Association for Prevention Teaching and Research offers further details by listing 19 domains based on the four main components of the framework (2009). The component relating to EBP requires that the curriculum provide information regarding descriptive epidemiology and the etiology of disease, as well as recommendations, implementation, and evaluation of interventions aimed at improving population health. Clinical prevention services and health promotion topics include screenings, counseling, immunizations, and preventative interventions. The curriculum regarding health systems and health policy includes education regarding the types of health organizations that exist, financing of health care, members of the healthcare workforce, and the process and effects of health policy. Lastly, there is the area focusing on population health and community aspects of practice. This area covers health communication, environmental and occupational health issues, global health, cultural issues, and community services and organizations.

There are a variety of tools for evaluating population health, and there are also tools for developing targeted programs. The MEASURE Evaluation (USAID, 2012) is a website that offers tools for a variety of areas such as HIV/AIDS, child health, reproductive health, and gender and poverty issues. A helpful matrix for developing a program targeted to improve a population's health can be found on that site as well. The key components for a program development matrix are (USAID, 2012):

- Objective: Statements of desired, specific, realistic, and measurable program results
- Intermediate result: Benchmark progress result measured along the way to achieving the objectives
- Outcome: Indicator of changes in knowledge, attitudes, and practices that help demonstrate achievement of objectives
- Output: Indicator of activity or immediate result of program process
- Indicator: A variable that measures one aspect of a program, project, or outcome
- Data source: Where will you get this data? Will you collect it? Will your partner?
- Frequency: How often will this information be collected or reported?
- Baseline: What is the current level of this knowledge, attitude, or practice in the target area?
- End-of-project target: What level or change do you expect to see at the conclusion of the program?
- Discussion points: What issues, thoughts, concerns, and suggestions do you have about collecting this indicator information?
- Information user comments: Who needs this information? Where will it be reported? What decision makers have asked for it?

The PRECEDE-PROCEED model is another design for planning and evaluating population health programs (Green & Kreuter, 2005). PRECEDE stands for Predisposing, Reinforcing, and Enabling Constructs in Educational/Environmental Diagnosis and Evaluation. PROCEED stands for Policy, Regulatory, and Organizational Constructs in Educational and Environmental Development. Although this may seem overwhelming and complex, it is more easily understood as a roadmap for health promotion that includes the environment, as well as people's beliefs, abilities, skills, and behaviors (Crosby & Noar, 2011). In this approach, information is gathered during the PRECEDE steps; this information is then used as the framework for the PROCEED steps. It is a continuing process because the evaluation portion of PROCEED helps to inform and revise the steps in the PRECEDE portion of this model. See **FIGURES 8-4A** and **8-4B**.

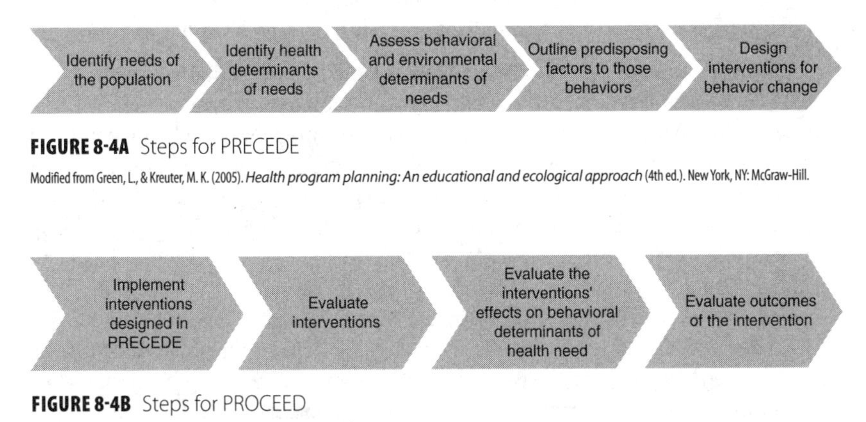

FIGURE 8-4A Steps for PRECEDE

Modified from Green, L., & Kreuter, M. K. (2005). *Health program planning: An educational and ecological approach* (4th ed.). New York, NY: McGraw-Hill.

FIGURE 8-4B Steps for PROCEED

Modified from Green, L., & Kreuter, M. K. (2005). *Health program planning: An educational and ecological approach* (4th ed.). New York, NY: McGraw-Hill.

Emergency Preparedness and the Nurse Practitioners

The NP as a primary care provider is on the front lines of detecting emergent illness. Routine surveillance measures such as the use of health indicator data serve as baseline data. Hospitals routinely collect statistics on emergency room visits and volume, nosocomial infections, and unexplained or untimely deaths. Healthcare providers, hospitals, clinics, and public health departments must submit reports on specific communicable diseases. As NPs you will be expected to file these reports pending assessment findings.

Man-made disasters are caused by human actions, deliberate or otherwise, and include biological or biochemical terrorism, chemical spills, transportation accidents, and armed conflicts. Complex emergencies occur when populations suffer significant casualties as the result of war and either civil or political conflict. Technological disasters are the result of industrial accidents, release of nuclear energy, and fire or explosion from hazardous substances.

In this post-9/11 world, a new set of expectations has emerged for healthcare providers. However, the emergence of diseases such as Zika virus, Ebola virus, SARS, avian flu, Hanta virus, West Nile virus, HIV/AIDS, and influenza add another dimension to these expectations. Emergency preparedness addresses not only being prepared for the event of biological, chemical, or nuclear/radiological terrorism, but it also relates to emergent infectious diseases and conditions or events such as earthquakes, floods, tornados, blizzards, or hurricanes that place the health of families and communities at risk.

Syndromic surveillance is one mechanism that can be used to detect uncommon and unusual health occurrences. This approach is based on an epidemiologic perspective and relies on the recognition of unusual patterns of illness. Biological terrorism can be expected if a set of health patterns appear that are out of the ordinary, as in the following:

- A cluster of diseases with similar clinical presentations and at a similar stage of illness
- A cluster of unexplained illness in a well-defined population
- Unusually severe disease or higher mortality than expected for a given agent
- A cluster of cases with an unusual mode of transmission
- Multiple or serial outbreaks
- A disease not typical for a specific age group
- A disease unusual for a season or region of the country
- Clusters of the same illness in various locations
- Clusters of morbidity or mortality in animals or livestock similar to humans

One of the most important resources available to all practitioners is the CDC website. Visit www.cdc.gov or www.bt.cdc.gov, and follow the emergency preparedness/terrorism link. Click on each of the Category A agents mentioned, and the most up-to-date information will be displayed. This website should be saved as a bookmark or on a favorites list. Another useful email alert group found via the CDC website is the Clinician Outreach and Communication Activity (COCA). Its goal is to help clinicians offer optimal care to patients by providing them with the most current and reliable information available on emerging health threats.

In the past decade, events such as Hurricane Katrina, tsunamis in Japan and Indonesia, earthquakes, and pandemic influenza have increased the demand for human and financial resources needed to answer the pleas for the relief of human suffering (Strong, personal communication, 2012). After 9/11, there has been an increased call for volunteers to become part of the resources available to respond to such events. A corps of volunteers is essential during these types of events, and volunteers can also be a valuable resource to promote the health and wellness of communities. Consider this short excerpt from Shery, a nurse volunteering to leave her own family and help others in need:

> After volunteering as a nurse in a small northeastern town of Sri Lanka a month after the devastating 2004 tsunami and volunteering a week after Hurricane Katrina in Biloxi, Mississippi, the similarities were striking and all too uncomfortable. The undercurrent of hopelessness and despondency was overwhelming, but the spirit in the response by the healthcare providers community was illuminating. Although the supplies were limited and communication was fragmented, it was the simplest words from another nurse who said "You mean I can go see my family now?" that eliminated all other concerns and frustrations. The relief that crossed her face spoke volumes; my small team and I were able to cover shifts to provide much needed relief for the regular healthcare staff who were trying to care for their families and friends. The healthcare community response was unmistakable after such devastation. It is one community to help each other and patients, putting others first during their time of need.

Priority setting is the initial stage of planning in a disaster, as well as in any approach to improving a population's health. Volunteers may end up doing more than merely providing health care. The needs are far greater in most cases. Consider this reflection:

> Upon arriving a week after a devastating natural disaster, our team took pause on what is the priority. The makeshift "emergency departments" were set up each day to treat nonlife-threatening injuries and wounds and caring for the acute illnesses. Through the second week, the prioritization shifted to treating patients for their chronic illnesses, realizing that when their house was left in rubble and the local pharmacy was only a cement foundation, the people needed their everyday medications. Our team looked out to a sea of faces, each person sharing the same story, "I don't know the name of my medicine." The temporary ED then turned into more than caring for injuries, rather a primary care clinic and a place for someone to share their story.

Nurse practitioners might want to consider volunteer service in times of local, state, or national disasters by joining a medical reserve corps (MRC). The MRC units are composed of licensed healthcare professionals or students and support staff to assist and "strengthen the public health infrastructure of their communities . . . work towards increasing disease prevention, eliminating health disparities, and improving public health preparedness" (Office of the Surgeon General, 2013). The Division of the Civilian Volunteer Medical Reserve Corps (DCVMRC) takes the lead in organizing and training volunteers of the MRC, which was initiated post-9/11 by President Bush in 2002. Housed in the U.S. Surgeon General's Office and directed by members of the U.S. Public Health Service, MRCs are designed to be prepared to assist and respond to public health, medical, and emergency events (Office of the Surgeon General, 2013):

1. Public health and medical
    - Surgeon general priorities (disease prevention, elimination of health disparities, health literacy)
    - Disease detection

- Health promotion
- Health education
- Health clinic support and staffing

2. Emergency preparedness and response
    - Mass dispensing and vaccinations
    - Pandemic flu planning
    - Preparedness campaigns
    - Shelter operations and support
    - First responder rehab
    - Mass casualty incident/emergency response

Denise is a nurse who has spent years working to improve the health of those less fortunate than we are in many other countries as well as our own.

DENISE'S STORY

We are all members of a global interdependent community, sharing the unique cultures of individual societies. The practice of health professionals should include not only the assessment and treatment of disease, but also the social, economic, and political variables that affect the health care of a population. Every NP should have the experience to care for people in their own environment, under the circumstances that they reside. As healthcare professionals we become ensconced in the environment of care that "we" find comfortable—an office, a hospital, a clinic. It is when we can integrate the care model into the patient's lives that we truly understand the variables that affect their health care.

Nurse practitioners who have participated in a global health experience have demonstrated improved comprehensive physical assessment skills and the ability to recognize infectious disease processes while displaying a higher sensitivity to cultural norms. NPs report an improved ability to work as a team, solving problems without the use of technology or laboratory equipment and dependent upon the knowledge and expertise of the entire team to determine the proper course of treatment. These health professionals work closely treating health problems that they may not have encountered in their practice, broadening their assessment skills.

For the past 12 years I have fostered a relationship with communities in the inner city of Kingston, Jamaica, an area known for poverty and violence. Teams of physicians and NPs work together to deliver care to this population, and we have become the primary care for many of the people living in these communities. The professionals who work in makeshift clinics spend upwards of 12 hours a day working outside under a tent or in a small community building or church, treating over 100 patients a day. Diabetes and hypertension have crossed all borders, but the challenge is trying to educate and prevent. Skin diseases, parasites, childhood and acute medical emergencies, and the need for gynecological and surgical intervention present themselves when caring for a segment of an entire population. Over the years we have built a trusting relationship, while allowing professionals to practice primary care at the purest level, and have made a difference in the overall care of these communities.

Global experiences are not limited to far-away exotic locations. Diverse populations can be found throughout the world in the most advanced cities as well as rural locations. It is the opportunity to expose health professionals to primary care by bringing that level of care to a patient in the environment in which he or she resides that labels it a "global experience." As members of the global community, it is our duty to care for each other.

Clearly there are many pertinent issues for the NP that have been briefly covered in this chapter as a supplement to comprehensive coursework. The NP/DNP is poised to take on a leadership role in assessing population health, designing interventions to improve community and population health, evaluating health outcomes of those interventions and programs, and implementing changes to improve programs. It is hoped that ideas for health promotion and disease prevention topics for individual patients, families, and communities, as well as national and even global communities, have been stimulated. It is up to the NP/DNP to make a difference in clinical prevention and population health.

Seminar Discussion Questions

1. Identify three priority issues for improving health in your community.
2. Describe the incidence and prevalence of a disease monitored in your state.
3. Discuss each of the three prevention levels as it pertains to the disease you chose.
4. Imagine starting your own clinical practice where you are able to practice to the full extent of your scope of practice.
   a. What population would you be providing care for, and why?
   b. What are three measures for evaluating improved health outcomes for your chosen population?
5. Using the PRECEDE-PROCEED model, draft a program plan and an evaluation of a health need.

References

American Association of Colleges of Nursing. (2006). *The essentials of master's education in nursing.* Washington, DC: Author.

Association for Prevention Teaching and Research. (2009). *Clinical prevention and population health curriculum framework.* Retrieved from http://c.ymcdn.com/sites/www.aptrweb.org/resource/resmgr/2011_ajpm/revised_cpph_framework_2009.pdf

Branson, B. M., Handsfield, H. H., Lampe, M. A., Janssen, R. S., Taylor, A. W., Lyss, S. B., & Clark, J. E. (2006). Revised recommendations for HIV testing of adults, adolescents, and pregnant women in health-care settings. *MMWR Recommendations and Reports, 55*(RR-14), 1–17.

Burke, R. C., Sepkowitz, K. A., Bernstein, K. T., Karpati, A. M, Myers, J. E., Tsoi, B. W., & Beiger, E. M. (2007). Why don't physicians test for HIV? A review of the US literature. *AIDS, 21*, 1617–1624.

Cawley, J. F. (July, 2012). Primary care and population health. *Advance for NPs and PAs, 3*(7), 16.

Centers for Disease Control and Prevention. (2009c). *Leading causes of death 1900–1998.* National Vital Statistics System. Retrieved from http://www.cdc.gov/nchs/data/dvs/lead1900_98.pdf

Centers for Disease Control and Prevention. (2012). *Principles of epidemiology in public health practice* (3rd ed.). Retrieved from http://www.cdc.gov/osels/scientific_edu/SS1978/Lesson1/Section10.html

Crosby, R., & Noar, S. (2011). What is a planning model? An introduction to PRECEDE-PROCEED. *Journal of Public Health Dentistry*, 71. doi:10.1111/j.1752-7325.2011.00235.x

Curley, A., & Vitale, P. (Eds.). (2012). *Population-based nursing: Concepts and competencies for advanced practice.* New York, NY: Springer Publishing.

de Chesnay, M., & Anderson, B. A. (2016). *Caring for the vulnerable: Perspectives in nursing theory, practice, and research* (4th ed.). Burlington, MA: Jones & Bartlett Learning.

Fos, P. (2011). *Epidemiology foundations: The science of public health.* San Francisco, CA: Jossey-Bass.

Fries, K., & Stewart, J. (2012). Partnering with those we serve: Using experiential learning activities to support community nursing practice. *Creative Nursing, 18*(3), 93–97.

Friis, R. H., & Sellers, A. T. (2004). *Epidemiology for public health practice* (3rd ed.). Sudbury, MA: Jones and Bartlett.

Green, L., & Kreuter, M. K. (2005). *Health program planning: An educational and ecological approach* (4th ed.). New York, NY: McGraw-Hill.

He, W., Goodkind, D., & Kowal, P. (2016). *An aging world: 2015*. U.S. Census Bureau, International Population Reports, P95/16-1, U.S. Government Publishing Office, Washington, DC.

Henry J. Kaiser Family Foundation. (2012). *The HIV/AIDS epidemic in the United States* (fact sheet). Menlo Park, CA: Author.

Hoyert, D. L., & Xu, J. Q. (2012). Deaths: Preliminary data for 2011. *National Vital Statistics Reports, 61*(6). Hyattsville, MD: National Center for Health Statistics.

Institute of Medicine. (2012). *Primary care and public health: Exploring integration to improve population health*. Washington, DC: National Academies Press. Retrieved from http://www.iom.edu/Reports/2012/Primary-Care-and-Public-Health.aspx

Keshavjee, S., & Farmer, P. (2012). Tuberculosis, drug resistance, and the history of modern medicine. *New England Journal of Medicine, 67*(10), 931–936.

Koh, H. K. (2010). Perspective: Healthy People 2020. *New England Journal of Medicine, 362*(18), 1653–1656.

Maurer, F. A., & Smith, C. S. (2009). *Community/public health nursing practice: Health for families and populations* (4th ed.). St. Louis, MO: Saunders Elsevier.

National Center for HIV/AIDS, Viral Hepatitis, STD, and TB Prevention. (2011). *U.S. Public Health Service syphilis study at Tuskegee*. Retrieved from http://www.cdc.gov/tuskegee/timeline.htm

National Institute on Aging. (2007). *Why population aging matters: A global perspective*. Washington, DC: Author.

Nurses' Health Study. (2012). *Homepage*. Retrieved from http://www.channing.harvard.edu/nhs

Office of the Surgeon General. (2013). *Strategic plan DCVMRC* (2011–2013). Retrieved from https://medicalreservecorps.gov/pageViewFldr/About/StrategicPlan1113

Sullivan-Marx, E., McGivern, D., Fairman, S., & Greenberg, S. (Eds.). (2010). *Nurse practitioners: The evolution and future of advanced practice* (5th ed.). New York, NY: Springer.

USAID. (2012). *MEASURE evaluation*. Retrieved from http://www.cpc.unc.edu/measure/tools/population-health-and-environment/population-health-and-environment-training-materials/PHE%20complete%20indicator%20matrix%20example.doc/view

U.S. Department of Health and Human Services. (2016a). *Guidelines for the use of antiretroviral agents in HIV-1-infected adults and adolescents*. Retrieved from https://aidsinfo.nih.gov/guidelines/html/1/adult-and-adolescent-treatment-guidelines/0/

U.S. Department of Health and Human Services. (2016b). *Guidelines for the use of prevention and treatment of opportunistic infections in HIV-infected adults and adolescents*. Retrieved from https://aidsinfo.nih.gov/contentfiles/lvguidelines/adult_oi.pdf

U.S. Department of Health and Human Services. (2017). *Guidelines for the use of antiretroviral agents in pediatric HIV infection*. Retrieved from https://aidsinfo.nih.gov/guidelines/html/2/pediatric-arv-guidelines/0

Van Leuven, K. (2012). Population aging: Implications for nurse practitioners. *Journal for Nurse Practitioners, 8*(7), 554–559.

World Health Organization. (2012). *Epidemiology*. Retrieved from http://www.who.int/topics/epidemiology/en

World Health Organization. (2013). *HIV/AIDS*. Retrieved from http://www.who.int/hiv/en

Additional Resources

Macha, K., & McDonough, J. (2012). *Epidemiology for advanced nursing practice*. Sudbury, MA: Jones & Bartlett Learning.

WHO, UNAIDS, & UNICEF. (2011). *Global HIV/AIDS response—Progress report 2011*. Retrieved from http://whqlibdoc.who.int/publications/2011/9789241502986_eng.pdf

CHAPTER 9

Electronic Health Record and Impact on Healthcare Outcomes

Stephen C. Burrows

Moving to Electronic Documentation/Electronic Health Record: Reasons for Doing So

Implementation of an electronic health record (EHR) has great potential to improve quality of care that paper medical records cannot provide. An EHR can offer many benefits for clinicians and their patients and provide functions that are not available without the technology in place. The reasons to convert from paper records to EHRs are many.

Greater Access to More Complete and Accurate Patient Information

An EHR allows clinicians access to the information necessary to deliver quality health care that ensures the "right care to the right patient at the right time—every time" (Clancy, 2009). King, Patel, Jamoom, and Furukawa (2014) examined the clinical benefits provided by EHRs to physicians by reviewing data from two large surveys of office-based physicians in the United States. With over 3,000 physician responses, King et al. concluded that "over three-quarters of EHR adopters reported that EHR use enhanced patient care overall" (2014, p. 400). Specifically, physicians were reported to state "to varying degrees, EHR adopters reported benefits of EHR use for specific measures of clinical quality, patient safety, and efficiency" (King et al., 2014, p. 400). Access to more complete information from evaluation and treatment strengthens the provider's clinical decision-making process by presenting a more complete picture of the patient's clinical picture. Legibility of handwriting is not an issue when information is entered into and accessed from an EHR.

Increased Care Coordination

EHRs provide better access to data than their paper counterparts. Sharing of patient information among physician, therapist, and other healthcare providers, hospitals, and health systems is greatly facilitated coordination of care. A number of studies have looked at the effectiveness of EHRs in the coordination of care (Goetz Goldberg, Kuzel, Feng, DeShazo, & Love, 2012; Goldzweig, Towfigh, Maglione, & Shekelle, 2005; O'Malley, Grossman, Cohen, Kemper, & Pham, 2010). O'Malley et al. found "that commercial ambulatory care EMRs facilitate care coordination within a practice by making data available at the point of care" (2010, p. 183). Goetz Goldberg et al. reported the greatest value and benefit to clinicians using EHRs as "increased organization, accessibility, and accuracy of patient documentation" (2012, p. e50). This was further evidenced by their findings regarding improvement in the quality of care performance measures "such as mammography screening and diabetes care, as demonstrated through performance reports shared with our research team" (p. e51).

Greater Efficiency

Paper charts no longer need to be located and transported to the clinician. Electronic charts are more easily located and often allow more than one person to work within a chart at the same time ("EMR Medical Software Information and Resources: Top Reasons to Implement an Electronic Medical Records Software System," n.d.). Walker et al. (2005) examined the value of electronic exchange of healthcare information between providers including the bidirectional exchange with laboratories, imaging centers, pharmacies, and others. With full national exchange in place, they estimated a net savings of "$77.8 billion annually, or approximately 5 percent of the projected $1.661 trillion spent on U.S. health care in 2003" (pp. W5-16). More modest savings can be seen in the ambulatory sector through a reduction in transcription costs as well as the cost for chart pull, storage, and refiling. Improved documentation can support more accurate reimbursement coding ("Improve Medical Practice Management with Electronic Health Records | Providers & Professionals | HealthIT.gov," n.d.).

Patient Participation and Empowerment

Providers and patients sharing access to electronic health information supports a collaborative environment of informed decision making and promotes patient participation in the management of chronic conditions. Providers can give patients "full and accurate information about all of their medical evaluations" and "create an avenue for communication with their patients" ("Increase Patient Participation in Care with Health IT | Providers & Professionals | HealthIT.gov," n.d.). Included with this more active role in their care, patients can receive electronic copies of their medical records after a clinical visit or hospital stay along with improved instructions, information, and education.

▶ Influencing Forces

The implementation and use of EHRs is one of the highest priorities for healthcare providers, organizations, and government agencies in the United States (Webster, 2010). In April 2004, then-president George W. Bush signed Executive Order 13335 ("Presidential Documents: Executive Order 13335 of April 27, 2004 Incentives for the Use of Health Information Technology and Establishing the Position of the National Health Information Technology Coordinator," 2004). This provided for the establishment of the Office of the National Coordinator for Health Information Technology (ONCHIT) and created the "leadership" as well as a national vision for the "development and nationwide implementation of an interoperable health information technology infrastructure to improve the quality and efficiency of health care" ("Presidential Documents: Executive Order 13335 of April 27, 2004 Incentives for the Use of Health Information Technology and Establishing the Position of the National Health Information Technology Coordinator," 2004, p. 160). Over the ensuing years, several strategies, committees, and contracts were created and awarded. While the expectation was that many physicians would jump on board the EHR train, very few did. In 2008, DesRoches et al. stated only "4% of physicians reported" were using a "fully functional electronic records system, and 13% reported having a basic system" (2008, p. 54). Decker, Jamoom, and Sisk (2012) found, as of 2011, only "24.2% of physicians in solo or two-physician practices had adopted a basic EHR, compared with 37.1% of groups of three to nine physicians and 60% of physicians in groups of 10 or more (p. 1111). Shamus and Stern (2011) reported among physical therapists "anecdotal evidence suggests only 13–15% of physical therapists" and "most of these cases appear to be in the inpatient environment" (p. 196). These rates of adoption suggest "that EHRs will reach maximum penetration by the year 2024," 10 years beyond President Bush's original goal of 2104 (Zandieh et al., 2008, p. 755). Recognizing this, Meaningful Use (MU) was created: "Yet we have not moved significantly to extend the availability of EHRs from a few large institutions to the smaller clinics and practices where most Americans receive their health care" (Blumenthal & Tavenner, 2010, p. 501).

In February 2009, then-president Barack Obama signed into law the American Recovery and Reinvestment Act (ARRA). Often called the "The Stimulus Act," it appropriated federal expenditures toward a variety of national projects across differing sectors of the U.S. economy. Included within ARRA was the Health Information Technology for Economic and Clinical Health Act (HITECH) providing $17.2 billion for incentives and $2 billion for grants toward "supporting the adoption and use of EHRs" which will "support [the] liftoff for the creation of a nationwide system of EHRs" (Blumenthal & Tavenner, 2010, p. 501). Equally important, HITECH's goal is not adoption alone but "meaningful use" of EHRs (Blumenthal & Tavenner, 2010, p. 501; Spicer, 2009; Wright, Feblowitz, Samal, McCoy, & Sittig, 2014).

Meaningful Use

Eligible providers (EPs) and eligible hospitals (EHs) may participate in Meaningful Use, and receive the incentive dollars through the "Medicare and Medicaid EHR Incentive Programs" by using certified EHR technology and demonstrating "that they are meaningfully using their EHRs by meeting thresholds for a number of objectives" ("How to Attain Meaningful Use," 2014).

The final rule establishing the three stages of Meaningful Use was announced by the Centers of Medicare & Medicaid Services (CMS) in July 2010 and is designed to support EPs and EHs with implementing and using EHRs in a "meaningful" way with the ultimate goal of improving the quality and safety of health care in the United States ("What Is 'Meaningful Use'?," n.d.). Each of the three stages has specific goals, priorities, and increasing requirements (**FIGURE 9-1**).

Stage 1

Stage 1 began in 2011 and includes the basic functionalities for EHRs. The requirements are focused on providers capturing patient data and sharing that data either with the patient or with other healthcare professionals.

"Data capture and sharing"

- Electronically capturing health information in a standardized format
- Using that information to track key clinical conditions
- Communicating that information for care coordination processes
- Initiating the reporting of clinical quality measures and public health information
- Using information to engage patients and their families in their care

Stage 2

Stage 2 began in 2014 and looks toward the use of advanced clinical processes. The requirements in this stage are focused on health information exchange between providers and promotes patient engagement by giving patients secure online access to their health information.

"Advanced clinical processes"

- More rigorous health information exchange (HIE)
- Increased requirements for e-prescribing and incorporating lab results
- Electronic transmission of patient care summaries across multiple settings
- More patient-controlled data

Stage 3

"Improved outcomes"

- Improving quality, safety, and efficiency, leading to improved health outcomes
- Decision support for national high-priority conditions
- Patient access to self-management tools
- Access to comprehensive patient data through patient-centered HIE
- Improving population health ("How to Attain Meaningful Use," 2014, "Meaningful Use, Meaningful Use definition, EHR Technology: HITECH Answers," n.d.)

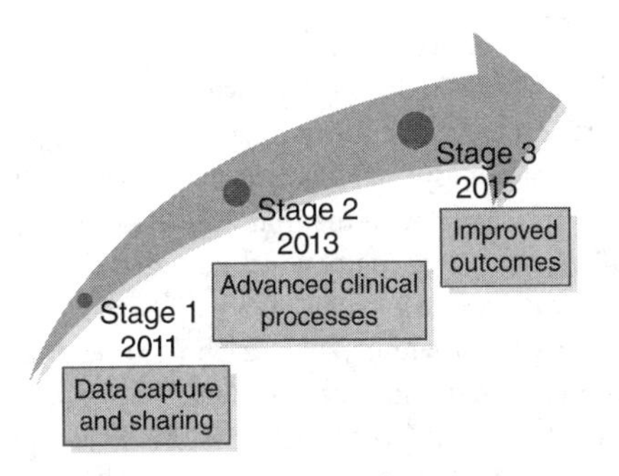

FIGURE 9-1 A Conceptual Approach to Meaningful Use

Reproduced from Centers for Medicare & Medicaid Services. (2010). Medicare & Medicaid EHR Incentive Program: Meaningful Use Stage 1 Requirements Overview. Retrieved from https://www.cms.gov/Regulations-and-Guidance/Legislation/EHRIncentivePrograms/downloads/MU_Stage1_ReqOverview.pdf

Until 2015, the EHR Incentive Program provides bonuses for eligible professionals and hospitals. After that time, EPs and EHs that do not meet meaningful use criteria through the use of EHR technology will be subject to a financial penalty. EPs and EHs will have their Medicare fee schedule reduced by 1%. This will be followed in 2016 by a 2% downward adjustment and 3% in 2017 and thereafter ("Are there penalties for providers who don't switch to electronic health records (EHR)? | FAQs | Providers & Professionals | HealthIT.gov," n.d.).

Each of the Meaningful Use stages has multiple clinically related measures with which EPs and EHs must meet to receive the bonus payments. By focusing not only on the implementation of certified EHRs but also on their meaningful use through the submission of the measures, the EHR Incentive Program is about "the effective use of EHRs to achieve health and efficiency" and to "improve the quality, safety, and efficiency of care while reducing disparities" ("What Is 'Meaningful Use'?," n.d.).

In 2008, the American Physical Therapy Association, House of Delegates demonstrated their support of the use of EHRs through the release of position statement HOD P06-08-13-11, "Support of Electronic Health Record in Physical Therapy," stating "the American Physical Therapy Association supports the use of electronic health record systems (EHRs) and promotes the widespread adoption of interoperable EHRs in all physical therapy practice settings" (American Physical Therapy Association, 2008).

The Electronic Health Record

Numerous terms are used to describe the concept of an EHR. However, basically it can be defined as providing "real-time, patient-centered records . . . available instantly and securely to authorized users" ("What is an electronic health record (EHR)? | FAQs | Providers & Professionals | HealthIT.gov," n.d.). Additionally, EHRs are thought of as a "longitudinal electronic record of patient health information generated by one or more encounters in any care delivery setting" ("Electronic Health Records | Health IT Topics | HIMSS," n.d.).

Often, the terms electronic medical record (EMR) and electronic health record (EHR) are used interchangeably. It is important to note that these terms describe completely different concepts albeit dependent on each other. Electronic medical records are often thought of as simply the digital version of the paper medical record from a single clinician's office. It is the "legal record created in hospitals and ambulatory environments" (Garets & Davis, 2006, p. 2) and contains important pieces of the patient's medical history including medical diagnoses, prescribed medication, provider generated treatment plans, immunization records, medication and food or environmental allergies, radiology imaging, and laboratory results (Garrett & Seidman, 2011). An EHR contains all of the items that are in an EMR plus others that focus on the patients entire health by "going beyond standard clinical data collected in the provider's office and inclusive of a broader view on a patient's care" by sharing "information with other health care providers, such as laboratories and specialists" (Garrett & Seidman, 2011). The National Alliance for Health Information Technology adds that EHRs contain functions that "conform to nationally recognized interoperability standards and that can be created, managed, and consulted by authorized clinicians and staff across more than one health care organization" (The National Alliance for Health Information Technology, 2008, p. 6).

Benefits of Using an EHR

1. Improved quality of patient care
   Kern, Barrón, Dhopeshwarkar, Edwards, and Kaushal (2013) looked at data from 4,403 ambulatory providers and the effect using an EHR might have on several quality indicators—hemoglobin A1c testing for diabetic patients, breast cancer screening, chlamydia screening, and colorectal cancer screening. They found the physicians who were using an EHR "provided significantly higher rates of recommended care than physicians using paper for [the] four quality measures. . . . The magnitude of the differences between EHR use and paper for these measures ranged from approximately 3 to 13 percentage points" (p. 500).
   Electronic health records also have the potential to improve quality of care by providing rapid access to more complete patient records and by providing enhanced decision support, clinical alerts, reminders, and medical information.
2. Reduction in medical errors
   Zlabek, Wickus, and Mathiason (2009) reported a 14% decrease in medication errors and a 38.9% decrease in near misses per 1,000 hospital days after computerized provider order entry (CPOE) was implemented in their hospital.
3. Improved care coordination and communication
   A number of studies have looked at the effectiveness of EHRs in the coordination of care (Goetz Goldberg et al., 2012; Goldzweig et al., 2005; O'Malley et al., 2010). O'Malley et al. (2010) found "that commercial ambulatory care EMRs facilitate care coordination within a practice by making data available at the point of care" (p. 183). Goetz Goldberg et al. (2012) reported the greatest value and benefit to clinicians using EHRs as "increased organization, accessibility, and accuracy of patient documentation" (p. e50). This was further evidenced by their findings regarding improvement in the quality of care performance measures "such as mammography screening and diabetes care, as demonstrated through performance reports shared with our research team" (p. e51).
4. Enhanced patient safety

EHRs are ideal for alerting providers to allergies, drug interactions, abnormal laboratory test findings, and redundant test orders. As an EHR becomes more comprehensive and "intelligent," it can trigger provider-alerts to health safety issues such as newly identified medication side effects, product recalls, and new strategies for disease management and preventive care. Such a system would allow a provider to "preemptively" notify patients of important health issues based on a continual automated process of cross-referencing of their medical histories with the latest medical findings. That could change health care from an encounter- and patient-complaint-driven system of care to a more proactive approach to complete health management.

5. Increased efficiencies and cost savings
   Kazley, Simpson, Simpson, and Teufel (2014) looked at national data representing individuals 18 years or older who were admitted for inpatient care. Examining data of over 5 million patients from 550 hospitals, they found a 9.66% reduction in the average cost per patient when treated in a hospital with advanced EHRs.
   Zlabek, Wickus, and Mathiason (2009) investigated the cost savings impact of EHR implementation. They examined data over a 2-year period (1 year pre-EHR and 1 year post-EHR implementation). Among a number of other factors, they found a 74.6% drop in monthly transcription costs for a total yearly reduction of $667,896 and a 26.6% reduction in the cost of copy paper for an annual savings of $11,815.
   In the ambulatory sector, Adler-Milstein, Salzberg, Franz, Orav, and Bates (2013) found an average reduction of $41.60 per member per month among Medicare beneficiaries when using an EHR. Due to their very nature, EHRs provide the time-saving efficiency of "collect data once, then use it many times" (American Physical Therapy Association, n.d.).
6. Increased population health
   Electronic health records have great potential for public and palpitation health through their ability to allow the aggregation of multiple sets of patient data and by "improving the reporting and investigation of diseases and conditions that are mandated for reporting to state and local public health agencies" (Friedman, Parrish, & Ross, 2013, p. 1561). Electronic health records also have the potential to provide estimates of "disease burden and its distribution in the population and population subgroups. Such estimates could facilitate program planning, targeting, implementation, and monitoring (Friedman et al., 2013, p. 1561).

Health Information Exchange

One of the ways in which full advantage of EHRs can be taken is through the electronic exchange of patient data. The goal of Meaningful Use is not to simply create isolated islands of clinical data but to form interconnected databases capable of leveraging each other's strengths. A health information exchange (HIE) is "the electronic movement of health-related information among organizations . . . to facilitate access to and retrieval of clinical data to provide safer, timelier, efficient, effective, equitable, patient-centered care" (Health Resources and Services Administration, n.d.-b). It is the vision of the U.S. federal government to create "an interoperable health IT ecosystem (that) makes the right data available to the right people at the right time across products and organizations in a way that can be relied upon and meaningfully used by recipients" (Office of the National Coordinator for Health IT, n.d., p. 2).

Barriers and Challenges to EHR Adoption

There are many obstacles to adoption of an EHR. These obstacles can be divided into a number of categories.

1. Financial

   The initial purchase cost of an EHR can be expensive. Estimates for the initial purchase of an EHR vary from $15,000 to $70,000 per provider with most averaging about $30,000 (Fleming, Culler, McCorkle, Becker, & Ballard, 2011; "How much is this going to cost me? | FAQs | Providers & Professionals | HealthIT.gov," n.d.). Costs for larger institutions (multiple-hospital health system) can reach over $600 million when all costs are considered (software licensing purchase, software/hardware upgrades, staffing, etc.) (Eastaugh, 2013, p. 51). Costs that haven't been completely considered can also provide a financial drain: "Hospital boards and managers too frequently consider only the initial cost of acquisition plus initial annual maintenance fees when considering EHR bids" (p. 36).

   In addition to these costs, there is inevitably a loss of productivity during the initial phases of implementation. Wang et al. (2003) estimate this to be a "temporary loss of productivity. . . . of 20% in the first month, 10% in the second month, and 5% in the third month, with a subsequent return to baseline productivity levels" (Wang et al., 2003, p. 398).
2. Technical
   a. Electronic health records are complex systems and require a certain level of computer skills by those who may be using the software. Many clinicians have "insufficient technical knowledge and skills to deal with EMRs, and that this results in resistance" (Boonstra & Broekhuis, 2010, p. 4). It is imperative that all users receive "proper technical training and support" prior to any EHR implementation (Boonstra & Broekhuis, 2010, p. 8).
   b. To overcome some of this fear, training is highly recommended. Bredfeldt, Awad, Joseph, and Snyder (2013) surveyed providers who were undergoing implementation and found "the providers valued advanced training on EHR tools and workflows, to the extent that they were willing to participate on Saturdays and return for additional content" (p. 8).
3. Complexity of selection and implementation process

   Selecting the most appropriate EHR can be a daunting task. It is estimated that there are over 400 software vendors from whom to select a product. Most clinicians are uncertain where to begin.
4. Organizational change barriers

   Implementation of a system as large and complex as an EHR represents tremendous change for any organization. There is bound to be moderate to significant disruption of workflow and processes (Carayon,

Smith, Hundt, Kuruchittham, & Li, 2009). Lin, Lin, and Roan (2012) pinpoint the attitude toward change: "Change, after all, causes people concern and is closely followed by a sense of anxiety, insecurity, inequity and threat" (p. 1967). Implementation of an EHR typically involved approaches to "change management" (Giniat, Benton, Biegansky, & Grossman, 2012; Health Management Technology, 2010; Henderson, Schoonbeek, & Auditore, 2013).

Converting to Electronic Health Record

When converting to electronic documentation, there are a number of imperative steps be taken to ensure a successful implementation. Preparing for a successful conversion requires both the right approach and mindset as much as the right technology selection.

Preparation

Setting Goal and Vision

First and perhaps foremost is having a clear vision of the end state being pursued. A few simple questions can help this process: What is it we are trying to achieve? Why are we implementing an EHR? What are the reasons to do so?

Having a shared vision means "goals and benefits are clearly defined, meaningful and measurable . . . [the] organization knows what success looks like and how to achieve it. Once the goals are set, it is essential to communicate that vision with all of those who will be involved in the process. Keep the vision visible; once it has been created, share it with various people and revisit it often" (Merrill, n.d.).

After gaining an understanding of the organization's vision, an EHR selection committee should be formed. This group consists of individuals from cross-institutional settings and brings "differing perspectives on how the EHR will be used . . . possess[es] a wide array of skills and knowledge . . . consist[s] of true end users and not just personnel who make IT purchasing decisions" ("Who should be on the electronic health record selection committee? | FAQs | Providers & Professionals | HealthIT.gov," n.d.).

Readiness Assessment

Evaluating an organization's readiness to adopt an EHR provides a window into the areas that need attending. This step helps clarify the state of readiness of all members of an organization for EHR adoption, how an organization is using current resources, and what steps you need to take for successful adoption of an EHR.

Available Resources

Understand resources available for the EHR implementation. This includes funding for purchase, upgrades to current technology infrastructure, and personnel. This applies to both current size and needs as well as any potential or future growth. Determine your facility's current number of sites and users.

Workflow Documentation

Although this step is too often overlooked or not completed fully, understanding the current processes and how they will be completed in an EHR is prerequisite to a successful implementation. Documenting current workflow consists of recording (in written or graphical form) who is involved in each step of how business occurs. This will also assist in identifying changes that could occur with implementation and with use.

Request for Proposal

Once these factors have been assessed, vendor seeking may begin. From the list of required functionality, current resources, and the organization's vision, potential vendors can be narrowed down. To better understand how each may fulfill the needs of an organization, a request for proposal (RFP) can be prepared. This document is provided to selected vendors and solicits responses to specific information about their product and what their specific approach is to EHR implementation. A thorough RFP is typically a lengthy document and asks the vendor to provide general company information (length of time in business, number of employees, number of implementations), current EHR functionality (in response to organizations' specific needs as identified during the readiness assessment), how the vendor's system will follow the organization's current workflow, how much customization is necessary and what is the cost, timeline for implementation and personnel involved, and the technologic requirements of the vendor's EHR. It is solid practice to request a vendor to provide a reference list of current customers who may be contacted and with whom a site visit may be scheduled. Vendor response to the RFP aids in narrowing the vendor candidates.

Communication Plan

Implementation of technology almost always entails change. Communicating the vision, plan, and expectations to all of the organization's members can ensure a successful outcome.

System/Product Selection

Choosing an EHR system that is "best" for an organization or facility can be an extremely daunting and overwhelming process. Ensuring a system will meet everyone's needs now and in the future is crucial. Often, users of an EHR will have one understanding of their "needs" and EHR capability will be different. Before choosing, understanding the users' requirements as well as the capability of different EHRs helps bring these two together. Key functionality needs to be identified and will be used to evaluate specific areas of the EHR. This step essentially assesses an EHR system's "fit" for an organization.

Vendor Demonstration

Once the RFP process has been completed and the potential EHRs have been narrowed to three or four options, onsite demonstrations of product functionality should be conducted. Potential vendors are invited to the organization to meet with the EHR selection committee and other key members of the organization. This is a vital step in understanding the functionality and capabilities of a potential EHR. Vendors should be asked to demonstrate how their product fulfills the organization's needs as set forth in the vision and goals as well as conforming to the current workflow and crucial needs in the RFP. It is most advantageous to use a standard set of scenarios that each vendor completes. In addition, having an objective scoring tool such as the American Academy of Family Physicians "Vendor Rating Tool" can provide subjective assessment of the EHR system being evaluated, to aid in the final decision.

Contracting

Once the product has been selected, contracting can begin. It is advisable to have vendor contracts reviewed by legal counsel. These documents list areas of vendor and provider accountability. "A carefully negotiated contract can minimize future problems with the EHR vendor and create an equally beneficial relationship for the vendor and provider" (American College of Surgeons, n.d.). Successful negotiation of an EHR contract will provide the fairest terms agreeable to both parties.

Implementation

Implementation involves the installation of the EHR system and other preparatory activities. The final project team is identified and an installation schedule developed. This stage comprises all of the necessary activities from contract signing until the actual "go-live."

Configuration

Prior to the EHR being used, the software must be installed and configured. The technology on which the EHR runs may need to be purchased or upgraded. This step includes the "creation and maintenance of the physical environment in which the system will operate" (HealthIT.gov, 2014). Often newer servers or other technology will need to be purchased and installed. Tasks may include setting up documentation templates for common types of visits or procedures; configuring data lists for diagnoses, medications, allegories, orders, etc.; and adding other customized items as identified during workflow analysis.

Training

Once the system is configured for the organization's needs, staff need to learn to use it. Depending on the size of the implementation, vendors may provide onsite classroom-based training. Other options include web-based training led by an instructor and self-guided scenarios. Training usually involves identifying a select number of "super users" who receive intense training and are then expected to train and assist other users (Health Resources and Services Administration, n.d.-a).

Testing

Ensuring that the EHR is configured correctly is essential prior to go-live. Testing of the EHR is "the process of executing a program or system with the intent of finding errors" (Jiantao Pan, n.d.) and ideally should be accomplished in a systemic manner. Testing plans are standard scenarios that, when followed, provide expected outcomes.

Many vendors will provide high-level testing plans. Customized plans based on the organization's configuration are also necessary to fully test the system.

Paper Chart Migration

Patient information recorded on paper needs to be transitioned to the EHR. This can seem like an overwhelming task given the amount of information contained in the paper charts; however, there are different methods to managing this task. Most organizations opt for an abstracting approach whereby only pertinent pieces of the patient's record are entered into the EHR (diagnosis, medications, allergies, procedures, etc.) and only for a finite period of time in the past (~7 years, depending on state laws). It is not recommended to create an electronic image of the entire patient record by scanning all of the paper pages as this can be extremely time consuming and uses significant technology resources (American Academy of Family Physicians, n.d.). It is then advised to only pull paper charts for a visit or two after go-live.

Go-Live

After all preparations have been completed, the EHR software will become "active" at the time of go-live. This can be a stressful time but can be minimized with some preparations. A smooth go-live requires that a number of details are addressed. Supporting the organization is key to a successful go-live. Many organizations designate a room or space as the "command center" and house support personnel in this one location to best support the end users on go-live day. In smaller organizations, this could be a corner of the staff lunch room. It is best to also provide "at the elbow" support of all users on the initial days or weeks. Many software vendors can provide onsite support but the cost may be a burden for small organizations. The previously identified "super users" can be utilized for this capacity.

Many organizations find it helpful to reduce patient schedules and load during a go-live. This will allow the organization to focus on a successful rollout. An alternative is to go live with a portion of providers or all providers using limited functionality.

Part of the aforementioned communication plan should include other key individuals and third parties such as other vendors (e.g., billing company) of the intended go-live date.

Post Go-Live

Once the hard work of implementing the EHR has been completed, there are additional steps to be taken to ensure its continued use and smooth operation.

- Ensure system backups are occurring and have been tested and validated. EHR data need to be backed up on a regular basis and the data's integrity ensured in the rare event of a system failure.
- Downtime procedures should be established should the EHR not be available. Most organizations become highly dependent on EHRs but still need to function should the system be unavailable. Paper copies of all patient forms, templates, etc., need to be available in the event of a system failure.
- Upgrades are handled differently by different EHR vendors. It is vital to understand your vendor's approach. Upgrades may occur in the background without affecting any users and therefore do not affect daily performance. Others may require downtime requiring the system to be unavailable.

Electronic Health Records Features and Functionality

In 2003, The Institute of Medicine released "Key Capabilities of an Electronic Health Record System" and determined there to be eight core functions of an EHR:

1. Health information and data
   Essentially, the EHR should "contain certain data about patients" in order that clinicians "make sound clinical decisions" (Committee on Data Standards for Patient Safety, 2003, p. 7).
2. Result management
   Electronically available test results provide distinctive advantages over those that are reported on paper. Once electronic, these results can be more easily accessed when they are needed thereby reducing lag time. Having searchable data also reduces redundant testing and provides better interpretation and easier detection of abnormalities.
3. Order management
   There has been much written regarding the benefits of computerized provider order entry (COPOE) (Bates & Gawande, 2003; Martin, 2004; O'Connor, 2004). COPOE provides medication dose and frequency, allergy checking, and other clinical decision support functions.
4. Decision support
   Discussed further in another part of this chapter, clinical decision support (CDS) provides clinicians, staff, patients, or other individuals with person-specific, actionable knowledge that is "intelligently filtered or presented at appropriate times, to enhance health and health care" (HealthIT.gov, 2013, para. 1). Clinical decision support utilizes alerts and reminders to providers and patients based on clinical guidelines that "improve health and healthcare delivery" (HealthcareITNews, 2014, para 2.
5. Electronic communication and connectivity
   Coordination of care, as detailed earlier in this chapter, can only be accomplished if all parties are connected electronically (Burton, Anderson, & Kues, 2004).
6. Patient support
   Evidence has shown that patients engaged in their care have "better outcomes . . . and, some evidence suggests, lower costs" (Health Affairs, 2013, p. 1). It is believed to be "shared decision making, in which patients and providers together consider the patient's condition, treatment options, the medical evidence behind the treatment options, the benefits and risks of treatment, and patients' preferences, and then arrive at and execute a treatment plan" (p. 2).
7. Administrative processes
   EHRs can assist with many of the nonclinical functions such as billing and claims, inpatient census, outpatient procedures, etc., to improve the efficiency of healthcare organizations (Committee on Data Standards for Patient Safety, 2003).
8. Reporting and population health
   As compared to patient health, population health is "the health outcomes of a group of individuals, including the distribution of such outcomes

within the group" (Kindig & Stoddart, 2003, p. 381). With the availability of electronic clinical data, organizations can improve populations of patients with "increase[d] . . . accuracy of the data reported" (Committee on Data Standards for Patient Safety, 2003, p. 11).

Technical Considerations

When adopting technology, there are a number of technical details to consider and concepts to keep in mind. This section will discuss architectural approaches to an EHR as well as the implementations options.

Architecture

Electronic health records will often be available via one of two methods.

In an application service provider (ASP) platform, software is "hosted" by the vendor and customers "rent the use of the application and access it over the Internet or via a private line connection" (PC Magazine, n.d.). Commonly known as "cloud computing," this is also called "software as a service" (SaaS). With this model, the organization needs to have a connection to internet to access the software. The vendor/host is responsible for all software updates, hardware maintenance and upgrades, and system availability. This can represent a significant reduction in cost for a smaller organization. Alternatively, with the client-server option, the organization hosts the EHR software on an in-house computer system (called a server). This can require large capital expenditures and internal IT staffing to ensure that the system is properly supported and maintained. Servers are typically out of date within 3 to 4 years and thus need replacing. This model is used in larger organizations that can afford the initial financial outlay and ongoing costs to update, maintain, and repair the internal network as needed.

Best-of-Breed Versus Integrated Systems

With the complexity of EHRs and other clinical information systems, coupled with the intricate needs and size of many larger organizations, not all EHR products are able to meet their customers' needs. Best-of-breed involves purchasing different software systems from more than one vendor to obtain the best "fit" for each function or department. For instance, healthcare organizations may purchase the clinical documentation system from one vendor, human resources module from another, and radiology from a third. This approach is followed when organizations have very specific needs and one vendor is unable to fulfill them. In order for information to be exchanged between these disparate systems, electronic interfaces need to be created. This can be a costly (both in time and resources) undertaking and often creates a discordant environment where information may not always be exchanged as expected.

Contrary to the best-of-breed system is an integrated system. With this model, all software is purchased from a single vendor and configures such that the complication of an interface is not necessary. Some refer to this as a "single database" or source of data. This can also simplify support in that a single vendor provides the convenience of a single point of contact for support and technical concerns.

Hardware Options

Selecting the correct hardware on which the EHR will run is an important decision in the success of the project. Many options are available and choosing the one that makes the most fit takes some research. Factors such as cost, current infrastructure (will a hardware upgrade be necessary for an option to be implemented?), available support, level of comfort with technology, as well as how the hardware fits into the current processes are all considered (HealthIT.gov, n.d.). Part of this decision centers on the workflow analysis (described earlier) and how the practitioners will be using the hardware. Will the clinicians prefer to use the EHR in a stationary location? Do they prefer mobility? Will they need to complete their work offsite? These are the type of questions that factor into the decision for hardware purchase. If mobility isn't a factor, fixed computer workstations can be the best option. However, it is important to consider the effect of a computer in the exam room as "many clinicians are concerned about how having a computer in the exam room will change their interaction with the patient" (American EHR Partners, n.d.-a). Placement of the hardware is a key factor in minimizing this effect. If the workstation is placed such that the clinician must face away from the patient, many patients feel this presents a barrier to their relationship and interaction with the clinician: "The computer can act as a barrier and it can be disconcerting for patients to be looking at the back of a computer monitor wondering what it is that you are writing" (AmericanEHR Partners, 2011, para 7.).

If the clinicians prefer mobility, the use of laptops or tablets can assist them in moving around the clinical areas. With the growth of wireless networks, these options provide much flexibility when using the EHR. Tablets have become particularly appealing because of their size and weight. Many vendors are customizing their software to run easily on a tablet. "Just like a paper chart, this device can be used to input data using a [touch] pen to select items from a checklist or to enter information using handwriting recognition" (American EHR Partners, 2011, para. 7.).

Seminar Discussion Questions

1. As a new student gathering information about your assigned patients via an EHR, what advantages can this approach provide you over traditional paper records?
2. Describe the ways in which electronic health records can eliminate redundant efforts. Provide detailed rationales.
3. When selecting an EHR system, why is it so vital to create and communicate a vision for its use? Which individuals should be involved in this process?
4. What are the ethical considerations related to interoperability and a shared EHR?
5. Discuss the advantages and disadvantages associated with implementing and using a regional and/or national EHR.

References

Adler-Milstein, J., Salzberg, C., Franz, C., Orav, E. J., & Bates, D. W. (2013). The impact of electronic health records on ambulatory costs among Medicaid beneficiaries. *Medicare & Medicaid Research Review, 3*(2), 1–16. doi:10.5600/mmrr.003.02.a03

American Academy of Family Physicians. (n.d.). *Migrating old records to your EHR—Health IT guides.* Retrieved from http://www.aafp.org/practice-management/health-it/product/old-records.html

American College of Surgeons. (n.d.). *Electronic health records: Negotiating the electronic health record vendor contact*. Retrieved from http://www.facs.org/fellows_info/bulletin/negotiatingehr.html

American EHR Partners. (n.d.-a). *Choosing the right hardware for your practice*. Retrieved from http://www.americanehr.com/blog/2011/06/choosing-the-right-hardware-for-your-practice/

American EHR Partners. (n.d.-b). *How to integrate computers into your practice for maximum patient benefit*. Retrieved from http://www.americanehr.com/blog/2011/04/how-to-integrate-computers-into-your-office-for-maximum-patient-benefit/

American Health Information Management Association. (n.d.). *Assessing and improving EHR data quality* (updated). Retrieved from http://library.ahima.org/xpedio/groups/public/documents/ahima/bok1_050085.hcsp?dDocName=bok1_050085

American Physical Therapy Association. (n.d.). *Understanding and adopting electronic health records (EHR): Part 1 - Decision*. Retrieved from http://www.apta.org/EHR/Guide/Decision/

American Physical Therapy Association. (2008). Support of Electronic Health Record in Physical Therapy, HOD P06-08-13-11.

Are There Penalties for Providers Who Don't Switch to Electronic Health Records (EHR)? | FAQs | Providers & Professionals | HealthIT.gov. (n.d.). Retrieved from http://www.healthit.gov/providers-professionals/faqs/are-there-penalties-providers-who-don't-switch-electronic-health-record

Bates, D. W., & Gawande, A. A. (2003). Improving safety with information technology. *New England Journal of Medicine, 348*(25), 2526–2534. Retrieved from http://search.ebscohost.com/login.aspx?direct=true&db=cmedm&AN=12815139&cpidlogin.asp?custid=s6328807&site=ehost-live&scope=site

Blumenthal, D., & Tavenner, M. (2010). The "meaningful use" regulation for electronic health records. *New England Journal of Medicine, 363*, 501–504. doi:10.1056/NEJMp1006114

Boonstra, A., & Broekhuis, M. (2010). Barriers to the acceptance of electronic medical records by physicians from systematic review to taxonomy and interventions. *BMC Health Services Research, 10*, 231. doi:10.1186/1472-6963-10-231

Bredfeldt, C. E., Awad, E. B., Joseph, K., & Snyder, M. H. (2013). Training providers: Beyond the basics of electronic health records. *BMC Health Services Research, 13*, 503. doi:10.1186/1472-6963-13-503

Burton, L. C., Anderson, G. F., & Kues, I. W. (2004). Using electronic health records to help coordinate care. *Milbank Quarterly, 82*(3), 457–481, table of contents. doi:10.1111/j.0887-378X.2004.00318.x

Carayon, P., Smith, P., Hundt, A. S., Kuruchittham, V., & Li, Q. (2009). Implementation of an electronic health records system in a small clinic: The viewpoint of clinic staff. *Behaviour & Information Technology, 28*(1), 5–20. doi:10.1080/01449290701628178

Clancy, C. M. (2009). *What is health care quality and who decides?* U.S. Department of Health and Human Services. Retrieved from http://www.hhs.gov/asl/testify/2009/03/t20090318b.html

Clinical Decision Support | Healthcare IT News. (n.d.). Retrieved from http://www.healthcareitnews.com/directory/clinical-decision-support-cds

Committee on Data Standards for Patient Safety. (2003). *Key capabilities of an electronic health record system letter report*. Washington, DC: National Academies Press.

Committee on Quality of Health Care in America. (2001). *Crossing the quality chasm: A new health system for the 21st century*. Washington, DC: National Academies Press. Retrieved from http://site.ebrary.com/lib/sacredheart/docDetail.action?docID=10032412

Decker, S. L., Jamoom, E. W., & Sisk, J. E. (2012). Physicians in nonprimary care and small practices and those age 55 and older lag in adopting electronic health record systems. *Health Affairs (Project Hope), 31*(5), 1108–1114. doi:10.1377/hlthaff.2011.1121

Delaune, M. F., & Bemis-Doughterty, A. (n.d.). *Documentation in physical therapy services*. Retrieved from http://www.apta.org/PTinMotion/2007/2/Documentation/

DesRoches, C. M., Campbell, E. G., Rao, S. R., Donelan, K., Ferris, T. G., Jha, A., . . . Blumenthal, D. (2008). Electronic health records in ambulatory care—A national survey of physicians. *New England Journal of Medicine, 359*(1), 50–60. doi:10.1056/NEJMsa0802005

Eastaugh, S. R. (2013). Electronic health records lifecycle cost. *Journal of Health Care Finance, 39*(4), 36–43. Retrieved from http://www.ncbi.nlm.nih.gov/pubmed/24003760

Electronic Health Records | Health IT Topics | HIMSS. (n.d.). Retrieved from http://www.himss.org/library/ehr/

EMR Medical Software Information and Resources: Top Reasons to Implement an Electronic Medical Records Software System. (n.d.). Retrieved from http://electronic-medical-record.blogspot.com/2007/09/top-reasons-to-implement-electronic.html

Fleming, N. S., Culler, S. D., McCorkle, R., Becker, E. R., & Ballard, D. J. (2011). The financial and nonfinancial costs of implementing electronic health records in primary care practices. *Health Affairs (Project Hope), 30*(3), 481–489. doi:10.1377/hlthaff.2010.0768

Friedman, D. J., Parrish, R. G., & Ross, D. A. (2013). Electronic health records and US public health: Current realities and future promise. *American Journal of Public Health, 103*(9), 1560–1567. doi:10.2105/AJPH.2013.301220

Garets, D., & Davis, M. (2006). Electronic medical records vs. electronic health records: Yes, there is a difference. A HIMSS Analytics White Paper. Retrieved from https://www.himssanalytics.org/docs/WP_EMR_EHR.pdf

Garrett, P., & Seidman, J. (2011). EMR vs EHR – What is the difference? | Health IT Buzz. Retrieved from http://www.healthit.gov/buzz-blog/electronic-health-and-medical-records/emr-vs-ehr-difference/

Giniat, E. J., Benton, B., Bieganksy, E., & Grossman, R. (2012). People and change management in an uncertain environment. *Healthcare Financial Management: Journal of the Healthcare Financial Management Association, 66*(10), 84–89. Retrieved from http://search.ebscohost.com/login.aspx?direct=true&db=mnh&AN=23088059&site=ehost-live&scope=site

Goetz Goldberg, D., Kuzel, A. J., Feng, L. B., DeShazo, J. P., & Love, L. E. (2012). EHRs in primary care practices: Benefits, challenges, and successful strategies. *American Journal of Managed Care, 18*(2), e48–e54. Retrieved from http://www.ncbi.nlm.nih.gov/pubmed/22435884

Goldzweig, C. L., Towfigh, A., Maglione, M., & Shekelle, P. G. (2005). Costs and benefits of health information technology: New trends from the literature. *Health Affairs (Project Hope), 28*(2), w282–w293. doi:10.1377/hlthaff.28.2.w282

Health Affairs. (2013). Health policy brief: Patient engagement. *Health Affairs* (February).

Health Management Technology. (2010). Change management: Toy story style. *Health Management Technology, 31*(3), 14–18. Retrieved from http://search.ebscohost.com/login.aspx?direct=true&db=c8h&AN=2010596056&site=ehost-live&scope=site

Health Resources and Services Administration. (n.d.-a). *How to implement your EHR system.* Retrieved from http://www.hrsa.gov/healthit/toolbox/healthitimplementation/implementationtopics/implementsystem/implementsystem_4.html

Health Resources and Services Administration. (n.d.-b). *What is health information exchange?* Retrieved from http://www.hrsa.gov/healthit/toolbox/RuralHealthITtoolbox/Collaboration/whatishie.html

HealthIT.gov. (n.d.-a). *Selecting an EHR system or upgrading an EHR system.* Retrieved from http://www.healthit.gov/providers-professionals/ehr-implementation-steps/step-3-select-or-upgrade-certified-ehr

HealthIT.gov. (n.d.-b). *System configuration.* Retrieved from http://www.healthit.gov/policy-researchers-implementers/safer/guide/sg004

HealthIT.gov. (n.d.-c). What is clinical decision support (CDS)? | Policy Researchers & Implementers | HealthIT.gov. Retrieved from http://www.healthit.gov/policy-researchers-implementers/clinical-decision-support-cds

Henderson, A., Schoonbeek, S., & Auditore, A. (2013). Processes to engage and motivate staff. *Nursing Management* (UK), *20*(8), 18–25. doi:10.7748/nm2013.12.20.8.18.e1150

How Much Is This Going to Cost Me? | FAQs | Providers & Professionals | HealthIT.gov. (n.d.). Retrieved from http://www.healthit.gov/providers-professionals/faqs/how-much-going-cost-me

How to Attain Meaningful Use. (2014). Retrieved from http://www.cms.gov/Regulations-and-Guidance/Legislation/EHRIncentivePrograms/Meaningful_Use.html

Hsiao, C.-J., Hing, E., & Ashman, J. (2014). Trends in electronic health record system use among office-based physicians: United States, 2007-2012. *National Health Statistics Reports, 75,* 1–18. Retrieved from http://www.ncbi.nlm.nih.gov/pubmed/24844589

Improve Medical Practice Management with Electronic Health Records | Providers & Professionals | HealthIT.gov. (n.d.). Retrieved from http://www.healthit.gov/providers-professionals/medical-practice-efficiencies-cost-savings

Increase Patient Participation in Care with Health IT | Providers & Professionals | HealthIT.gov. (n.d.). Retrieved from http://www.healthit.gov/providers-professionals/patient-participation

Institutes of Medicine, Quality of Health Care in America. (2001). *Crossing the quality chasm: A new health system for the 21st century.* Washington, DC: National Academies Press, p. 360.

Jiantao Pan. (n.d.). *Software testing.* Retrieved from http://users.ece.cmu.edu/~koopman/des_s99/sw_testing/

Kazley, A. S., Simpson, A. N., Simpson, K. N., & Teufel, R. (2014). Association of electronic health records with cost savings in a national sample. *American Journal of Managed Care, 20*(6), 183–191.

Kern, L. M., Barrón, Y., Dhopeshwarkar, R. V., Edwards, A., & Kaushal, R. (2013). Electronic health records and ambulatory quality of care. *Journal of General Internal Medicine, 28*(4), 496–503. doi:10.1007/s11606-012-2237-8

Kindig, D., & Stoddart, G. (2003). What is population health? *American Journal of Public Health, 93*(3), 380–383. doi:10.2105/AJPH.93.3.380

King, J., Patel, V., Jamoom, E. W., & Furukawa, M. F. (2014). Clinical benefits of electronic health record use: national findings. *Health Services Research, 49*(1 Pt 2), 392–404. doi:10.1111/1475-6773.12135

Kohn, L. T., Corrigan, J. M., & Donaldson, M. S. (2000). *To err is human: Building a safer health system.* Washington, DC: National Academies Press. Retrieved from http://site.ebrary.com/lib/sacredheart/docDetail.action?docID=10038653

Lin, C., Lin, I.-C., & Roan, J. (2012). Barriers to physicians' adoption of healthcare information technology: an empirical study on multiple hospitals. *Journal of Medical Systems, 36*(3), 1965–1977. doi:10.1007/s10916-011-9656-7

Martin, G. T. (2004). Leading up to CPOE. Benefits begin long before full implementation. *Healthcare Informatics, 21*(2), 96–98.

Meaningful Use, Meaningful Use Definition, EHR Technology: HITECH Answers. (n.d.). Retrieved from http://www.hitechanswers.net/ehr-adoption-2/meaningful-use/

Medscape.org. (n.d.). *Do your EHR manners turn patients off?* Retrieved from http://www.medscape.com/viewarticle/809237

Merrill, M. (n.d.). *Top 10 factors for successful EHR implementation.* Retrieved from http://www.healthcareitnews.com/news/top-10-factors-successful-ehr-implementation?single-page=true

The National Alliance for Health Information Technology. (2008). Defining key health information technology terms. Washington, DC: Department of Health and Human Services.

O'Connor, K. J. (2004). CPOE: Show me the benefits! *Journal of Healthcare Information Management, 18*(1), 11–12.

O'Malley, A. S., Grossman, J. M., Cohen, G. R., Kemper, N. M., & Pham, H. H. (2010). Are electronic medical records helpful for care coordination? Experiences of physician practices. *Journal of General Internal Medicine, 25*(3), 177–185. doi:10.1007/s11606-009-1195-2

Office of the National Coordinator for Health IT. (n.d.-a). About ONC | Newsroom | HealthIT.gov. Retrieved from http://www.healthit.gov/newsroom/about-onc

Office of the National Coordinator for Health IT. (n.d.-b). Connecting health and care for the nation: A 10-year vision to achieve an interoperable health IT infrastructure (pp. 1–13).

Office of the National Coordinator for Health IT, & Consortium, N. L. (n.d.). Meaningful use definition and meaningful use objectives of EHRs | Providers & Professionals | HealthIT.gov. Retrieved from http://www.healthit.gov/providers-professionals/meaningful-use-definition-objectives

PC Magazine. (n.d.). *ASP definition from PC Magazine Encyclopedia.* Retrieved from http://www.pcmag.com/encyclopedia/term/38037/asp

Presidential Documents: Executive Order 13335. (2004). Incentives for the use of health information technology and establishing the position of the national health information technology coordinator. Washington, DC.

Shamus, E., & Stern, D. (2011). *Effective documentation for physical therapy professionals* (2nd ed., p. 338). New York, NY: McGraw-Hill.

Spicer, S. S. (2009). HITECH stimulus for physicians. *North Carolina Medical Journal, 70*(4), 354–357. Retrieved from http://www.ncbi.nlm.nih.gov/pubmed/19835259

Walker, J., Pan, E., Johnston, D., Adler-Milstein, J., Bates, D. W., & Middleton, B. (2005). The value of health care information exchange and interoperability. *Health Affairs (Project Hope),* e5–e18. doi:10.1377/hlthaff.w5.10

Wang, S. J., Middleton, B., Prosser, L. A., Bardon, C. G., Spurr, C. D., Carchidi, P. J., . . . Bates, D. W. (2003). A cost-benefit analysis of electronic medical records in primary care. 12.6 Identify properties of electrical, sound, light, and heat energy. (5), 397–403. doi:10.1016/S0002-9343(03)00057-3

Webster, P. C. (2010). Electronic health records a "strong priority" for US government. *CMAJ: Canadian Medical Association Journal = Journal de l'Association Medicale Canadienne, 182*(8), e315–e316. doi:10.1503/cmaj.109-3218

What Is an Electronic Health Record (EHR)? | FAQs | Providers & Professionals | HealthIT.gov. (n.d.). Retrieved from http://www.healthit.gov/providers-professionals/faqs/what-electronic-health-record-ehr

What Is "Meaningful Use"? (n.d.). Retrieved from http://www.hrsa.gov/healthit/meaningfuluse/MUStage1CQM/whatis.html

Who Should Be on the Electronic Health Record Selection Committee? | FAQs | Providers & Professionals | HealthIT.gov. (n.d.). Retrieved from http://www.healthit.gov/providers-professionals/faqs/who-should-be-electronic-health-record-selection-committee

Wright, A., Feblowitz, J., Samal, L., McCoy, A. B., & Sittig, D. F. (2014). The Medicare electronic health record incentive program: Provider performance on core and menu measures. *Health Services Research, 49*(1 Pt 2), 325–346. doi:10.1111/1475-6773.12134

Zandieh, S. O., Yoon-Flannery, K., Kuperman, G. J., Langsam, D. J., Hyman, D., & Kaushal, R. (2008). Challenges to EHR implementation in electronic- versus paper-based office practices. *Journal of General Internal Medicine, 23*(6), 755–761. doi:10.1007/s11606-008-0573-5

Zlabek, J. A, Wickus, J. W., & Mathiason, M. A. (2009). Early cost and safety benefits of an inpatient electronic health record. *Journal of the American Medical Informatics Association: JAMIA, 18*(2), 169–172. doi:10.1136/jamia.2010.007229

CHAPTER 10

Palliative Care and Chronic Disease Management

Marylou Siefert, Jean Boucher, and Elizabeth Ercolano

▸ Introduction

This chapter provides a brief overview of palliative care. The relationship between palliative care, the nursing role, quality of life for patients with serious illness and their families, and information pertinent to the goals of care and transitions of care are discussed. Additionally, some key national organizations that are instrumental in providing palliative care resources and guidelines are described and presented. Symptom management in palliative care is reviewed; resources are provided for further information and up-to-date symptom management guidelines. Finally, a case study is presented to pull the elements of palliative care together in the context of advance practice nursing.

▸ Palliative Care Definition and Background

Palliative care is both a philosophy and a structure for the delivery of care. There are many definitions of palliative care; common themes through most definitions are (1) the addressing of symptoms to relieve and prevent suffering and improve one's quality of life in the face of serious illness, (2) the inclusion of the patient and family caregivers, (3) facilitation of autonomy, and (4) access to information and choice with a team approach to the delivery of care. These themes do ***not*** preclude treatment of the underlying condition or illness (World Health Organization, 2015). The overall goal of palliative care is to provide symptoms management, prevent and treat suffering, and maintain or improve one's quality of life for the patient and the family

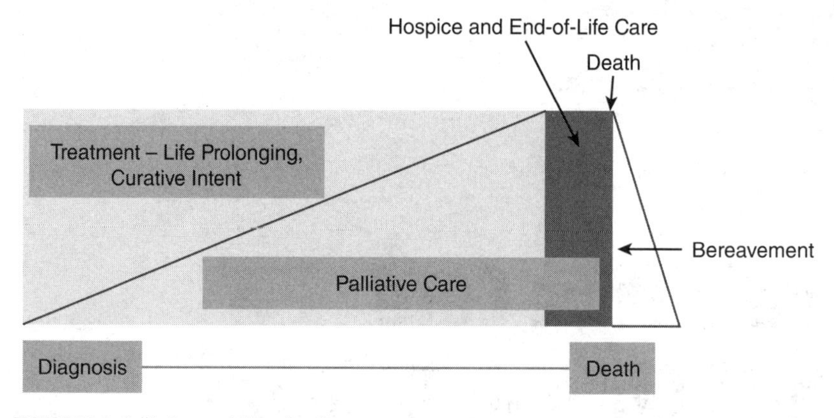

FIGURE 10-1 Palliative and Hospice Care

Data from Parikh, R. B., Kirch, R. A., Smith, T. J., & Temel, J. S. (2013). Early specialty palliative care—translating data in oncology into practice. *The New England Journal of Medicine, 369*(24), 2347–2351.

members (Center to Advance Palliative Carey [CAPC], (n.d.); Centers for Medicare & Medicaid Services [CMS], 2008; National Consensus Project [NCP] for Quality Palliative Care, 2013) at any time in one's life.

Although palliative care grew out of the hospice movement, it is not the same as hospice care. Hospice care has a defined focus on end-of-life care; it is provided to patients with serious illnesses with a limited prognosis, who are not receiving treatment with a curative or life-prolonging intent. Palliative care is often misunderstood and thought to be the same as hospice care by both healthcare professionals and the general public (*Oxford Textbook of Palliative Nursing*, 2010). Many healthcare professionals and the general public hold the same misconception that all palliative care is hospice care and that one is the same as the other. Misconceptions and misunderstandings about palliative care can be detrimental to the successful implementation and delivery of palliative care and thus detrimental to patients and their families such that one's quality of life is compromised. Healthcare professionals and patients and families are often hesitant to discuss palliative care because of the misconception that it must be end-of-life care and that other disease-focused treatments cannot be administered concurrently with palliative care. While hospice care falls under the larger umbrella of palliative care, hospice care is not representative of the whole of palliative care; rather hospice care can be understood as including elements of palliative care or as a type of palliative care provided as patients near death with a focus on end-of-life care (see **FIGURE 10-1**). Both palliative care and hospice care show improved patient outcomes in terms of symptom management, satisfaction, and death at patient's place of preference; cost savings can be achieved with reduced hospital admission costs; and some evidence suggests life may be prolonged (Meier, 2011). Palliative care can be provided at any time during one's life or disease trajectory, does not preclude treatment of an underlying illness or disease with a curative or life-prolonging intent, and does not and should not only be provided as end-of-life care.

Goals of Care

One principal component of palliative care is goal-setting discussions with patients and their caregivers. A goal-oriented process encourages communication and decision making, reduces patient uncertainty, and promotes the identification of health outcomes a patient desires to achieve (Waldrop & Meeker, 2012). Discussion about goals encourages patients and families to identify facilitators that will help patients reach their goals and barriers that may prevent goal attainment. Identification of specific and measurable health-related goals that are congruent with and address the patient's and family's quality of lift (QOL) needs is associated with greater success in goal achievement. Research, however, has found that often patients and their healthcare providers are reluctant to have conversations about goals of care particularly in the context of advanced disease with a poor prognosis or when physical and emotional symptoms overwhelm patients (Wright et al., 2008). Therefore, it is most helpful for advanced practice nurses to engage patients and their caregivers in discussions about their care preferences and goals of care early in the delivery of palliative care services.

Care Transitions

Care transitions represent changes in treatment approaches and philosophy due to progression or remission of a disease. Care transitions also represent changes in the level of complexity of healthcare services. For most patients, care transitions are associated with uncertainty, worry, and related physical, functional, and social adjustments (Bakitas, 2017). Advanced practice nurses play a central role in supporting patients and their caregivers through care transitions to reduce uncertainty, increase knowledge, and promote their self-management. Transition times are opportunities for advanced practice nurses to reassess the goals of care and promote key palliative care objectives of symptom management, advocate for patients and families, and facilitate consults with the palliative care interdisciplinary team (McCorkle et al., 2015).

Quality of Life

For the purposes of this chapter, quality of life will be defined using the conceptual model of QOL developed and extensively used and tested by Ferrell and colleagues Ferrell, 1996; Ferrell, Dow, & Grant, 1995; Ferrell, Grant, Padilla, Vemuri, & Rhiner, 1991). Ferrell and colleagues (1991, 1995) defined QOL as including four domains—the physical, psychological, social, and spiritual areas of one's life. Each of the four domains contains different concepts, concerns, types of distress, and symptoms that fall within each domain (**FIGURE 10-2**). The areas within each domain may vary slightly depending on a specific illness or symptom. For example, for the patient with breast cancer, the model has been revised slightly to include menstrual change/fertility within the physical domain in the QOL model (Ferrell et al., 1996). Another example of a difference in the model is the inclusion of strength and fatigue in the physical domain in the QOL model for pain (Ferrell et al., 1991).

Quality of life is a multidimensional concept and when one dimension of QOL is affected, other dimensions are also affected. For example, when the physical domain or dimension of QOL is affected by pain, the psychological and social domains may also be affected. One may not only be distressed by the physical presence of pain but may thus also experience psychological distress by feeling anxious or depressed about the meaning of the pain. One may also feel unable to engage with friends or family socially due to the unpleasant and uncomfortable nature of the pain. Persons

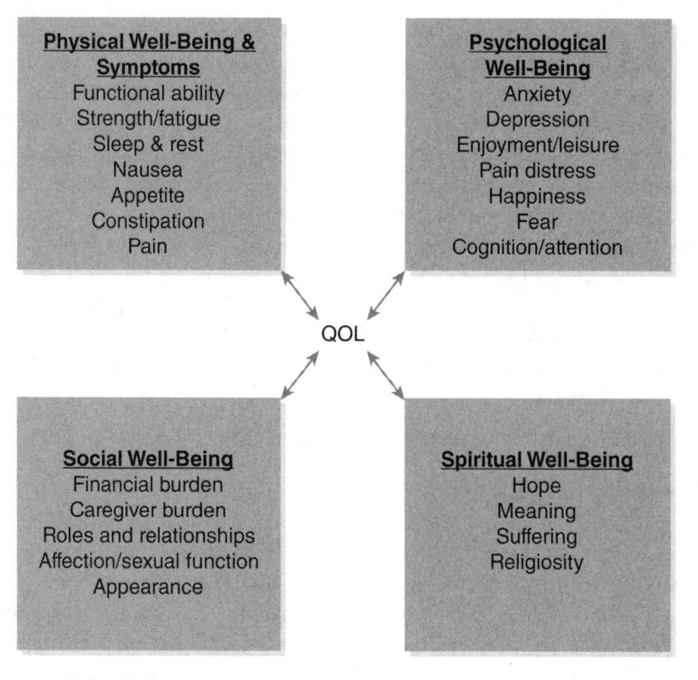

FIGURE 10-2 Quality of Life (QOL) Model

Reproduced from Ferrell, B.R., & Grant, M. (2000). Quality-of-life model. Duarte, CA: City of Hope National Medical Center. Reprinted with permission. Available online at http://prc.coh.org

with pain can therefore feel socially isolated because they are unable to enjoy time with friends and family due to the distress associated with both the physical and psychological symptoms associated with the pain. The lack of social engagement can thus also negatively impact their psychological distress; therefore, it is understandable why one area of distress in the QOL model can have a profound impact in other areas of QOL. Research has shown that when advanced practice nurses (APRNs) provide interventions to address symptoms in more than one area of QOL, patients showed stronger outcomes than if only one area of QOL was targeted by nurses (McCorkle et al., 2009).

National Organizations

There are a number of national palliative care–focused organizations and each has a slightly different focus, mission, and goals. However, they each foster and support the implementation and delivery of high-quality palliative care through the provision of various resources and activities. A few of these organizations that the APRN will find helpful are highlighted here. The reader is encouraged to seek further information from and about any of the organizations and the affiliates listed here as well as others they may find helpful. The websites are included in the text, and information is regularly updated for each of the organizations described here.

The National Coalition Project for Hospice and Palliative Care (The Coalition) (http://www.nationalcoalitionhpc.org/) was founded in 2001 and originally consisted of four member organizations. The Coalition was originally founded to communicate, coordinate, and collaborate around issues related to hospice and palliative care. Today,

The Coalition is comprised of nine national hospice and palliative care organizations and has subsequently grown to include tens of thousands of interdisciplinary healthcare professional members from the nine member organizations. The current goals of The Coalition are:

> To *coordinate* and communicate a shared vision to the public about the importance of high-quality palliative care in multiple settings including hospice, hospitals, and in the community.
>
> To *educate* the public and policy makers about the need for high-quality palliative care for those patients and families diagnosed with serious illness and the need for high-quality hospice care for those at the end of life.
>
> To *collaborate* on public policies to improve the care of seriously ill patients and their families.
>
> To *facilitate* the National Consensus Project's efforts to establish and implement high-quality palliative care guidelines in all settings (National Coalition for Hospice and Palliative Care, n.d.)

The National Consensus Project (NCP) is a task force of The Coalition that began in 2002 and whose purpose is to develop guidelines through an evidence-based review process, and to promote and implement these guidelines in order to assist in the delivery of consistent high-quality palliative care (http://keyweb24.com/nchpc/about-and-history/). The NCP has developed and disseminated three versions of the Clinical Practice Guidelines for Quality Palliative Care in 2004, 2009, and 2013. The National Quality Forum (NQF) has used these guidelines as a framework for the NQF Preferred Practices and they have been used to guide policy, healthcare providers, and consumers in defining and understanding quality palliative care (National Coalition for Hospice and Palliative Care). In January 2017, The Coalition announced that the Hospice and Palliative Nurses Foundation (HPNF) (one of the nine member organizations of The Coalition) was awarded a grant from the Gordon and Betty Moore Foundation to support The Coalition's efforts to develop community-based guidelines for quality palliative care modeled on the NCP Clinical Practice Guidelines for Quality Palliative Care (2013). The websites for The Coalition, its member organizations, and task forces provide a vast amount of additional information and resources that are updated regularly for those who desire more detailed information about the abovementioned efforts, recommendations, and guidelines.

The Center to Advance Palliative Care (CAPC) was established in 1999 as a National Program Office of the Robert Wood Johnson Foundation. Since 2006 it has been supported by a consortium of foundations and individuals, and in 2015 became a membership organization; it is affiliated with the Icahn School of Medicine at Mount Sinai in New York City. CAPC is a major resource supporting the development and quality of palliative care through education, collaboration, and providing public awareness of palliative care. The website (https://www.capc.org/) provides a wealth of information for providers, institutions, payors, and policy makers.

The End of Lifer Nursing Education Consortium (ELNEC) is an education project originally founded with a large grant from the Robert Wood Johnson Foundation in 2000 and is currently funded by a large number of institutions and organizations including the National Cancer Institute (NCI). ELNEC provides education about palliative care to nurses and other healthcare professionals. It has provided education in palliative care with a distinct focus on end-of-life care nationally and internationally in over

90 countries. Course content is comprehensive, uses a train-the-trainer model, and has grown to include not only the original core course but specialty focused courses such as those for APRNs, pediatric, critical care, and geriatric nurses, among other courses. The reader is encouraged to thoroughly review the ELNEC website (http://www.aacn.nche.edu/elnec/about/fact-sheet) with regularly updated resources and course information available there.

Nurses and Palliative Care

Nurses make up the largest group of healthcare professionals. The latest estimates of the U.S. Department of Labor Bureau of Labor Statistics indicate there are 2,857,180 nurses (excluding nurse practitioners, midwives, and anesthetists) and 150,230 nurse practitioners employed in The Country (https://www.bls.gov/oes/current/oes291141.htm#(3)). In the hospital setting, nurses are the primary frontline professional caregivers. Although much nursing time is spent with documentation and indirect care away from the patient, nurses spend a significant amount of time with patients and families (Hendrich, Chow, Skierczynski, & Lu, 2008; Paice, 2015; Westbrook, Duffield, Li, & Creswick, 2011). Nurses spend more time and advocate for patients especially when palliative care services at end of life are needed (Paice, 2015; Thacker, 2008) and are well positioned as healthcare professionals to assess, intervene, and refer patients to other healthcare professionals as needed and appropriate for palliative care services. Advance practice nurses are by definition and in their advanced practice role able to *not only* assess and intervene on a basic nursing level but are also allowed to diagnose, treat, and prescribe within the scope of the state statutes governing nursing practice. According to the American Nurses Association (2017):

> Nursing is the protection, promotion, and optimization of health and abilities, prevention of illness and injury, facilitation of healing, alleviation of suffering through the diagnosis and treatment of human response, and advocacy in the care of individuals, families, groups, communities, and populations.

The ANA statement about nursing fits perfectly with the core tenets and definitions of palliative care. Nurses, and specifically APRNs, are and have been the ideal healthcare providers to deliver and coordinate palliative care services to patients and their families. Nurses have played a pivotal role in palliative care since its beginnings as it grew from the hospice movement. The hospice movement was started in Great Britain in the 1960s by Dame Cicely Saunders, who was first a nurse and a social worker before becoming a physician. In the early 1970s Florence Wald, MSN, FAAN, former Dean at the Yale School of Nursing, was instrumental in opening The Connecticut Hospice, the first hospice in the United States, in New Haven, in 1971. Nurses are educated to be clinicians, leaders, educators, administrators, and researchers and are therefore in an excellent position to contribute to palliative care at all levels (Paice, 2015). For the NP, adequate palliative care requires knowledge of the evidence to support palliative care interventions, the ability to conduct an excellent and comprehensive assessment, to intervene early to relieve and prevent distress related to symptoms, and to address QOL needs for patients and their families. Obviously it is not expected that nurses would or should be able to provide all palliative care without the expertise of their colleagues in other disciplines. Just as QOL is multidimensional, palliative care is intended to include an interdisciplinary healthcare team with expertise in other areas in addition to nursing, including those disciplines and professionals who attend to the spiritual needs of patients and their families. Palliative care teams typically include nurses, physicians, social workers, and spiritual or religious professionals. Teams often also include pharmacists, psychologists, dieticians, and volunteers.

Symptom Management

The symptom experience can negatively impacts one's QOL; the experience includes not only the number, type, and severity of symptoms but also the associated distress with the symptoms. In people with cancer, where the majority of the symptom management research has been conducted and reported, it is has been well established that multiple co-occurring symptoms are associated with increased distress, decreased function, and decreased survival (Cleeland, 2007; Degner & Sloan, 1995; Kurtz, Kurtz, Stommel, Given, & Given, 2000). In the context of serious illness, patients usually experience more than one symptom from the illness and the treatments, thus increasing the symptom burden and impact on one's QOL. Patients with illnesses other than cancer, such as cardiac disease, dementia, and HIV/AIDS, also experience a high symptom burden. The essence of palliative care, which aims to relieve suffering, is symptom management. In the elderly or aging population comorbidities can also contribute to the existence of multiple co-occurring symptoms. In addition to pharmacologic management for symptoms, psychosocial care is also needed, and thus interdisciplinary care is needed to optimally address symptom distress. Common symptoms especially in palliative care for end-of-life care include respiratory symptoms such as dyspnea, pain, anorexia, other gastrointestinal-related symptoms, anxiety, depression and fatigue, and loss of function. Many other symptoms can exist especially at end of life and the authors refer the readers to the symptom management literature for end-of-life care for a more complete discussion of end-of-life symptoms. The management of all symptoms is beyond the scope of this chapter, and we will highlight some of the more common symptoms for patients who receive palliative care services. For the purposes of this chapter we will review some of the evidence-based practices for the assessment and treatment of anorexia, dyspnea, fatigue, anxiety, and depression. We also refer the reader to other sources for up-to-date clinical practice guidelines and evidence-based practices for symptom management (see **BOX 10-1**).

Anorexia/Cachexia

Anorexia and cachexia are common in many advanced illnesses. Both are experienced together by up to 80% of all patients with cancer (Tarricone, Ricca, Nyanzi-Wakholi, & Medina-Lara, 2016) and are associated with a negative impact on QOL and survival. Anorexia is a loss of appetite and desire to eat associated with a reduced intake (Wholihan, 2015). Cachexia is due to a lack of nutrition and involves muscle wasting, weight loss, is associated with fatigue and is common in advanced cancer and other illnesses (Wholihan, 2015). Anorexia and cachexia are difficult to treat. Causes can vary from the illness to different treatments. A careful and thorough assessment includes a patient history of involuntary weight loss, other comorbid conditions or deficiencies, a physical exam to assess for wasting and weakness, skin conditions, and gastrointestinal problems. Laboratory tests may be helpful to identify deficiencies. Interventions are not always successful. When possible, remove underlying causes.

BOX 10-1 Symptom Management and Palliative Care Resources

Putting Evidence into Practice (ONS)
https://www.ons.org/practice-resources/pep

Clinical Practice Guidelines for Dyspnea (American Thoracic Society)
https://www.thoracic.org/professionals/

National Comprehensive Cancer Network (NCCN) Palliative Care Clinical Practice Guidelines
https://www.nccn.org/professionals/physician_gls/f_guidelines.asp#supportive

City of Hope Pain and Palliative Care Resource Center
http://prc.coh.org/

National Coalition for Hospice and Palliative Care and the National Consensus Project
http://www.nationalcoalitionhpc.org/

World Health Organization—Palliative Care
http://www.who.int/mediacentre/factsheets/fs402/en/

Hospice and Palliative Nurses Association (most resources are limited to members only)
http://hpna.advancingexpertcare.org/

End-of-Life Nursing Education Consortium (ELNEC)
http://www.aacn.nche.edu/elnec

Center to Advance Palliative Care
https://www.capc.org/

Referrals to dieticians may be considered. Individualized interventions are most appropriate. There is some evidence for appetite stimulants (Dev, Del Fabbro, & Bruera, 2007); however, these are not always helpful especially in advanced illness. When considering the impact of anorexia and cachexia for patients, the NP must take a moment to consider the social and cultural importance that is often placed on food and mealtimes. Eating is frequently a social event, even when dining at home, and includes more than simply eating for nourishment. Meal planning, preparation, and sharing in the meal are not enjoyed by those affected by anorexia and cachexia.

Dyspnea

Dyspnea is a very common, distressing symptom experienced by patients with respiratory illnesses such as lung cancer and chronic obstructive pulmonary disease (COPD), cardiac disease, and other serious and advanced illnesses. It severely impacts functionality and QOL (Mularski et al., 2013; Sung et al., 2017; Weingaertner et al., 2014; Yancy, Lopatin, Stevenson, De Marco, & Fonarow, 2006). Dyspnea is a subjective and multidimensional symptom experience and is defined by the American Thoracic Society (Mularski et al., 2013) as the "sustained and severe resting breathing discomfort that occurs in patients with advanced, often life-limiting illness and overwhelms the patient and caregivers' ability to achieve symptom relief" (p. S100). The experience causes anxiety for patients and their caregivers and is a common cause of emergency department visits. A dyspnea crisis occurs with a changing severity of the underlying dyspnea, a chaotic environment with caregiver stress, and the patient's own physical, psychosocial, and spiritual distress; it is characterized by fear, anxiety, and increased shortness of breath (Mularski et al., 2013). The assessment of dyspnea is best accomplished with a self-report by the patient as with all symptoms, because the self-report is the most valid and reliable form of assessment. Patients can respond to a yes or no query ("Are you short of breath?") to determine the presence of dyspnea. However, it is recommended to perform an assessment that encompasses more than a yes or no to obtain an accurate assessment of this multidimensional symptom and to use at least a numeric rating scale such as a 1–10 analog scale to assess the severity of dyspea so that the patient's response to treatment can also be assessed (Dorman, Byrne, & Edwards, 2007; Pang et al., 2014). In addition to assessing the actual dyspnea, the NP must assess the patient's functional status and anxiety.

Respiratory rate, oxygenation, and extent of disease may not correlate with the patient's experience or report of dyspnea (Blouin, Fowler, & Dahlin, 2008; Dudgeon, 2015; Myers & Dudgeon, 2011). The causes of dyspnea can range from various physiological reasons including neurological disturbances and severe anemias, to infiltration, obstruction, or compression of the respiratory tract, cardiac insufficiency, and other symptoms such as pain and anxiety. Be sure to think about the patient's goals of care, and risk versus benefit, when ordering tests. When weighing the risk and benefit of diagnostic tests used to determine the causes of dyspnea, the NP must always consider the importance of respecting the patient's wishes for care and if the results of the tests will change the course of treatment and provide benefit to the patient.

Management of dyspnea and respecting patients' goals of care can be challenging; when possible, reverse the underlying cause and always provide symptom management (Blouin et al., 2008). Pharmacologic interventions that can be beneficial in reducing the sensation of dyspnea and its related distress include the use of opioids, bronchodilators, steroids, and anxiolytic agents; oxygen use may be beneficial in the setting of hypoxia. Nonpharmacologic interventions include providing a calm environment, breathing exercises such as pursed lip breathing, attending to caregiver and patient anxiety, and using a fan or open window to provide a sense of air flow (National Comprehensive Cancer Network [NCCN], 2017). The readers are directed to clinical practice guidelines that are regularly updated at the American Thoracic Society website (https://www.thoracic.org/statements/health-care.php) and the National Comprehensive Cancer Network Guidelines for Palliative Care (NCCN, 2017).

In addition to causing anxiety for patients, caregivers who observe their loved ones experience of dyspnea can also experience distress and anxiety. It is important to consider the caregivers' distress and related needs; and provide support including resources for coping, information and education about the patient's dyspnea, and ways to treat the dyspnea, to help alleviate caregiver distress.

Fatigue

Fatigue is the most commonly reported symptom by those with cancer, reported by 80%–100% of patients (even in fairly healthy patients), and is prevalent and distressful in other diseases as well, such as cardiac disease and respiratory illnesses (Brissot, Gonzalez-Bermejo, Lassalle, Desrues, & Doutrellot, 2006; Mitchell et al., 2014; Siefert, 2010; Stridsman, Müllerova, Skär, & Lindberg, 2013). Fatigue is worse in those with advanced COPD, with respiratory symptoms or heart disease and COPD, and in heart disease without COPD (Stridsman et al., 2013). Fatigue is a subjective sense of tiredness and may have a sudden or gradual onset and has a high inverse correlation with functional status. Fatigue may occur as a single symptom; however, it is also associated with other symptoms such as insomnia, depression, and pain. Fatigue may be caused by the underlying disease and/or its treatments, but often the etiology of fatigue is not known or well understood. Some medications can contribute to fatigue, as do other symptoms such as insomnia. A complete history and assessment should include a careful assessment of contributing factors and other symptoms, and lab tests if appropriate, to rule out anemias or other physiologic causes of anemia. The assessment of fatigue is most accurate by obtaining a patient self-report using an analog (1–10) scale. However, since fatigue often occurs with other symptoms and is associated with QOL and functional status, a full symptom assessment including QOL should be considered. Treatment of underlying causes when possible should be considered, and if other symptoms are contributing to the fatigue, such as insomnia, they should also be treated. If it is considered safe and appropriate, instruct the patient and caregiver about activities such as short periods of walking. Instruction should also include good sleep hygiene techniques combined with daytime activity conservation and management techniques such as priority setting and readjustment of priority tasks and activities, and monitoring of activities and fatigue (Mitchell et al., 2014).

Fatigue in the cancer population has been well studied and reported over the past decade in patients with various cancer diagnoses, receiving chemotherapy and or radiation therapy, and in the post treatment period. It is well established that short periods of activity such as a home-based or supervised exercise or activity program, even 10 to 20 minutes a day of activity such as walking, can help mitigate fatigue in patients who are physically able to participate in an exercise program (Mitchell et al., 2014). The optimal dose and intensity of an exercise or activity program has not been determined; however, it is recommended that if tolerated patients maintain or start some type of physical activity as tolerated and safe.

Anxiety

Anxiety is subjective feelings of uneasiness and apprehension. Although anxiety is a normal response to life events, anxiety typically co-occurs with pain and dyspnea and may peak as patients experience care transitions they feel unprepared to handle. Anxiety has been associated with decreased learning, impaired decisions, and patients' inability to perform or complete illness-related tasks. Advanced practice nurses in the palliative care setting need to routinely assess for anxiety in order to intervene early to reduce and control its effects on patients' QOL. Advanced practice nurses can take the lead in identifying and acting upon evidence-based psychosocial approaches that can best target anxiety. The interdisciplinary team approach to anxiety management supports a range of evidence-based modalities with proven efficacy to treat anxiety, including cognitive-based therapies, mindfulness-based interventions, psychoeducation interventions, and psychopharmacology (Ercolano, 2017).

Depression

It is expected that in the course of the illness trajectory, most individuals experience short-lived sadness or feelings of helplessness or hopelessness that are intermittent. Not all instances of advanced disease will result in clinical depression. Prolonged sadness greater than 2 weeks, however, may indicate a clinical depression, which is also accompanied by sleep disturbance, body aches, appetite changes, concentration problems, social isolation, and thoughts of hurting oneself or others (Pasacreta et al., 2016).

Anxiety and depression often coexist with overlapping physical, emotional, and mental symptoms. In the course of progressive disease, the decline of physical function, loss of social roles, and increasing pain may exacerbate symptoms of depression. In the palliative care, non-psychiatric setting brief screening measures are now routinely used to assess for depressive symptoms or clinical depression. These brief screening measures, including the Hospital Anxiety and Depression Scale, Beck Depression Inventory, or the Physicians Health Questionnaire 9, will alert advanced practice nurses to underrecognized or untreated depression and provide a foundation for referrals to other disciplines with specific expertise in psychosocial management. For example, behaviorally oriented interventions that encourage expression of feelings, reduce social isolation, and help with negative cognitive distortions have demonstrated efficacy. Psychopharmacology has shown efficacy in both the treatment of depression and pain in advanced disease and may be used as an adjunct to psychotherapies or other behavioral therapies (Ercolano, 2017).

Conclusion

Palliative care is a growing field in health care that has evolved from the earlier hospice movement. Palliative care is, at its essence, excellent symptom management at any time during a serious illness to relieve suffering and maintain or improve the quality of life for patients and their families. Similar to hospice care, excellent palliative care requires a multidisciplinary approach. Nurses play a key role in the implementation and delivery of palliative care to patients and their families.

CASE STUDY

Mr. Mendez is a 76-year-old Latino gentleman admitted to the hospital for his third acute episode of COPD exacerbation in the past few months. The patient has symptoms of severe dyspnea requiring continuous oxygen at home. The patient uses a walker to ambulate, but notes he becomes quite fatigued after ambulating from the bedroom to his bathroom. Mr. Mendez's wife states that he has lost his appetite with a noticeable weight loss of 12 pounds that has occurred in the last 3 months. Mr. Mendez requires home care support with the visiting nurse including assistance with medication management and a home health aide for his activities of daily living. Mr. Mendez is homebound, has visits occasionally with his church minister at home, and has two children who live within an hour driving distance from his home.

Mr. Mendez has been told by his clinicians in the hospital that his COPD condition has progressed to a severe state based on his symptoms and diagnostic testing (chest x-ray and pulmonary function testing). The patient has no advanced care directives or plan in place. Mr. Mendez is worried about his wife managing his illness at home, which causes her anxiety and is concerned about what will happen to her when he is no longer around. The interdisciplinary care team including the nurse, physician, social worker, and case manager determine that Mr. Mendez has a life-limiting illness that requires consideration of a palliative care consult to discuss the patient's goals of care for advanced care planning including transition of care.

(continues)

CASE STUDY

(continued)

1. What would be the next steps to take with regard to introducing palliative care to the patient and family?

According to the palliative care best practices based on the National Consensus Project Domains (2013) and National Quality Forum Preferred Practices (2006), the steps include processes and structure of care that involve a comprehensive care plan with goals of care conversations about advanced care planning, decision making, and consideration of the patient's goals, preferences, and values.

A comprehensive plan of care includes an assessment of the patient and family. An interdisciplinary team can include medicine, nursing, social work, chaplain, pharmacist, physical therapy, occupational therapy, nutrition, and other allied care services (National Consensus Project Domains, 2012; National Quality Forum Preferred Practices, 2006). Quality assessment includes timely and thorough communication of the patient's goals of care, including preferences, values, and clinical information for assuring continuity of care during transition of care (You, Fowler, & Heyland, 2014). Goals of care conversations include setting up a meeting to discuss with Mr. Mendez and his family about his goals or wishes, preferences, and values regarding his current medical condition. Important aspects include providing a systematic approach in asking the patient what he understands about his illness, and asking permission to discuss the nature of his condition including in what detail he would like to know about his prognosis and illness using simple language in small chunks (avoiding medical jargon), building rapport, listening, and providing empathy. The patient should be asked about his wishes, preferences, and values that are important to him. The patient and family also need to be asked about their fears and concerns. Important goals, wishes, values, and preferences should be taken into consideration in developing the plan of care. The plan of care should be discussed regarding advanced care planning (ACP), including advanced care directives and surrogate designations. The ACP discussion involves asking and documenting the patient and family wishes about care setting for palliative and end-of-life care including advanced care directives. Education on the process of the disease, prognosis, and benefits and burdens of potential interventions need to be discussed with the patient and family to make informed decisions about Mr. Mendez's care. Patients and families, such as Mr. Mendez's, should be asked about introducing palliative care and hospice care programs as options (National Consensus Project Domains, 2012; National Quality Forum Preferred Practices, 2006).

2. What are the important aspect of care that need to be addressed based on palliative care best practices?

Based on National Consensus Project Domains (2013) and National Quality Forum (NQF) Preferred Practices (2006), aspects of care include assessment of physiological, psychological, social, and spiritual components by the interdisciplinary team. Physiological aspects of care involve the patient's activities of daily living, symptom management, and maintaining physical comfort. Management of Mr. Mendez's dyspnea, fatigue, and loss of appetite includes timely assessment using standardized scales in a safe and effective manner to a level acceptable to patient and family, with documentation.

Psychological aspects of care involve Mr. Mendez's fears, worries, and concerns. Psychological reactions involve the patient and family including stress, anticipatory grief, and coping. Symptom management of the patient's anxiety or other related symptoms should be addressed with safe, effective interventions. The family will also need a plan of care that involves grief and bereavement for at least 13 months after

CASE STUDY (continued)

Mr. Mendez's death. Untoward behavioral disturbances or maladaptive coping may require psychological consultation for evaluation and counseling (National Consensus Project Domains, 2012; National Quality Forum Preferred Practices, 2006).

Social aspects of care involve ongoing communication by the interdisciplinary team with the patient and family to identify social needs and respond to assessments of religious, spiritual, and existential concerns. Information on spiritual care services and counseling should be provided while encouraging Mr. Mendez to talk to his own clergy minister for support.

Cultural aspects of care should be assessed with patient and family. Mr. Mendez may have certain preferences based on an assessment of his preferences in decision making, disclosing information, dietary preferences, language, family communication, and supportive measures such as complementary and alternative medicines. The interdisciplinary team needs to ask Mr. Mendez and his family about what they need to know about their cultural preferences and values as important patient factors in his care (National Consensus Project Domains, 2012; National Quality Forum Preferred Practices, 2006).

Ethical/legal considerations (Ferrell & Coyle, 2010; Prince-Paul & Daly, 2010) include aspects of care that involve respecting the patient's goals, preferences, and choices within the limits of applicable state and federal laws and current acceptable standards of medical care. An advanced care directive that documents the surrogate/decision maker in accordance with state law should be in place. Documentation of patient/surrogate preferences for goals of care should be transferrable across hospital, community, and emergency service settings. Such documentation ensures that the patient/surrogate wishes are maintained when transitions of care occur across acute, short-term, long-term, and home care settings. Documentation within health records needs to also adhere to the Health Insurance and Portability and Accountability Act (HIPAA) regulations to ensure patient privacy (National Consensus Project Domains, 2012; National Quality Forum Preferred Practices, 2006).

3. What is the role of the nurse in caring for Mr. Mendez and his family?

The role of the nurse involves providing physiological, psychological, sociocultural, and ethical/legal aspects of care to Mr. Mendez as previous outlined in this case study. The nurse works within an interdisciplinary team that provides care focused on communication with patient and family about providing care that meets their goals while reducing symptom burden, alleviating stress, and enhancing comfort and well-being.

Goals of care (GOC) discussions offer important ways in which persons can communicate with healthcare providers, including nurses, and family members about their wishes in advanced care planning about the type of care desired while honoring personal choices, values, and beliefs (Kaldijian, Curtis, Shinkunas, & Cannon, 2008). Despite a perceived societal culture of persons not wanting to have GOC conversations with clinicians, including advanced care planning and end-of-life care, studies have shown that patients want to have these conversations sooner, including hearing about options and using a systematic, interprofessional team approach (Bach, Arnold, & Tulsky, 2011; Gesme & Wiseman, 2011; Legare et al., 2011). Studies have shown that earlier conversations reduce stress, anxiety, and depression in the relatives of the elderly (Detering et al., 2010) including use of early palliative and less aggressive care that resulted in patients with non-small-cell lung cancer living almost 3 months longer

(continues)

CASE STUDY

(continued)

(Temel et al., 2010). Evidence supports the provision of early communication regarding serious illness and GOC conversations including EOL preferences for improved care outcomes involving better quality of life, less life-sustaining treatments near death, consistency of care with patient preferences, and improved bereavement outcomes for families (Bernacki & Block, 2014).

Nurses require training on effective communication skills within an interdisciplinary team approach. Evidence reveals barriers to communication of GOC conversations include inadequate healthcare provider training, documentation and exchange of patient values and goals, and misperceptions of increasing anxiety and depressions in patients (Bernacki & Block, 2014). Barriers identified by hospital-based clinicians involve patient-related and family-member factors in difficulty accepting a poor prognosis, difficulty understanding the limitations and complications of life-sustaining treatments, disagreements among family member on GOC, and patient incapacity to make decisions. Such barriers require a tailored approach to address individualized approaches to GOC conversations that involve a team approach by healthcare providers. An interprofessional team approach of healthcare providers can be effective (Reeves et al., 2008), including physicians and nurses, by improving communication training to initiate and participate in GOC conversations within their professional role and scope of practice (Schroder, Heyland, Jiang, Rocker, & Dodek 2009). Such preparation includes effective communication skills on best practice approaches involving assisting patients with understanding their illness, building rapport, providing empathy, listening, and discussing prognosis (Bernacki & Block, 2014).

Systematic approaches to GOC conversations that can be used with patients such as Mr. Mendez and family include use of cognitive maps or mnemonic tools that are useful to implement within a healthcare provider team approach with patients and families. An important cognitive map communication mnemonic for use as a process for sharing in a GOC conversation meeting is the use of S.P.I.K.E.S: Setting, Perception, Invitation, Knowledge, Emotions, Summary (Bailey et al., 2000). The setting includes a private quiet area where the healthcare interdisciplinary team, patient, family, and/or surrogate decision maker can meet. The setting should allow for the ability to communicate with seating, proper eye contact, and verbal interaction. Patient perception can be addressed by asking patients what has been told to them about the medical situation, including thoughts and understanding of their illness. This invitation also includes asking the patient permission about discussing the medical condition as more global or in greater detail based on what the patient wants to know about the condition. Knowledge includes giving information in small chunks while ascertaining understanding periodically, using simple language in layperson terms (avoiding medical jargon) while acknowledging the uncertainty of the prognosis. Addressing emotions includes asking about patient fears and worries while providing empathy and pauses for emotions as important. A summary of the goals of care and plan for future conversation or next steps should occur at the conclusion of the meeting (You et al., 2014).

The R.E.M.A.P. framework can be a useful tool for nurses in transitions in GOC conversations (Childers, Back, Tulsky, & Arnold, 2017). Reframe can be used in asking about feelings regarding how the patient and family think things are going. Expect emotion and empathize; ask permission to talk about what the patient and family are worried about, while recognizing their concerns and what this means to them. Map out patient goals or values, including what is most important to persons like Mr. Mendez and his family, such as future goals and future concerns. Aligning with

CASE STUDY (continued)

goals or values includes listening and verbalizing back to patients about what is most important, including a plan proposing to help with those important goals (Vitaltalk.org, 2017).

The NURSE statements are another useful cognitive map for nurses to respond to emotion in articulating empathy. Naming the emotion can include stating, "It sounds like you are frustrated." The understanding statement acknowledges, "Help me understand what you are thinking" and respecting the person in stating, "You really have been trying to follow the instructions" or through praise in "I think you have done a great job with this." Supporting includes a powerful statement such as "I will do my best to make sure you have what you need" while exploring in asking, "Could you say more about what you mean when you say that. . .?" (Vitaltalk.org, 2017).

Lastly, the nurse can provide continuity of care through assessment, education, and support that impacts quality of palliative care (Ferrell & Coyle, 2010). The End-of-Life Nursing Education Curriculum (ELNEC, 2013) addresses the role of the nurse in palliative care involving aspects of care, as summarized previously, guided within the context of a quality of life framework developed by Ferrell and Coyle (2010). Nurses also have a therapeutic presence (Krammer, Hanks-Bell, & Cappleman, 2011) to address existential concerns about personal meaning, maintaining hope (Ersek & Cotter, 2010; Ferrell & Coyle, 2010), spiritual needs, and realistic expectations for patients such as Mr. Mendez and his family (Ferrell & Coyle, 2010).

References

American Nurses Association (ANA). (2017). retrieved on June 3, 2017 from http://www.nursingworld.org/EspeciallyForYou/What-is-Nursing

Back, A., Arnold, R., & Tulsky, J. (2009). *Mastering communication with seriously ill patients*. Cambridge, England: Cambridge University Press.

Baile, W. F., Buckman, R., Lenzi, R, et al. (2000). SPIKES—a six-step protocol for delivering bad news: Application to the patient with cancer. *Oncologist, 5*, 302–311.

Bernacki, R. E., & Block, S. D. (2014). American College of Physicians high value care task force. Communication about serious illness care goals: A review and synthesis of best practices. *JAMA Internal Medicine, 174*(12), 1994–2003.

Centers to Advance Palliative Care (CAPC): About Palliative Care (n.d.) retrieved June 13, 2017 from: https://www.capc.org/about/palliative-care/

Centers for Medicare & Medicaid Services (CMS). (2008). Medicare and Medicaid programs: hospice conditions of participation; final rule. *Federal Register. Vol 73*. Washington, DC: Author. Last accessed June 2, 2017 from: http://www.gpo.gov/fdsys/pkg/FR-2008-06-05/pdf/08-1305.pdf

Childers, J., Back, A., Tulsky, J., & Arnold, R. (2017). REMAP. *Journal of Oncology Practice*. doi:10.1200/JOP.2016.018796. [Epub ahead of print]

Detering, K. M., Hancock, A. D., Reade, M. C., et al. (2010). The impact of advance care planning on end of life care in elderly patients: Randomised controlled trial. *BMJ, 340*, c1345.

Ersek, M., & Cotter, V. (2010). The meaning of hope in the dying. In B. R. Ferrell & N. Coyle (Eds.), *Oxford textbook of palliative nursing* (3rd ed.) (chap. 29, pp. 579–595). New York, NY: Oxford University Press

Ferrell, B. R., & Coyle, N. (Eds.). (2010). *Oxford textbook of palliative nursing* (3rd ed.). New York, NY: Oxford University Press.

Gesme, D. M., & Wiseman, M. (2011). Advance care planning with your patients. *Journal of Oncology Practice, 7*(6), e42–e44.

Kaldjian, L. C., Curtis, A. E., Shinkunas, L. A., & Cannon, K. T. (2011). Goals of care toward the end of life: A structured literature review. *American Journal of Hospital Palliative Care*. doi:2550111

(continues)

CASE STUDY

(continued)

Krammer, L. M., Hanks-Bell, M. J., & Cappleman, J. (2011). Therapeutic presence. In J. Panke & P. Coyne (Eds.), *Conversations in palliative care* (3rd ed.) (chap. 17). Philadelphia, PA: Hospice and Palliative Nurses Association.

Légaré, F., Stacey, D., Gagnon, S., et al. (2011). Validating a conceptual model for an inter-professional approach to shared decision making: A mixed methods study. *Journal of Evaluation in Clinical Practice, 17*(4), 554–564.

National Consensus Project (NCP) for Quality Palliative Care. (2013). *Clinical practice guidelines for quality palliative care* (3rd ed.). Retrieved from http://www.nationalconsensusproject.org/Guideline.pdf

National Quality Forum. (2006). *A national framework and preferred practices for palliative and hospice care quality.* Washington, DC: Author. Retrieved from http://www.qualityforum.org/publications/2006/12/A_National_Framework_and_Preferred_Practices_for_Palliative_and_Hospice_Care_Quality.aspx.

Prince-Paul, M. J., & Daly, B. (2010). Ethical considerations in palliative care. In B. R. Ferrell & N. Coyle (Eds.), *Oxford textbook of palliative nursing* (3rd ed.) (chap. 62, pp. 1157–1171). New York, NY: Oxford University Press.

Reeves, S., Zwarenstein, M., Goldman, J., et al. (2008). Interprofessional education: Effects on professional practice and health care outcomes. *Cochrane Database System Reviews, 1*, CD002213.

Schroder, C., Heyland, D., Jiang, X., Rocker, G., & Dodek, P. (2009). Canadian researchers at the end of life network. Educating medical residents in end-of-life care: Insights from a multicenter survey. *Journal of Palliative Medicine, 374*, 1196–1208.

Temel, J. S., Greer, J. A., Muzikansky, A., et al. (2010). Early palliative care for patients with metastatic non-small-cell lung cancer. *New England Journal of Medicine, 363*, 733–742.

Vitaltalk.com. (2017). Retrieved from http://vitaltalk.org/guides/responding-to-emotion-respecting/

You, J. J., Fowler, R. A., & Heyland, D. K. (2014). On behalf of the Canadian Researchers at the End of Life Network (CARENET). Just ask: Discussing goals of care with patients in hospital with serious illness. *Canadian Medial Association Journal, 186*(6), 425–432. doi: 10.1503/cmaj.121274

References

Bakitas, M. A. (2017). On the road less traveled: Journey of an oncology palliative care researcher. *Oncology Nursing Forum, 44*(1), 87–95.

Blouin, G., Fowler, B. C., & Dahlin, C. (2008). The national agenda for quality palliative care: Promoting the National Consensus Project's domain of physical care and the National Quality Forum's preferred practices for physical aspects of care. *Journal of Pain & Palliative Care Pharmacotherapy, 22*(3), 206–212.

Brissot, R., Gonzalez-Bermejo, J., Lassalle, A., Desrues, B., & Doutrellot, P. L. (2006). Fatigue and respiratory disorders. *Annales De Readaptation Et De Medecine Physique: Revue Scientifique De La Societe Francaise De Reeducation Fonctionnelle De Readaptation Et De Medecine Physique, 49*(6), 320.

Cleeland, C. S. (2007). Symptom burden: Multiple symptoms and their impact as patient-reported outcomes. *Journal of the National Cancer Institute (Monographs), 37*, 16–21.

Degner, L. F., & Sloan, J. A. (1995). Symptom distress in newly diagnosed ambulatory cancer patients and as a predictor of survival in lung cancer. *Journal of Pain & Symptom Management, 10*(6), 423–431.

Dev, R., Del Fabbro, E., & Bruera, E. (2007). Association between megestrol acetate treatment and symptomatic adrenal insufficiency with hypogonadism in male patients with cancer. *Cancer, 110*(6), 1173–1177.

Dorman, S., Byrne, A., & Edwards, A. (2007). Which measurement scales should we use to measure breathlessness in palliative care? A systematic review. *Palliative Medicine, 21*(3), 177–191.

Dudgeon, D. (2015). Dyspnea, terminal secretions, and cough. In B. R. Ferrell, N. Coyle, & J. Paice (Eds.), *Oxford textbook of palliative nursing* (4th ed., pp. 247–261). New York, NY: Oxford University Press.

Ercolano, E. (2017). Psychosocial concerns in the postoperative oncology patient. *Seminars in Oncology Nursing, 33*(1), 74–79. doi:10.1016/j.soncn.2016.11.007

Ferrell, B., Grant, M., Padilla, G., Vemuri, S., & Rhiner, M. (1991). The experience of pain and perceptions of quality of life: Validation of a conceptual model. *Hospice Journal, 7*(3), 9–24.

Ferrell, B. R. (1996). The quality of lives: 1,525 voices of cancer. *Oncology Nursing Forum, 23*(6), 909–916.

Ferrell, B. R., & Coyle, N. (Eds.). (2010). *Oxford textbook of palliative nursing* (3rd ed.). New York, NY: Oxford University Press.

Ferrell, B. R., Dow, K. H., & Grant, M. (1995). Measurement of the quality of life in cancer survivors. *Quality of Life Research, 4*(6), 523–531.

Ferrell, B. R., Grant, M., Funk, B., Garcia, N., Otis-Green, S., & Schaffner, M. L. (1996). Quality of life in breast cancer. *Cancer Practice, 4*(6), 331–340.

Hendrich, A., Chow, M. P., Skierczynski, B. A., & Lu, Z. (2008). A 36-hospital time and motion study: How do medical-surgical nurses spend their time? *Permanente Journal, 12*(3), 25–34.

Kurtz, M. E., Kurtz, J. C., Stommel, M., Given, C. W., & Given, B. A. (2000). Symptomatology and loss of physical functioning among geriatric patients with lung cancer. *Journal of Pain and Symptom Management, 19*(4), 249–256.

McCorkle, R., Dowd, M., Ercolano, E., Schulman-Green, D., Williams, A.-l., Siefert, M. L., . . . Schwartz, P. (2009). Effects of a nursing intervention on quality of life outcomes in post-surgical women with gynecological cancers. *Psycho-Oncology, 18*(1), 62–70. doi:10.1002/pon.1365

McCorkle, R., Jeon, S., Ercolano, E., Lazenby, M., Reid, A., Davies, M., . . . Gettinger, S. (2015). An advanced practice nurse coordinated multidisciplinary intervention for patients with late-stage cancer: A cluster randomized trial. *Journal of Palliative Medicine, 18*(11), 962–969. doi:10.1089/jpm.2015.0113

Meier, D. E. (2011). Increased access to palliative care and hospice services: Opportunities to improve value in health care. *Milbank Quarterly, 89*(3), 343–380. doi:10.1111/j.1468-0009.2011.00632.x

Mitchell, S. A., Hoffman, A. J., Clark, J. C., DeGennaro, R. M., Poirier, P., Robinson, C. B., & Weisbrod, B. L. (2014). Putting evidence into practice: An update of evidence-based interventions for cancer-related fatigue during and following treatment. *Clinical Journal of Oncology Nursing, 18*(6), 38–58. doi:10.1188/14.CJON.S3.38-58

Mularski, R. A., Reinke, L. F., Carrieri-Kohlman, V., Fischer, M. D., Campbell, M. L., Rocker, G., . . . White, D. B. (2013). An official American Thoracic Society workshop report: Assessment and palliative management of dyspnea crisis. *Annals of the American Thoracic Society, 10*(5), S98–S106. doi:10.1513/AnnalsATS.201306-169ST

Myers, J., & Dudgeon, D. (2011). Dyspnea. In S. Y. a. E. Bruera (Ed.), *Oxford American Handbook of Hospice and Palliative Medicine* (pp. 169–180). New York, NY: Oxford University Press.

National Coalition for Hospice and Palliative Care. *About Us*. Retrieved from http://www.nationalcoalitionhpc.org/about/

National Coalition for Hospice and Palliative Care. *National Coalition for Hospice and Palliative Care Home of the National Consensus Project*. Retrieved from http://keyweb24.com/nchpc/

National Coalition for Hospice and Palliative Care. *National Consensus Project*. Retrieved from http://keyweb24.com/nchpc/about-and-history/

National Comprehensive Cancer Network. (2017). *Clinical Practice Guidelines in Oncology (NCCN Guidelines®): Palliative Care*. Retrieved from https://www.nccn.org/professionals/physician_gls/pdf/palliative.pdf

Paice, J. (2015). Introduction to palliative nursing care. In B. Ferrell, N. Coyle, & J. Paice (Eds.), *Oxford textbook of palliative nursing* (4th ed., pp. 3–10). New York, NY: Oxford University Press.

Pang, P. S., Collins, S. P., Sauser, K., Andrei, A.-C., Storrow, A. B., Hollander, J. E., . . . Mebazaa, A. (2014). Assessment of dyspnea early in acute heart failure: Patient characteristics and response differences between Likert and visual analog scales. *Academic Emergency Medicine: Official Journal of the Society For Academic Emergency Medicine, 21*(6), 659–666. doi:10.1111/acem.12390

Pasacreta J. V., Minarik P. A., Nield-Anderson L., & Paice, J. (2016) A. Anxiety and depression. In B. Ferrell, N. Coyle, & J. Paice (Eds.), *Oxford textbook of palliative nursing* (4th ed., pp. 366–384). New York, NY: Oxford University Press.

Siefert, M. L. (2010). Fatigue, pain, and functional status during outpatient chemotherapy. *Oncology Nursing Forum, 37*(2), e114–e123. doi:10.1188/10.ONF.114-123

Stridsman, C., Müllerova, H., Skär, L., & Lindberg, A. (2013). Fatigue in COPD and the impact of respiratory symptoms and heart disease—a population-based study. *COPD, 10*(2), 125–132. doi:10.3109/15412555.2012.728642

Sung, M. R., Patel, M. V., Djalalov, S., Le, L. W., Shepherd, F. A., Burkes, R. L., . . . Leighl, N. B. (2017). Evolution of symptom burden of advanced lung cancer over a decade. *Clinical Lung Cancer, 18*(3), 274–280, e276. doi:10.1016/j.cllc.2016.12.010

Tarricone, R., Ricca, G., Nyanzi-Wakholi, B., & Medina-Lara, A. (2016). Impact of cancer anorexia-cachexia syndrome on health-related quality of life and resource utilisation: A systematic review. *Critical Reviews in Oncology/Hematology, 99*, 49–62. doi:10.1016/j.critrevonc.2015.12.008

Thacker, K. S. (2008). Nurses' advocacy behaviors in end-of-life nursing care. *Nursing Ethics, 15*(2), 174–185. doi:10.1177/0969733007086015

Waldrop, D. P., & Meeker, M. A. (2012). Communication and advanced care planning in palliative and end-of-life care. *Nursing Outlook, 60*(6), 365–369. doi:10.1016/j.outlook.2012.08.012

Weingaertner, V., Scheve, C., Gerdes, V., Schwarz-Eywill, M., Prenzel, R., Bausewein, C., . . . Simon, S. T. (2014). Breathlessness, functional status, distress, and palliative care needs over time in patients with advanced chronic obstructive pulmonary disease or lung cancer: A cohort study. *Journal of Pain and Symptom Management, 48*(4), 569–581, e561. doi:10.1016/j.jpainsymman.2013.11.011

Westbrook, J. I., Duffield, C., Li, L., & Creswick, N. J. (2011). How much time do nurses have for patients? A longitudinal study quantifying hospital nurses' patterns of task time distribution and interactions with health professionals. *BMC Health Services Research, 11*(1), 319. doi:10.1186/1472-6963-11-319

Wholihan, D. (2015). Anorexia and cachexia. In B. R. Ferrell, N. Coyle, & J. Paice (Eds.), *Oxford textbook of palliative nursing* (4th ed., pp. 167–174). New York, NY: Oxford University Press.

World Health Organization. (2015). *Palliative care*. Retrieved from http://www.who.int/mediacentre/factsheets/fs402/en/

Wright, A. A., Zhang, B., Ray, A., Mack, J. W., Trice, E., Balboni, T., . . . Prigerson, H. G. (2008). Associations between end-of-life discussions, patient mental health, medical care near death, and caregiver bereavement adjustment. *JAMA, 300*(14), 1665–1673. doi:10.1001/jama.300.14.1665

Yancy, C. W., Lopatin, M., Stevenson, L. W., De Marco, T., & Fonarow, G. C. (2006). Clinical presentation, management, and in-hospital outcomes of patients admitted with acute decompensated heart failure with preserved systolic function: A report from the Acute Decompensated Heart Failure National Registry (ADHERE) Database. *Journal of the American College of Cardiology, 47*(1), 76–84.

PART 4

The Professional Nurse Practitioner

CHAPTER 11

Concepts of the Professional

Julie G. Stewart

As the student NP prepares for graduation, or the employed NP considers a workplace change, factors that can enhance the work environment can assist in choosing a successful practice setting. Having a supportive workplace environment has been shown to improve work efficiency, enhance the ability to provide high-quality patient care, contribute to cost effectiveness, and promote the retention of NPs in successful collaborative practices in a variety of healthcare settings. To prepare the graduate NP for professional practice, it is important to review the core concepts related to being a professional.

Professionalism

Historically, the title of *professional* has been reserved for lawyers, the clergy, and physicians. In the early 1900s, Abraham Flexner (1910) wrote *The Flexner Report*, which was a critical assessment of medical education of that time. Many reformations were made in response to this assessment. After Flexner studied a wide variety of disciplines, he then became an expert on what constituted a profession. These characteristics have been revised and expanded by various disciplines; however, there are several attributes that define the core characteristics of professionalism. These are autonomy, ethics, specialized knowledge, and service and altruism (Chitty & Black, 2011).

In their book *The Making of Nurse Professionals*, Crigger and Godfrey (2011) focused on virtue ethics as the core framework for professionalism in nursing. In this view, an individual responds to specific situations in a manner that is appropriate to that particular situation. When performed in an admirable manner, the moral message that this was "good" is reinforced so the person will conduct the action similarly in future situations. This viewpoint emphasizes that the nurse has a choice in how to interact with patients and in society at large. This experiential development process is transformational and moves toward encompassing professional ideals and ethics when good choices are reinforced. Occasionally, "doing good" for the patient may not be what the patient believes is best, and this is when the integrity of the nurse professional, based on an ethical code, must prevail. For NPs, these types of situations occur fairly frequently in daily practice: patients who want narcotics for prolonged periods of time without a known etiology of pain, the neighbor who calls and asks for an antibiotic prescription without being evaluated as a patient of that practitioner's practice setting, and so forth. We can all come up with numerous examples of when the patient view and the NP view of "doing good" do not coincide.

Crigger and Godfrey (2011) state that the virtues that are significant for nursing professionals are compassion, humility, integrity, and courage. It is hoped that nurse practitioner students have developed these virtues during their nursing education and career. It is imperative that these virtues are transferred and developed during the transformative process in the NP educational experience in order to make the best choices in the provision of excellent health care to patients, and to be responsive to the moral and ethical code of professionalism required to succeed.

Adams and Miller (2001) investigated nurse practitioner behaviors indicative of professionalism. Over 500 NPs were recruited to complete the Professionalism in Nursing Behaviors Inventory questionnaire at the 1998 American Academy of Nurse Practitioners annual conference held in Arizona. The Professionalism in Nursing Behaviors' Inventory was adapted for NPs by the authors in 1998 and is composed of 48 items that cover demographic information and nine categories of behaviors:

1. Educational preparation
2. Autonomy
3. Adherence to the American Nurses Association (ANA) code of ethics
4. Theory
5. Competency maintenance
6. Participation in research
7. Participation in publication
8. Participation in community service
9. Participation in professional organizations

Findings in the self-regulation and autonomy category included that 74% of the NPs regularly performed self-evaluation. Furthermore, the majority of NPs were making autonomous clinical decisions, were accountable for patient outcomes, and were independently determining what their job positions entailed. This is particularly noteworthy as the study was performed in 1998.

Interestingly, in the United Kingdom, professionalism for nurses describes skills, attitudes, values, and behaviors that are similar to those who practice medicine (UK Department of Health, 2006). It includes concepts such as the maintenance of competence for a unique body of knowledge and skill set, personal integrity, altruism, adherence to ethical codes of conduct, accountability, a dedication to self-regulation, and the exercise of discretionary judgment (UK Department of Health, 2006). Professionalism is also described as a moral understanding among health professionals when providing health care to individuals and the community as a whole. Healthcare professionals determine how to use medical knowledge, have the right to practice with considerable autonomy, and have the privilege of self-regulation.

In an ethnographic study, a researcher observed advanced practice nurses (APNs) who relocated to an area with high needs for healthcare services who started the only partnership with general practitioners (MDs) in the country (McMurray, 2010). The study relates the accounts of APNs' struggles to be accepted as professionals. The author's discussions are quite thought provoking and worth a short review here. McMurray provides a background on nurses struggling to be seen as more than the performers of "dirty" tasks—those directed to be done by the physician, but not esoteric enough for the physician to perform. In addition, there is reference to the hierarchical model of health care, with medicine being in charge of the division of labor and indeed, even proclaiming its right to "challenge the legitimacy of other occupations" (McMurray, 2010, p. 805). The relationship of nurses and physicians is noted to have been one of subservience—the nurse being the "handmaiden"—as well as the feminist view of nurses' work being "women's work."

McMurray goes on to describe the vast amount of interpersonal and social expertise nurses need to deal with "the messy and dirty work of emotions, bodies, fluids, relations, attending, nurturing, and being there" (2010, p. 806). As noted in an earlier chapter, the attributes of emotions, nurturing, and being there are part of the theoretical basis that gives meaning to what nurses and NPs do. The study uncovered what it meant to be an APN, how difficult it was to combine "the nurturing skills of nursing with the curative knowledge of medicine" (p. 810). Upon graduation, finding an appropriate place for an APN to practice to the full scope of his or her knowledge was difficult; therefore, this unique small group of APNs went where they were needed most and hired general practitioners to work *with* them instead of the APNs working *for* them.

It is interesting to note how the objective observer collecting research material was able to clearly describe that the biggest issue causing the rift between professions was related to diagnosing. Diagnosing was noted to be the specialized knowledge of the physician group, and barriers to practice in the UK are the same as seen in the United States. These included limited prescribing rights, difficulties with signing progress notes, insurance reimbursement inequalities, difficulty admitting patients to the hospital, and having referrals and consults occasionally denied unless there was an attending physician in charge of the patient instead of an APN. The researcher found the process of APNs becoming accepted as professionals to be one that has not yet been fully embraced. McMurray uses the term "occupational equivalent" to sum up how the APNs worked with GPs on a similar level—with *equivalent* being the operative term; obviously not the same as *equal*.

Qualities uncovered in research about NPs highlight the core values of professionalism. In a study conducted with NPs in New Zealand and Australia (Carryer, Gardner, Dunn, & Gardner, 2007), professionalism was identified as one of the core roles of the NP. In addition, dynamic practice and clinical leadership were also identified as core components of the role of the NP. When discussing the transition from nurse to nurse practitioner, the study findings cause the authors to dispute that nurses leave nursing behind when they learn medical aspects of patient care. Instead, Carryer et al. state that tasks are not the defining characteristics of a profession; rather, it is the "philosophical approach guiding practice that defines the nature of the discipline" (2007, p. 1824).

Various models revolving around professionalism in nursing exist, all incorporating the basic tenets of the more generalized definitions of what constitutes a profession. Later in this section, Harriet Fields, EdD, RN, discusses professional behaviors that she developed while at Columbia University and that she articulates as she teaches nursing and health policy. Adams and Miller (2001) developed a wheel of professionalism that has at its base education in a university setting, and the spokes of the wheel include publication and communication; adherence to a code of ethics for nurses; theory development, use, and evaluation; community service orientation; continuing education/competence; research development, use, and evaluation; self-regulation (autonomy); and professional organization participation.

A nurse leader who spent many years studying nursing as a profession, Lucie Kelly, RN, PhD, FAAN, developed eight characteristics of professional practitioners (Chitty & Black, 2011). Kelly's criteria are (1981, p. 157):

1. The services provided are vital to humanity and the welfare of society.
2. There is a special body of knowledge that is continually enlarged through research.
3. The services involve intellectual activities; individual responsibility (accountability) is a strong feature.
4. Practitioners are educated in institutions of higher learning.
5. Practitioners are relatively independent and control their own policies and activities (autonomy).
6. Practitioners are motivated by service (altruism) and consider their work an important component of their lives.
7. There is a code of ethics to guide the decisions and conduct of practitioners.
8. There is an organization (association) that encourages and supports high standards of practice.

Autonomy

Autonomy is often discussed as it relates to the professional practice of NPs. However, autonomy can have different meanings for individuals, and autonomy does not necessarily mean practicing on one's own without collaborating with others.

In a concept analysis of autonomy, Keenan (1999) sought to provide an operational definition for autonomy in response to the increased need for NPs whose roles require autonomous practice. Defining attributes of autonomy included independence, capacity for decision making, judgment, knowledge, and self-determination. Keenan's operational definition of autonomy was, "the exercise of considered, independent judgment to effect a desirable outcome" (1999, p. 561).

Being able to make decisions regarding one's patients is a requirement for effective patient care. Chumbler, Geller, and Weier (2000) examined the relationship between NP clinical productivity (amount of patients seen per week) and clinical decision-making levels. Clinical decision making was defined as practice autonomy. A survey was mailed to all NPs practicing in Wisconsin ($n = 628$), with a final sample size of 293 NPs. Outpatient clinical productivity was the dependent variable, and the independent variable to measure clinical decision making was a seven-item questionnaire (tasks routinely performed by NPs), with responses rated in Likert-type categories, developed by the authors. Among the study's significant findings was that NPs who had greater decision-making authority (greater autonomy) had greater outpatient clinical productivity ($r = .265$, $P < .001$). This study did not include the extent to which prescriptive privileges correlated to outpatient productivity, nor did it consider the complexity of patient characteristics.

The concept of autonomy cannot be simply related to outpatient clinical productivity. A study focusing on primary care NPs in Florida (Bahadori & Fitzpatrick, 2009) explored levels of autonomy by using the Dempster Practice Behavior Scale (DPBS). The 30-item tool used a 5-point Likert scale with questions related to the NPs' practices. Findings were that these primary care NPs had high levels of autonomy, skill, competence, decision making, and accountability. Although this sample was reflective of NPs in one state, it is noteworthy to mention that at this time, Florida is one of the most restrictive states for NPs' legislative scope of practice. A national survey to validate these findings would be useful to affect legislation and policy makers.

Jeffrey Bauer, PhD, is well-known as a medical economist and health futurist. In an article identifying nurse practitioners as a cost-effective resource for health reform, Bauer (2010) encourages policy makers to allow NPs to be independent practitioners and be used to the full extent of their scope of practice. He clearly identifies that the multitude of gaps in our increasingly complex healthcare system, which is in dire need of solutions, can be provided by NPs who provide cost-effective, safe, quality health care.

Ethics

Every profession has a code of ethics, which is a social contract for society and is fundamental for providing guidance to the profession in ethical as well as legal situations. There are nine provisions listed in the Code of Ethics for Nurses developed by the American Nurses Association, first in 1985 and updated in 2001 (ANA, 2001). Every nursing student is expected to incorporate these obligations of the nursing profession, and to act in accord with this code. The International Council of Nurses (ICN) also has a code of ethics that was initially developed in 1953. The organization encourages all nurses to share the code as widely as possible. The preamble to the elements of the code states:

> Nurses have four fundamental responsibilities: to promote health, to prevent illness, to restore health and to alleviate suffering. The need for nursing is universal. Inherent in nursing is a respect for human rights, including cultural rights, the right to life and choice, to dignity and to be treated with respect. Nursing care is respectful of and unrestricted by considerations of age, colour, creed, culture, disability or illness, gender, sexual orientation, nationality, politics, race or social status. Nurses render health services to the individual, the family and the community and coordinate their services with those of related groups. (ICN, 2012)

An area that lacks significant study is related to applied ethics and nurse practitioners, particularly outside of the acute care setting. In daily interactions with patients, families, colleagues, institutions, and even our sociopolitical world, dilemmas are often presented to the NP who needs to respond in an ethical and culturally sensitive manner. Studies have identified issues that are frustrating and can cause moral distress and/or ethical dilemmas for NPs. These include topics around the constraints from patients' lack of adequate healthcare coverage, unrealistic demands by patients, limited time to spend with patients due to scheduling pressures, restrictive drug formularies, allocation of resources, and abortion (Fox & Chesla, 2008; Laabs, 2005).

Diane C. Viens, DNSc, CFNP, undertook a qualitative study titled "The Moral Reasoning of Nurse Practitioners" (1995). In her thought-provoking article, Viens discusses the limitations of the biomedical ethics approach for NPs facing moral dilemmas in the outpatient setting. In addition, she pinpoints issues related to gender bias that critics identified in Kohlberg's model of moral development; in particular, Carol Gilligan as critic, whose model of moral development (Gilligan, 1982; Gilligan, Ward, & Taylor, 1988) suggests that females and males have differing approaches to moral reasoning. Often NPs have difficult patient situations requiring the ability to make clinical decisions based on moral values held by the NPs. For most NPs these types of decisions are faced daily in clinical practice. The NP participants in this study valued caring and the patient–NP relationship as essential components of successful practice. Another qualitative study found that forming a personal and caring relationship with patients is a foundation for a trusting patient–healthcare provider relationship, which leads to better health outcomes for patients (Fox & Chesla, 2008). Terms that were uncovered to describe this positive relationship include *partnership, mutual respect, empathetic attunement, negotiation, flexibility, patience, encouragement, personableness, authentic,* and *open*.

Peterson and Potter (2004) recommended a specific code of ethics for nurse practitioners. The authors related the overlap of nursing and medicine that forms the unique role of nurse practitioner. The proposal presented discussed the code of ethics for nurses, the code of ethics for physicians, and the standards for practice for NPs. Building upon the standards would be the framework for the code of ethics for NPs. Due to the continued issues revolving around scope of practice in various states, as well as the development of the consensus model, this has not yet been developed.

Service/Altruism

In an effort to explore and stimulate critical thinking and professional self-reflection, at this author's university, family NP students who accompany faculty to developing countries to provide health care to underserved or unserved needy populations are required to write two comprehensive SOAP notes on at least two different patients focusing on the plan of care. One of the plans covers what was actually done, offered while in the guest country; the other is to be a treatment plan that would be reflective of what would be done for the same patient if he or she was in the United States with good health insurance. The teaching "moment" is remarkable. In addition, students who take the opportunity to work in a community health clinic are also encouraged to share patient experiences that they find frustrating, being unable to offer treatment plans per expert guidelines because the patient does not have adequate—or any—health insurance. Deciding what diagnostic testing is truly required, and at what expense, is frequently illuminating for NP students who had been working as RNs in an acute care setting, where most often care is provided without thought to the cost or absolute necessity, and students may find that care is sometimes provided as a proactive defense against malpractice claims.

Following is an example of using the qualities discussed thus far and how we, as faculty, try to instill these qualities in our students.

FACULTY/STUDENT HEALTHCARE MISSION

We are sitting very tightly together in a cramped small bus that is taking us to a Mayan village that expects us to see about 150 children who are coming to the malnutrition center today. The roads are quite bumpy and curvy as we head up the mountain looking at trash on the sides of the road but with amazingly beautiful scenery in the background. Such a dichotomy . . . the nursing students and the NP students are anxious as they are unaware of what this clinic will be like—will the interpreters be there—will the children be very sick—will they even want to come and be seen by us? The other faculty member, the two host mission workers, and I try to reassure them that we will be welcomed with open arms. We are here by their request, and we are their guests during our time here. I remind my NP students that they are nurses—the skills they already possess will take care of most of the types of needs for the day. We only have a limited supply of medications, mostly vitamins, acetaminophen, topicals, a few antibiotics, and antiparasitics. As we turn the corner we all see the very long line of the Mayan village's young children, wearing the colorful clothing worn by the indigenous. Many of the children are obviously malnourished, but almost every face beaming with smiles for us.

As we were getting set up, I took a few students with me to get a general idea of where everything is and how things would work for us. As part of our outdoor "tour" began, we saw the very small area that contained the brand new bathroom stalls (which were leaking water everywhere) that the host was very proud of so we made sure to acknowledge the monies and effort this must have taken; however, this 5-foot-square area also housed the chickens and a guard dog, the chicken being plucked, another chicken being cooked, and yet another cooked chicken being deboned—all on the ground next to the leaking toilets. Our group learning discussion later that evening after a very busy clinic taking care of small undernourished children with horribly decaying teeth and superficial burns, and of course everyone (almost) had symptoms of parasites, revolved around basic public health principles and the education we could provide to help improve health that did not require complex medication regimens. Also part of the discussion was how to incorporate cultural considerations and professionalism as well as kindness and understanding as we offer suggestions to our patients. Our patients were most often 10- to 12-year-old girls who were in charge of the younger children all day while mom attended to household chores and dad was out working in the fields. These were the patients we were directing our educational efforts to—needing them to understand how to take care of themselves as well as the many younger children they were in charge of. The most obvious answer to most of the problems we were seeing was clean water for drinking, cooking, bathing, and cleaning. It was the one thing we really could not provide.

Later that night a rapid knocking on my bedroom door had me scurrying to find out what was wrong. A student said someone needs you—someone's niece in another village got burned with hot water and you need to go see her, they are waiting outside with a jeep. I ran down the stairs with many questions running through my mind. A nonmedical friend offered to accompany me since it was dangerous to be out alone in the evening. As we hopped in the car with only a first aid kit in hand, the driver raced over the bumps, and off we went into the night, having no clue what we would find. I asked why they didn't bring the girl to a hospital ER. They said her family could not afford that, and they hoped we could do something. When we arrived, we had to make

(continues)

FACULTY/STUDENT HEALTHCARE MISSION

(continued)

our way through a tiny pathway, and we could see the open cooking area with two small rooms alongside it. A shelter made out of tin. The girl turned out to be a teenager who was lying on a single bed with her thin nightgown falling off her. She was moaning and holding her ear and pointing to her throat. Only one of us could fit in the tiny room, and I had to climb onto the bed and crawl up to see her using a flashlight. Although it didn't seem to be a bad burn, she told the translator she was having a lot of pain in her ear and it ran down her throat to her chest. Apparently the hot liquid had splashed into her ear and she felt it go down her throat. Now I was faced with some difficult clinical decision making. Once the translator told us there was no 9-1-1 in the area if her throat started to swell, and that they had no medical equipment for me to look in her ear or down her throat, I said I felt she needed a more thorough assessment (her moaning was pitiful). We said we would like to take her to the private hospital in the next town, and that we would pay for the visit and any medication she might need if we did not have it. Visibly relieved, we took the girl to this private hospital—tiny but clean. The doctor also acted as the triage nurse and admitting person! After a thorough inspection, he gave her some pain medicine, a prescription for some ear drops and Silvadene cream for her skin burns, and a wonderful education on how to care for herself as well as things to be concerning enough for her to then return to the ER. What a surprise to find out the entire visit and medications cost us about $40 U.S.!

Leadership

Joyce (2001) conducted a study that looked at the perception of leadership attributes among nurse practitioners. The attribute of "professional" was identified in those who display leadership qualities. In addition, the characteristics of integrity; of being competent, accountable, and resourceful; having confidence in one's judgment, managing time well, and the ability to raise the bar for setting standards were identified as describing the "professional."

Practice models for NPs need to incorporate core values of professionalism and leadership. One example of a model of practice for acute care NPs was developed at Strong Memorial Hospital in Rochester, New York (Ackerman, Norsen, Martin, Wiedrich, & Kitzman, 1996). Although the model was developed for the then-new role of acute care NP, the conceptual strands encompassed with it are pertinent to all NP practice types. The concepts of scholarship, collaboration, and empowerment are threaded throughout the domains of the model, which are direct, comprehensive care; support of systems, education, and research; and publication and professional leadership. The concept of scholarship integrates the need to maintain a high standard of clinical competence to provide excellent patient care. Collaboration encompasses the belief that the unique skills of a variety of healthcare providers are needed to provide excellence in patient care. Attributes that underscore the concept of collaboration for NPs in this model include cooperation, autonomy, assertiveness, responsibility, communication, and coordination. This framework is dependent on mutual regard and respect. The Strong model described empowerment as the atmosphere that sustains advanced practice. This concept is central to the model. The NP is responsible for, and has the authority to, identify and analyze patient problems, develop and implement a plan of action, as well as evaluate and be accountable for these decisions.

As noted in all of these models, it is important for all student NPs and practicing NPs to join their professional organization and to become active in it. The American College of Nurse Practitioners (ACNP) and the American Academy of Nurse Practitioners (AANP) have merged so that NPs can speak and be heard with one common voice. The merger of the two long-standing organizations helps the student by not having to choose which organization is best. This merger helps to create a myriad of positive benefits including increased visibility, stronger representation regarding health policy issues, and unity when working with other professional organizations on matters pertinent to NPs and our patients.

Clearly, the student NP must use reflective processes during didactic and clinical educational experiences to develop this new professional role and to understand the full scope of what it means. The AANP includes descriptors for integrity and professionalism, which are trust and transparency, accountability, ethical commitment, reliability, respect, personal and professional accountability, unity within the profession/discipline, and inclusivity.

Nurses have been identified as the most trusted profession in the United States by the Gallup poll for many years (Gallup, 2012). That people trust nurses to provide ethically based care, be an integral part in improving patient outcomes, increase access to care, and help to reduce costs of health care puts nurses in the forefront of health care today. Nurse practitioners are in a position to be an advanced practice role model who continues to build on the characteristics of professionalism. The NP/DNP has a responsibility not only to individual patients, but also to the profession, and to generate knowledge to advance nursing practice (Dahnke & Dreher, 2011).

Seminar Discussion Questions

1. What constitutes a "profession"? What are the most commonly referred to professional disciplines?
2. What does professionalism as a nurse practitioner mean to you?
3. Discuss your personal beliefs of the three most important components or identifiers of professionalism as an NP.
4. Discuss examples of daily clinical situations that have posed moral dilemmas for you and/or your preceptor and how you approached these with patients and families.

References

Ackerman, M. H., Norsen, L., Martin, B., Wiedrich, J., & Kitzman, H. J. (1996). Development of a model of advanced practice. *American Journal of Critical Care, 5*(1), 68–73.

Adams, D., & Miller, B. K. (2001). Professionalism in nursing behaviors of nurse practitioners. *Journal of Professional Nursing, 17*(4), 203–210.

American Nurses Association. (2001). *Code of ethics for nurses.* Retrieved from http://nursingworld.org/MainMenuCategories/EthicsStandards/CodeofEthicsforNurses

Bahadori, A., & Fitzpatrick, J. J. (2009). Level of autonomy of primary care nurse practitioners. *Journal of the American Academy of Nurse Practitioners, 2*, 513–519.

Bauer, J. (2010). Nurse practitioners as an underutilized resource for health reform: Evidence-based demonstrations of cost-effectiveness. *Journal of the American Academy of Nurse Practitioners, 22*, 228–231.

Carryer, J., Gardner, G., Dunn, S., & Gardner, A. (2007). The core role of the nurse practitioner: Practice, professionalism and clinical leadership. *Journal of Clinical Nursing, 16*(10), 1818–1825. doi:10.1111/j.1365-2702.2006.01823.x

Chitty, K., & Black, B. (2011). *Professional nursing: Concepts and challenges* (6th ed.). Maryland Heights, MO: Saunders.

Chumbler, N. R., Geller, J. M., & Weier, A. W. (2000). The effects of clinical decision making on nurse practitioners' clinical productivity. *Evaluation & the Health Professions, 23*(3), 284–304.

Crigger, N., & Godfrey, N. (2011). *The making of nurse professionals: A transtheoretical approach.* Sudbury, MA: Jones and Bartlett.

Dahnke, M., & Dreher, H. M. (2011). *Philosophy of science for nursing practice: Concepts and application.* New York, NY: Springer.

Flexner, A. (1910). *Medical education in the U.S. and Canada.* The Carnegie Foundation.

Fox, S., & Chesla, C. (2008). Living with chronic illness: A phenomenological study of the health effects of the patient-provider relationship. *Journal of the American Academy of Nurse Practitioners, 20*(3), 109–117.

Gallup. (2012). *Honesty/ethics in professions.* Retrieved from http://www.gallup.com/poll/1654/honesty-ethics-professions.aspx

Gilligan, C. (1982). *In a different voice: Psychological theory and women's development.* Cambridge, MA: Harvard University Press.

Gilligan, C., Ward, J. V., & Taylor, J. M. (Eds.). (1988). *Mapping the moral domain.* Cambridge, MA: Harvard University Press.

International Council of Nurses. (2012). *Code of ethics.* Geneva, Switzerland: Author.

Joyce, E. (2001). Leadership perceptions of nurse practitioners. *Lippincott's Case Management, 6*(1), 24–30.

Keenan, J. (1999). A concept analysis of autonomy. *Journal of Advanced Nursing, 29*(3), 556–562.

Kelly, L. (1981). *Dimensions of professional nursing* (4th ed.). New York, NY: Macmillan.

Laabs, C. (2005). Moral problems and distress among nurse practitioners in primary care. *Journal of the American Academy of Nurse Practitioners, 17*(2), 76–84.

McMurray, R. (2010). The struggle to professionalize: An ethnographic account of the occupational position of advanced nurse oractitioners. *Human Relations, 64*(6), 801–822. doi:10.1177/0018726710387949

Peterson, M., & Potter, R. L. (2004). A proposal for a code of ethics for nurse practitioners. *Journal of the American Academy of Nurse Practitioners, 16*(3), 116–124.

UK Department of Health. (2006). Professionalism—The big conversation by Karen Middleton. *Voicepiece.* Retrieved from http://ahp.dh.gov.uk/2012/02/27/voicepiece-karen-middleton-chief-health-professions-officer

Viens, D. (1995). The moral reasoning of nurse practitioners. *Journal of the American Academy of Nurse Practitioners, 7*(6), 277–284.

Additional Resources

Deming, W. E. (1994). *The new economics for industry, government, education* (2nd ed.). Cambridge, MA: The MIT Press.

DeNisco, S., & Barker, A. (2012). *Advanced practice nursing: Evolving roles for the transformation of the profession* (2nd ed.). Burlington, MA: Jones & Bartlett Learning.

CHAPTER 12

Health Policy and the Nurse Practitioner

Julie A. Koch

The need for political activism in the healthcare arena has never been greater. Since the 1960s, nurse practitioners (NPs) have been advocating for the profession and the improvement of social policies impacting health care. Over the past 50 years, NPs have gained ground in efforts to eliminate barriers in the delivery of care and to enhance patient access to their services, but additional work is needed. At the time of this writing, NPs within 22 states and the District of Columbia had been granted full practice authority (American Association of Nurse Practitioners [AANP], 2017b), the ability to practice to the full extent of training and education; additional states had similar legislation in various stages of development or approval. Yet, those with full practice authority still may face barriers to providing optimal care for their patients, and a number of issues still warrant attention on an institutional, regional, or national level.

The push for practicing to the full extent of one's academic and experiential preparation is vitally important as the nation's population ages and the number of primary care physicians stagnates. The growth both in the number and proportion of older Americans is unprecedented; because of longer life spans and the number of aging baby boomers, the population of Americans age 65 years and older will double over the next 25 years to approximately 72 million (Centers for Disease Control and Prevention [CDC], 2013). And by 2030, these effects may become readily apparent as older adults will account for approximately 20% of the U.S. population (CDC, 2013). Based on existing data, it can be assumed that these older adults will face the challenges of living with chronic health conditions. Currently, approximately two-thirds of older Americans have multiple chronic conditions; medical treatment for this population accounts for 66% of the country's healthcare budget (CDC, 2013), presenting a strong economic incentive for cost-effective health care. Yet, an increasing number of thought leaders have recognized that physicians alone will not be able to meet the healthcare needs of older adults. The Association of American Medical

Colleges' (AAMC) comprehensive national analysis projected that the nation will face a shortage of 12,000 to 31,000 primary care physicians by the year 2025 (AAMC, 2015). This projected shortage was further impacted by the Affordable Care Act of 2010 (ACA), which provided healthcare access for millions of previously uninsured older and younger Americans. The White House Office of the Secretary noted that prior to the 2016 open enrollment period, 17.6 million previously uninsured individuals had gained healthcare coverage (The White House President Barack Obama Office of the Press Secretary, 2016). The increased number of individuals with access to healthcare services through their newly acquired insurance coverage placed an additional strain on primary care physician practices. Yet, the lack of access to primary care providers and the need to provide cost-effective quality care to the U.S. population can be addressed by the more than 222,000 NPs who have been educationally and experientially prepared to fill this gap (AANP, 2017a).

As NPs prepare to meet the healthcare needs of the American population, it is paramount to recognize where we have come from in order to understand the ramifications of where we are going and where we need to be to meet the needs of the nation's health care. This chapter reviews the history of health policy related to nurse practitioners, examines the current regulatory structure impacting health care today, addresses current health policy issues (including a view of the quest for full practice authority), and identifies strategies to enhance the NP's role in political activism, meeting the healthcare needs of Americans nationwide.

History of the NP and Related Health Policy

The foundation of nurse practitioner healthcare advocacy can be linked to Florence Nightingale, a visionary of public policy on numerous healthcare issues: promoting clean water, good nutrition, decent lodging, and adequate ventilation to reduce infection rates. Astutely political, as a woman living in the 1800s, Nightingale was unable to vote; yet, she was able to move healthcare reform issues through leadership, innovative thought, and perseverance. She lobbied the British Parliament to educate nurses who would serve in public workhouses and was passionate in her opinion that individuals who were sick should avoid hospitalization, advocating for home health services provided by nurses and physicians. The fact that Nightingale was able to obtain the support of high-level medical experts, cabinet ministers, and senior governmental officials has been attributed to her careful preparation and attention to detail. The most prominent sanitarians of the time, statisticians, engineers, and water experts alike were willing to work with her to advance health policies because they shared her vision and respected her methods (McDonald, 2006).

Building upon Nightingale's legacy of using innovative thoughts and actions to improve health care, Loretta C. Ford developed the first NP program in 1965 at the University of Colorado Schools of Medicine and Nursing (National Women's Hall of Fame, 2017). Dr. Ford, along with pediatrician Henry K. Silver, recognized that a shortage of family care physicians and pediatricians was impacting the ability to provide health care in rural and underserved areas. The pair obtained a small grant from the University of Colorado and implemented the nation's first pediatric nurse practitioner program. The curriculum combined clinical practice, education, and research to address the social, psychological, environmental, and economic aspects of patient care. Through her innovative thought and actions, Dr. Ford transformed the nursing profession, enhanced access to care for the general public, and led the future movement for nurse practitioners.

By the early 1970s, more than 65 programs were preparing nurse practitioners across the nation and approximately 10,000 NPs were practicing (AANP, n.d.). Since national NP organizations were in their infancy at that time (the National Association of Pediatric Nurse Practitioners [NAPNAP] was established in 1973), grassroots movements were essential in the attainment of formal reimbursement of NP services. In 1974, the first federal legislation was introduced; the bill was intended to amend the Social Security Act so that NPs' services would be covered under Medicare and Medicaid (Bartol, 2015). Over the next 20 years or so, at least 10 pieces of federal legislation that gradually established the role of the NP and provided reimbursement for NP services were adopted (Bartol, 2015). In 1985, the American Academy of Nurse Practitioners (AANP) was established, and the organization quickly began a concerted effort to affect pertinent national legislation (AANP, n.d.). The ultimate culmination of these early health policy efforts was the Balanced Budget Act of 1997, signed by President Clinton, which granted provider status to NPs and authorized them to bill Medicare directly for providing services to its recipients, regardless of setting (Bartol, 2015).

These early grassroots movements, followed by structured advocacy set forth in part by national organizations, resulted in significant changes in the landscape of NP practice. Yet, additional policy changes are still needed. With education advancing to the doctoral level, NPs are now being prepared to position themselves as leaders who impact, guide, and develop health policies that address accessible, quality care for all Americans and in turn advance NPs' professional status.

Formal Health Policy Education for NPs

Consistent with the beliefs of the Advanced Practice Registered Nurse (APRN) Joint Dialogue Group (2008), today's doctorally prepared NPs need to have the knowledge and skills to respond to the increased need for healthcare providers and be positioned as leaders in the development of health policies affecting patients and professional practice. Instead of reacting to potentially detrimental policy proposals, the NP can and should be at the forefront contributing to the policy-making process. While the scope of health policy education is far more comprehensive than can be covered in this chapter, the intention is to cover essential elements of health policy as they pertain to NPs, with the goal of stimulating discussion and action plans for current issues.

Recognizing that practice-focused doctoral programs, designed to prepare experts in specialized, innovative, evidence-based advanced nursing practice, differ from traditional PhD programs, the American Association of Colleges of Nursing (AACN) created a task force to develop curricular expectations for DNP education. In October 2006, the AACN released *The Essentials of Doctoral Education for Advanced Nursing Practice*, commonly referred to as The DNP Essentials. The DNP Essentials outline health policy related objectives for DNP graduates. Essential V: Health Care Policy for Advocacy in Health Care cites that DNP graduates should be prepared to:

1. Critically analyze health policy proposals, health policies, and related issues from the perspective of consumers, nursing, other health professions, and other stakeholders in policy and public forums.

2. Demonstrate leadership in the development and implementation of institutional, local, state, federal, and international health policy.
3. Influence policy makers through active participation on committees, boards, or task forces at the institutional, local, state, regional, national, and international levels to improve healthcare delivery and outcomes.
4. Educate others, including policy makers at all levels, regarding nursing, health policy, and patient care outcomes.
5. Advocate for the nursing profession within the policy and healthcare communities.
6. Develop, evaluate, and provide leadership for healthcare policy that shapes healthcare financing, regulation, and delivery.
7. Advocate for social justice, equity, and ethical policies within all healthcare arenas. *(The Essentials of Doctoral Education for Advanced Nursing Practice, October 2006, p. 14. Reprinted with permission of the American Association of Colleges of Nursing.)*

Recognizing that today's nurse practitioners have the opportunity to address the scope of practice issues identified by the Institutes of Medicine of the National Academies (IOM) and positively impact the nation's health, the National Organization for Nurse Practitioner Faculties (NONPF) developed a set of NP core competencies. The health policy competencies, which are reflective of the DNP Essentials, were published in 2014 and updated in 2017. The *Nurse Practitioner Core Competencies Content* includes suggestions for curricular content relative to the core competencies (NONPF, 2017). Under the policy competency area, NONPF has noted that the NP graduate:

1. Demonstrates an understanding of the interdependence of policy and practice.
2. Advocates for ethical policies that promote access, equity, quality, and cost.
3. Analyzes ethical, legal, and social factors influencing policy development.
4. Contributes in the development of health policy.
5. Analyzes the implications of health policy across disciplines.
6. Evaluates the impact of globalization on healthcare policy development. *(NONPF. Nurse Practitioner Core Competencies Content, 2017, pp. 9–10. Reprinted with permission from the National Organization of Nurse Practitioner Faculties)*
7. Advocates for policies for safe and healthy practice environments.

These outcomes and competencies reflect the DNP graduate's ability to assume broad leadership in political activism and policy development. The health policy objectives have been incorporated within DNP programs throughout the nation and are still being instituted today.

Advancing NP Practice through Health Policy

In order to advance the profession, it is imperative that doctorally prepared NPs have a foundational knowledge of healthcare legislation and regulation. These two areas of health policy significantly impact the profession's movement toward full practice authority.

Healthcare Legislation

Understanding the key processes in the health policy arena can assist the doctorally prepared NP to keep abreast of current issues and take steps to initiate change that will further advance the profession. Nurse practitioners can play a major role leading health policy change, from the introduction of a policy issue through petitioning legislators for a vote to support a specific healthcare bill.

Policy issues warranting the NP's attention can range from patient-related issues (e.g., funding for immunizations and smoking cessation programs) to practice-specific issues (i.e., restrictions to scope of professional practice). Once an issue is identified that warrants legislative change, the doctorally prepared NP should prepare a brief synopsis, frequently called an "elevator speech" or "sound bite" that can be presented to others who share the same vision for moving the issue forward. Short messages that convey the key points succinctly are useful when communicating with other professionals, the media, and politicians. This process of agenda setting has the greatest chance for success when it is founded in statistics and pertinent factual information, yet provided in language that is easily understood by those not employed in health care.

Getting the appropriate organization to work on the bill will help to move it forward. Most NP organizations have lobbyists who know how and who to reach with the message; lobbyists can advise the NP organization if there are other interests competing with their efforts or if the timing is right to introduce a specific bill, thus maximizing the potential for passage. This underscores the need for NPs to be involved with local, state, and national NP organizations. In addition to lobbying, these organizations can initiate grassroots advocacy movements, educating their members about pending legislation and asking them to contact their legislators and other government officials. NPs can participate in letter-writing campaigns or meet with their legislators on an individual basis or as part of a larger group. Legislators are often willing to meet with NP constituents who reside in their legislative districts during periods when they are not in session, and NP organizations can schedule session meetings as part of their grassroots advocacy. House session calendars are available on each state's general assembly website, and these sites also serve as a valuable resource for NPs, identifying legislators by district/region (which can be searched by constituent's zip code), specifying the committees that they serve on, and providing contact information. Websites of state and local NP organizations often include political action agenda items, and there is a wealth of federal and state legislative information, as well as policy toolkits, on the AANP's website. The NAPNAP also has resources available for its members that will be reviewed later in this chapter.

Although a bill can be drafted by an individual or an organization, it can only be introduced once a legislator in the Senate or House of Representatives has sponsored it. Legislators usually sponsor bills that are important to them and their constituents; so, it is integral for the individual NP or NP organization to convey the issue's impact on constituents to key legislators. Having previously established relationships with legislators provides an opportunity for NPs to further advocate for bill sponsorship.

Drafted bills are sent to the appropriate clerk who assigns a title and number. Once printed, the bill's legislative author will garner support for the bill as it is sent to the appropriate committee(s) to view and discuss. Legislators with a strong degree of political clout are more likely to gather significant support at the stage of committee review. During the committee review period, there may be public hearings where

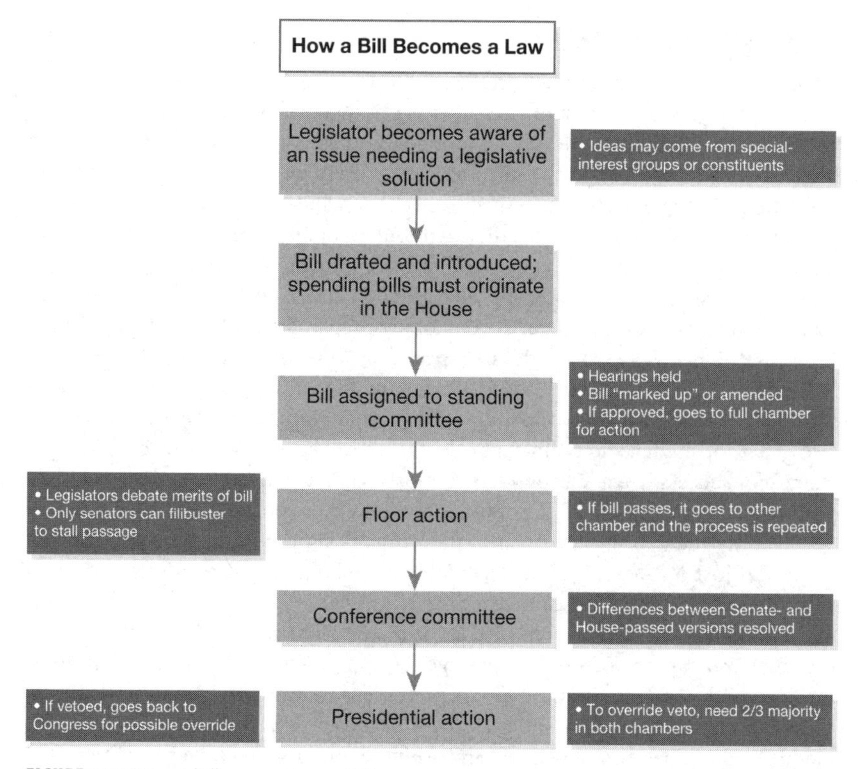

FIGURE 12-1 How a bill passes through Congress

NPs and others with interest in the topic can provide short testimonials. If the bill is viewed favorably, it may be passed on to other involved committees and be discussed and approved. If the proposed bill does not fail along the way, the process moves on to the state assemblies, and the governor can sign it or veto the bill. The process is similar for federal bills and laws, with the president being the one to veto or approve a bill (**FIGURE 12-1**).

Healthcare Regulation

Once a federal bill has been signed into law, agencies create regulations or rules under the authority of Congress to help carry out public health policies. Proposed rules are published daily by the National Archives and Records Administration (NARA) in the *Federal Register* (https://www.federalregister.gov). Interested parties are invited to provide comments on the website and/or attend a scheduled hearing or public meeting to provide input into the regulatory process. Once the agency has reviewed and considered all related information and associated comments, an implementation plan is developed and the rule is published in the *Federal Register*; the rule becomes effective 30 days after publication.

For NPs across the nation, many policies related to practice are regulated by the U.S. Department of Health and Human Services (DHHS). The overall mission of DHHS is "to enhance the health and well-being of Americans by providing for effective health and human services and by fostering sound, sustained advances in the sciences underlying medicine, public health, and social services" (DHHS, n.d.). The DHHS develops a strategic plan to further define its mission, goals, and the methods for evaluating progress in meeting selected goals for a 4-year period. Because the GPRA (Government Performance and Results Act) Modernization Act requires federal agencies to consult with Congress and to solicit and consider views of external parties, while developing its strategic plan, DHHS engages the public through the DHHS Open Government website (http://www.hhs.gov/open), the *Federal Register*, conference calls or email notices to key stakeholders, and social media postings. Feedback from all sources is used to finalize the DHHS's strategic plan.

For fiscal years 2014–2018, DHHS has four overarching strategic goals that align with its mission (DHHS, 2015):

Goal 1: Strengthen health care.

Goal 2: Advance scientific knowledge and innovation.

Goal 3: Advance the health, safety, and well-being of the American people.

Goal 4: Increase efficiency, transparency, and accountability of HHS programs.

Eleven divisions (see organizational chart within **FIGURE 12-2**), which administer an array of health and human services focusing on the strategic goals, operate within the DHHS. Within these 11 divisions, the DHHS is responsible for providing healthcare coverage to more than 100 million people; assuring the safety and effectiveness of food, drugs, vaccines, and medical devices; providing the largest funding source for medical research in the world; and eliminating disparities in health (DHHS, 2014).

Ten regional DHHS offices directly serve state and local organizations; regional directors maintain close contact with state, local, and tribal partners, ensuring that DHHS programs and policies address the needs of the community. The work of the Region VI's Senior Program Manager Officer for the Office of Minority is featured in a Health Policy Exemplar later in this chapter.

Current Health Policy Issues

Keeping abreast of current health policy issues is essential to the advocacy initiatives of socially conscious healthcare providers. Topics that continue to generate interest among doctorally prepared NPs include scope of practice, healthcare reform, access to care, and reimbursement.

Scope of Practice

Scope of practice issues continue to serve as barriers for NPs who strive to practice to the full extent of their educational and experiential preparation. Back in 2008, The Robert Wood Johnson Foundation (RWJF) and the Institutes of Medicine (IOM) launched a 2-year initiative to respond to the need to advance the nursing profession; a joint committee was charged with the task of producing a report outlining an action-oriented blueprint. As a result of this joint effort, in 2010, the IOM issued *The Future of Nursing: Leading Change, Advancing Health*, which called for the removal of policies, regulations, and laws that prevent APRNs, including NPs, from providing the full scope of services that they have been trained and educated to provide (Institute of Medicine [IOM], 2010).

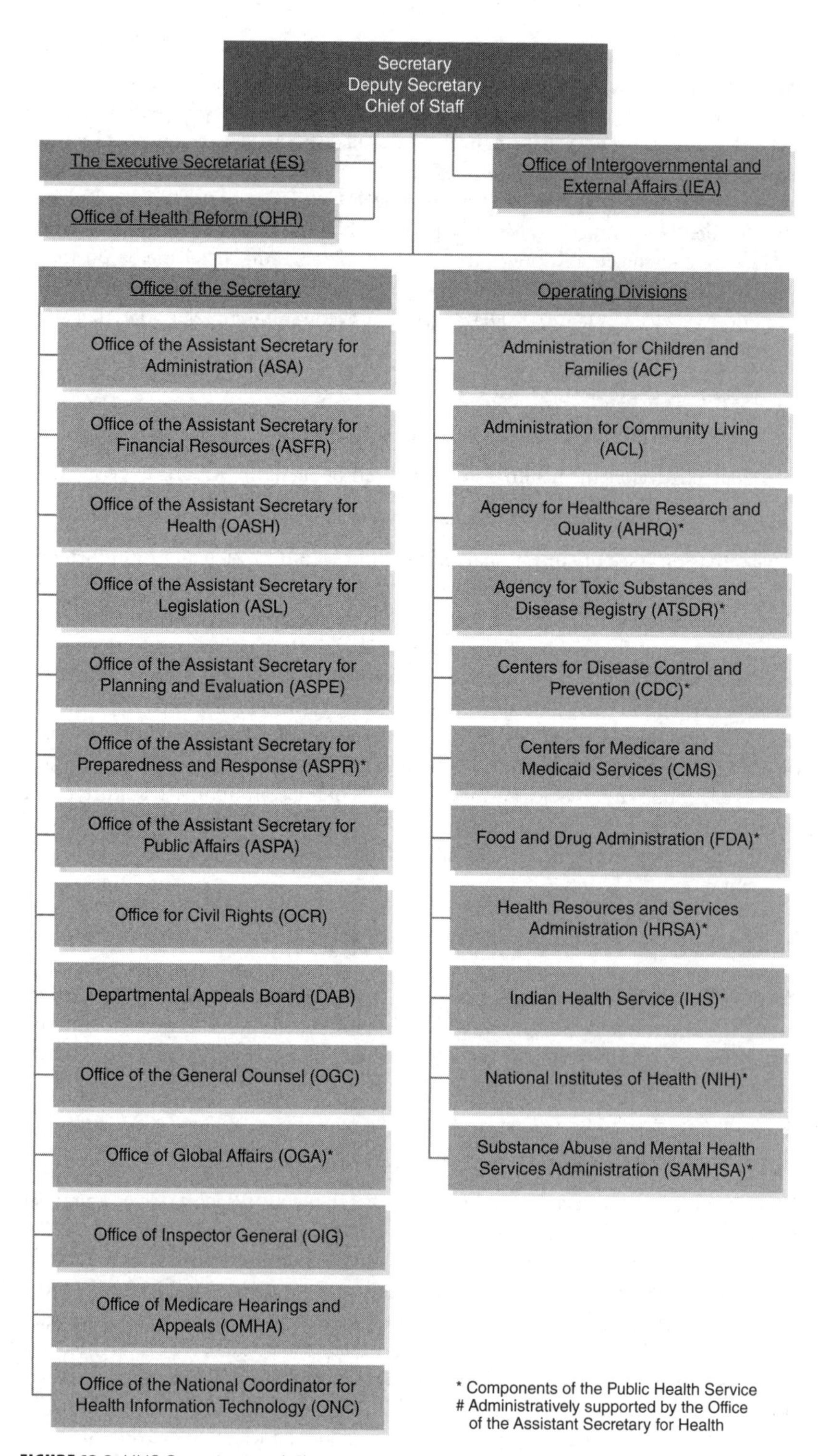

FIGURE 12-2 HHS Organizational Chart

Reproduced from U.S. Department of Health & Human Services. (2017). HHS Organizational Chart. Retrieved from https://www.hhs.gov/about/agencies/orgchart/index.html

As a follow up to the IOM's publication, in 2017, the RWJF published a brief outlining the barriers to APRN practice, including the patchwork of laws and regulations that restrict patients' access to APRN services and the cost of collaborative practice agreements. The authors of the RWJF brief noted that state practice acts, institutional policies, and federal statutes and regulations that require physician oversight or otherwise restrict APRN practice continue to limit access to care, create disruptions in care, increase the cost of care, and undermine efforts to improve the quality of care; the authors cited that a growing body of research suggests removing practice restrictions on NPs has the potential to actually reduce cost and improve access to care without compromising the quality of that care (RWJF, 2017). Within the brief, it was also noted that physician oversight in collaborative agreements can be financially burdensome for APRNs and confusing for policy makers and members of the public, who may mistakenly think that the agreements facilitate true collaborative care (RWJF, 2017).

The Consensus Model for APRN Regulation: Licensure, Accreditation, Certification, & Education (LACE), an APRN Joint Dialogue Group Report, was completed through work of the APRN Consensus Work Group and the National Council of State Boards of Nursing APRN Advisory Committee. The APRN Joint Dialogue Group described the APRN regulatory model; defined APRN practice, roles, and population foci; and presented strategies for implementation including the requisite education, certification, and licensure in terms of role and population foci (ARPN Joint Dialogue Group, 2008). Although the authors determined that APRNs could specialize in a specific area (e.g., endocrinology or oncology), they must be licensed in one of the four roles (CRNA, CNM, CNS, or CNP) with a population focus (see **FIGURE 12-3**). Furthermore, certification must meet the standards provided within the LACE guidelines, ensuring entry-level competency of the APRN. The Joint Dialogue Group noted that the boards of nursing within individual states need to be the regulatory body that issues licenses and provides oversight of APRNs. The group's goal was to ultimately have consistency in licensure, accreditation, certification, and education in all states, work that is still in progress.

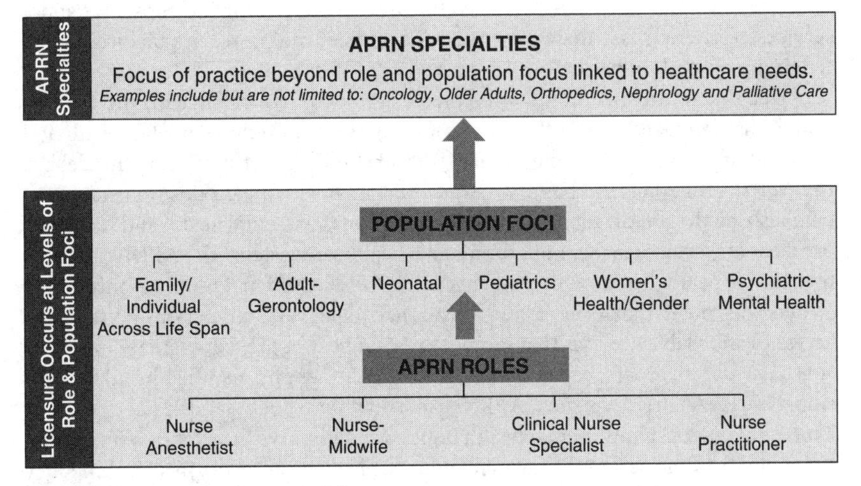

FIGURE 12-3 APRN Regulatory Model

Reproduced from APRN Joint Dialogue Group Report, July 7, 2008, p. 10. Reprinted by permission of American Association of Colleges of Nursing.

To date, each state has been able to define APRN legal scope of practice, recognize the APRN roles and titles, as well as define the criteria for entry into practice, and the certification examinations that are acceptable. The scope of practice for nurse practitioners across the nation, by state, can be found on the AANP website (https://www.aanp.org/legislation-regulation/state-legislation/state-practice-environment). Because each state can define the scope of practice in statutes, some of which are detailed and others more general, it is essential that NPs review the most current scope of practice legislated by the state in which they practice. NPs have the authority to diagnose, treat, and prescribe medications without the requirement of physician collaboration or oversight in 22 states and the District of Columbia (Phillips, 2017). In the remaining 28 states, there is some form of physician collaboration or supervision required, despite the IOM's recommendations to allow APRNs to practice to the full extent of their education and training. But, on a more positive note, in December 2016, the Department of Veterans Affairs (VA) published a final rule (81 FR 90198) that granted veterans direct access to care from three of the four APRN specialties (CNMs, CNSs, and NPs) (VA, 2016). The final rule authorizes NPs to practice to the full extent of their education and preparation without physician supervision in all areas, with the exception of prescribing controlled medications (which are still subject to individual state restrictions under the Controlled Substances Act). The AANP applauded the movement to provide our nation's veterans with direct access to the services provided by NPs, CNSs, and CNMs, but encouraged the VA to include CRNAs in future rules. Reflecting back on the processes outlined within the "Healthcare Legislation" and "Healthcare Regulation" sections of this chapter, it is important to note that the VA is currently evaluating full practice authority for CRNAs and comments on this issue were accepted through January 13, 2017.

Affordable Care Act/American Health Care Act

Few current issues incite as much passionate debate as healthcare reform. At the time of this writing, the repeal of the Affordable Care Act headlined prominent news networks on a weekly basis. Topics within heated discussions of the American Health Care Act include altering fees for pre-existing conditions, discriminating coverage rates by age, waiving the need to cover mental health and substance abuse services, restricting essential women's health services, and imposing Medicaid work requirements and rollbacks.

Healthcare organizations have voiced significant concerns with the AHCA, noting that language within the current proposal would reduce mental health and substance use coverage for millions of Medicaid enrollees. In the midst of this debate, the American Psychiatric Nurses Association (APNA) issued a position statement emphasizing the importance of threading provisions for mental health and substance use disorder services throughout the nation's healthcare system. The APNA's stance is that "whole health begins with mental health" (APNA, 2017, p. 1), and organizational leaders have noted that local, state, and national policies and regulations must ensure access to affordable services that promote mental health, prevent mental illness and substance use disorders, and provide care and treatment by qualified health professionals (APNA, 2017). As such, APRN leaders within APNA stand ready to provide expert guidance on how mental health policies can improve the overall wellness and productivity of the nation. The work of one such leader is featured in a Health Policy Exemplar later in this chapter.

Medicare Access and CHIP Reauthorization Act

Today's NPs are also entrenched in health policies that impact reimbursement for services. As part of the Medicare Access and CHIP Reauthorization Act of 2015 (MACRA), Medicare billing and reimbursement have been transformed from a fee-for-service schedule to a pay-for-performance program that focuses on quality, value, and accountability; the Quality Payment Program framework is intended to reward providers for better care, rather than the delivery of more services. The Merit-Based Incentive Payment System (MIPS) provides a performance score (rated from 0–100) for providers based on four categories (quality, resource use, clinical practice improvement activities, and meaningful use of electronic health records) which will be used to determine the provider's Medicare reimbursement for each payment year. Additional details about the Quality Payment Program, and its potential financial impact for NP practices, can be found at Centers for Medicare and Medicaid Services (CMS) website at https://qpp.cms.gov/. Links to the executive summary, final rule, and official DHHS press release can be found on the AANP's website: https://www.aanp.org/legislation-regulation/federal-legislation /macra-s-quality-payment-program.

Additional Health Policy Issues Impacting NPs

A number of other regulatory issues impacting the professional practices of NPs across the nation are available on the AANP website (https://www.aanp.org /legislation-regulation/federal-legislation/issue-briefs); primarily, these posted limitations relate to the provision of or reimbursement for services provided to patients enrolled in the Medicare program. Although NPs have been recognized as Part B Medicare providers who may bill for services under their own provider numbers for nearly 20 years, they still face a number of restrictions in their provision of care. The AANP has noted that by amending current statutes or directing the Centers for Medicare and Medicaid Services (CMS) to revise outdated rules and regulations, Congress should remove obsolete limitations that do not recognize NPs' advanced education and clinical preparation to furnish the full scope of services they are licensed to provide (AANP, 2015b).

One of the key recommendations within the IOM's 2010 report, *The Future of Nursing: Leading Change, Advancing Health,* was a call for revising the requirements for hospital participation in the Medicare program to ensure that NPs and other APRNs are eligible for clinical privileges (including admitting privileges). Although CMS has taken steps in recent regulations to improve opportunities for NPs to obtain clinical privileges and appointment to medical staff, without a requirement that establishes objective procedures for reviewing applications, concerns remain that hospitals will continue to deny NPs full access and privileges. Furthermore, Medicare conditions also limit clinical privileges within skilled nursing facilities (SNFs). Current regulations state that a physician must perform the admission examination and the first and subsequent alternating monthly assessments of Medicare recipients. Yet NPs have been providing care to Medicare recipients in SNFs for more than 25 years, and studies have demonstrated that NPs have increased the cost-effective quality of care provided to patients within that setting (AANP, 2015a).

For outpatient services, NPs are authorized to perform a face-to-face assessment for patients who need home health, but current legislation requires that a physician documents that the encounter has taken place, even if the physician has not participated in the assessment, is not present in the facility when the assessment was completed, and has not ever seen the patient. As another example, NPs are able to serve as attending providers and recertify Medicare patients' eligibility for hospice care, but they are still unable to provide the initial certification for care. NPs are also required under current legislation to send their diabetic patients who need therapeutic shoes to a physician who must certify the need, often resulting in a delay in receiving the necessary therapy. Furthermore, under the current statute, the certifying physician must not only document the need for therapeutic shoes, but must also treat the patient's diabetic condition after the certification, resulting in additional costs for duplication of services.

It is important to note that several of these regulatory barriers to NP practice could easily be addressed by simply using provider neutral language (i.e., "provider" rather than "physician") or correcting the interpretation of the term "physician" to be consistent with current Medicare payment policies that authorize Part B payment to NPs for services within their scope of practice. This minor change would enable NPs to certify Medicare beneficiaries for hospice and home health services and to conduct admission examinations for SNFs. Ideally, NPs should be recognized as primary care providers in all programs and settings. The AANP notes that the IOM's definition of primary care ("the provision of integrated, accessible health care services by clinicians who are accountable for addressing a large majority of personal health care needs, developing a sustained partnership with patient and practicing in the context of family and community" [IOM, 1994]) should serve as a benchmark for any legislation to expand access to primary care services (AANP, 2015b).

Get Involved

After gaining political competency within a DNP program, it is imperative that NPs remain politically engaged after graduation. Whether the DNP graduate opts to get involved in local activities or state and national NP organizations, it is the responsibility of the NP to remain aware of current issues that affect scope of practice, reimbursement, and patient and community health. Several options for political advocacy are available, but many NPs will benefit from the health policy resources available through membership in a national, state, or local NP organization.

As noted earlier in this chapter, the AANP has a plethora of health policy information on their website; white papers, toolkits, sample letters to legislators, and AANP and roundtable statements are available to download free of charge. Government affairs updates are posted weekly. The State Policy Toolkit includes AANP's state policy priorities, policy issue briefs, and state policy maps. The Federal Policy Toolkit contains sections on talking points, issue briefs, finding one's Senator or Representative, and tips on meeting or writing key legislators. It should be recognized that although proposed rules are published daily in the *Federal Register*, searching for and viewing pertinent topics can be a laborious, time-consuming process. National organizations have the personnel resources available to monitor legislation as it is being developed and send calls to action out to members. Calls to action include contact information for legislators and drafted letters that can be personalized.

Membership within a professional organization helps to support the development and maintenance of the above noted health policy resources, but dues are also used to offset the cost of lobbyists who serve the political interests of the organization. In addition to membership funds, the AANP also has a Political Action Committee (AANP-PAC) that provides members the opportunity to contribute support to candidates for national office whose actions or stated beliefs are congruent with the mission, principles, and purposes of AANP.

The NAPNAP also provides its members with health policy resources. The organization's website includes an advocacy center which has links to current campaigns, including key child health and practice legislation, and contact information for elected officials. Within their webpages, NAPNAP notes that they participate in more than 15 high-level collaboratives, focusing on advanced practice nursing and the health of our nation's children; NAPNAP also supports 49 state chapters, providing an online state advocacy center, monthly conference calls to discuss challenges and successes, and a mentoring program with leadership development opportunities (http://www.napnap.org/advocacy).

In addition to these national resources, the majority of state organizations can apprise the NP of current news, upcoming bills, and issues specific to NP practice within that state. Like federal legislation, state laws require processes that afford all interested parties reasonable opportunity to submit data, comments, or arguments, but many NPs do not take advantage of this opportunity. It would be appropriate for the NP to determine if the state organization has legislative committees in place to monitor and participate in the development of new or revised regulations that impact practice.

Professional organizations also offer experiences that directly connect members with their legislators. Although the following paragraphs contain information about face-to-face experiences supported by national organizations, it is important to recognize that individual state NP organizations often coordinate similar services within state capitals. Therefore, NPs are once again encouraged to become active members of their state's NP organizations and to familiarize themselves with the resources available within these groups as well.

The AANP offers two major events that promote political advocacy. Their Annual Health Policy Conference is held late winter in Washington, D.C. The conference includes an introduction to Capitol Hill, a government affairs update, presentations by the organization's health policy committee, interactions with NP elected officials representing various states across the nation, presentations on key legislative issues, and a day-long visit to Capitol Hill. The AANP also provides a Health Policy Fellowship program, a 4-week onsite experience at the AANP Government Affairs office in Alexandria, Virginia. Selected fellows provide support for health policy leadership development activities. Research activities may include reviewing literature, gathering information, collecting and analyzing data, and preparing reports. Fellows also attend relevant congressional briefings, political fundraisers, and policy meetings. Additional details about the major events can be found on the AANP website.

The NAPNAP sponsors an advocacy scholar, supporting his or her attendance at the AANP's Annual Health Policy Conference. The organization also coordinates its own annual Capitol Hill Day to raise awareness about child health priorities and the role of pediatric-focused APRNs. As noted on the organization's website (https://www.napnap.org), NAPNAP coordinates all meeting logistics, hosts an interactive training session, and provides participants with necessary advocacy materials and talking points for meetings with elected officials and their staffers. When NAPNAP members would like to meet with their elected officials during a visit to Washington,

D.C., that does not coincide with Capitol Hill Day, they can receive materials to share with legislators, helpful tips, and talking points for their meeting by contacting healthpolicy@napnap.org.

Armed with the resources available to support political activism, the NP will be in an excellent position to contribute to policy-making processes. The following strategies can be used as part of an overall goal of moving forth legislation to advance the profession and/or enhance health care:

- Become an active member of local, state, and/or national NP organizations.
- Become familiar with the resources available on NP organization websites.
- Volunteer to serve on legislative committees within these organizations.
- Become familiar with processes for passing legislation.
- Identify state and federal legislators who represent their residence and place of employment.
- Review "dos and don'ts" of meeting with legislators.
- Establish collegial relationships with key legislators.
- Develop "elevator speeches" or "sound bites" for topics of interest.
- Garner support or identify other like-minded individuals through a variety of resources, including social media and NP organization meetings.
- Contact legislators to garner their support and recognize those who do.
- Recognize parties who may oppose a specific bill.
- Prepare to provide testimony to legislative committees when appropriate.

Ideally, politically competent NPs will assume prominent roles in political activism and policy development. Doctorally prepared NPs are also prime candidates for leadership positions in government agencies or powerful consumer groups. Those with an earnest desire to further serve the public should also consider running for political office.

Nurse Practitioner Health Policy Exemplars

Health policies affect each and every NP; therefore, it is imperative that NPs have the tools to stay current in what is happening in their own state as well as nationally. The NP can become a leader in helping to move issues regarding health disparities, disease prevention, and practice issues to actualize the IOM's recommendation to become "full partners, with physicians and other health care professionals, in redesigning health care in the United States" (IOM, 2010, p.4). The following exemplars highlight the work of NPs who have made significant contributions through their healthcare policy actions.

Exemplar #1

Captain James L. Dickens, DNP, RN, FNP-BC, FAANP, is an accomplished senior federal healthcare officer with extensive expertise in global policy development. He currently serves in the U.S. Department of Health and Human Services Regional Office, Office of the Secretary, Region VI Dallas, as the Senior Program Manager Officer for the Office of Minority Health (OMH). He is a decorated veteran and recipient of numerous commendations, including the Meritorious Service Medal, the second-highest honor in the U.S. Public Health Service. Captain Dickens received this award in recognition of his work as the Officer in Charge of the Commissioned Corps Ebola Response Monrovia Medical Unit Team 2 in Liberia; he served as one of only four officers who led all operations, overseeing local Ebola virus response efforts while maintaining the safety and welfare of all deployed officers during an 8-month mission.

In his current role, as Senior Program Manager Officer for OMH, Captain Dickens manages programs to address disease prevention, health promotion, and risk reduction. He assesses state program plans, operating procedures, and policy and legislative proposals to determine their impact on minority, special, and at-risk populations. He has worked to develop and promote policies, programs, and practices aimed at eliminating health disparities, including the implementation of a systematic process within DHHS Region VI for requesting and awarding grants that target improving health equity for minority, racial, and ethnic populations. He works closely with the Office on Women's Health, Regional Resource Coordinator for HIV/AIDS, Office of Family Planning, and the Medical Reserve Corps to achieve programmatic goals, objectives, and activities that are aligned with the mission of DHHS and the Office of the Assistant Secretary for Health (OASH). His work has required him to maintain relationships with internal and external stakeholders on key public health and minority health objectives to leverage support for those issues that affect racial/ethnic and vulnerable populations.

Within his work at HHS, Captain Dickens sees himself as a champion for equity in all health policies, and he recognizes the distinct difference between equity and equality. Captain Dickens has noted that *every* American should have access to health care (equality); but more importantly, resources (e.g., transportation to or child care during appointments; access to affordable healthy food choices; insurance coverage for preventive and episodic services) should be distributed to effectively support the unique situation of those in need (equity). Based on that viewpoint, he works to address disparities and eliminate real and perceived barriers to health care. He envisions that future health policies could result in a "non-controversial health care system that's viewed as a right of every American, rather than a privilege . . . universal health care with a one payer system."

Reflecting back on his career, Captain Dickens is most proud of his work chairing the initial meetings for Texas nursing coalition groups in response to recommendations within the IOM's *Future of Nursing* and the RWJF's Campaign for Action. Those meetings of the Texas team convened stakeholders and initiated conversation that saw no boundaries: "There were no issues off the table." That working group is still meeting today and addressing barriers to professional practice. Captain Dickens continues to work diligently with those colleagues to obtain full practice authority for APRNs within the State of Texas, and ultimately throughout the nation.

Exemplar #2

Susan (Susie) M. Adams, PhD, APRN, PMHNP, FAANP, FAAN, has been instrumental in influencing mental health policy through her scholarly work in academia and professional organizations for more than two decades. Dr. Adams directed Vanderbilt School of Nursing's Psychiatric Mental Health Nurse Practitioner (PMHNP) Program, one of the first in the nation, for nearly 20 years prior to assuming a newly created position focusing on community engagement for behavioral health. She has long-standing ties to a network of community agencies providing integrative services for women with mental health and substance use disorders. She has been a strong advocate for policies that ensure that these women will receive the care they so desperately need. She currently maintains a private general mental health practice and provides medical-assisted detoxification services within a substance abuse treatment center and residential recovery program in collaboration with the Vanderbilt Addictions Psychiatry Department. Dr. Adams has published articles on mental healthcare policy in the *Journal of the American Psychiatric Nurses Association*; is an invited national conference speaker on the treatment of mood disorder, substance use disorders, and integrated health services; and is well recognized for her contributions to the field of advanced practice mental health nursing.

In addition to preparing the next generation of NPs who advocate for and serve the needs of those with mental health disorders, Dr. Adams has influenced health policy through her significant contributions to several national task groups. She served two terms on the National Task Force on Quality Nurse Practitioner Education, sponsored by NONPF and AACN, which produced the *2013* and *2016 Criteria for Evaluation of Nurse Practitioner Programs*. She was an expert panel member on fetal alcohol spectrum disorders, developing a national interdisciplinary educational module sponsored by the Association of Reproductive Health Professionals. Dr. Adams also served as the American Nurses Association's representative on the IOM Committee's 2015 report titled *Psychosocial Interventions for Mental and Substance Use Disorders: A Framework for Establishing Evidence-Based Standards*. She is currently serving as an expert panel member for the National Academy of Medicine, formerly the IOM, writing a white paper and call to action for healthcare providers on the U.S. opioid epidemic. She has recently been appointed to represent APRNs on the Providers' Clinical Support System for Medical Assisted Treatment (PCSS-MAT) for addiction coordinated by the American Academy for Addiction Psychiatry in collaboration with other national professional organizations; the task force has been charged with establishing national policies to address the opioid epidemic and other substances of abuse.

Within her current activities, Dr. Adams reports that she is focused on shaping policies that support harm reduction and innovative treatment strategies specific to the opioid epidemic. Ultimately, she notes, "We need to focus attention and resources on prevention of addictions at an early age." And, she cites evidence from the National Center on Addiction and Substance Abuse that reveals 1 in every 25 individuals who begins using any addictive substance (including alcohol) at age 21 and older will become addicted, but more ominously 1 of 4 who begins using before age 18 become addicted (National Center on Addiction and Substance Abuse, 2011). Thus, her advocacy for policies addressing early intervention is well founded.

Reflecting on her passion of advocating for those with mental health and substance use disorders, Dr. Adams recognizes that every APRN has at least one healthcare topic of concern, on issues that may range from childhood to end-of-life care. She would like to see every APRN involved in healthcare advocacy at the grassroots level to influence policy on their area of interest. She notes that according to annual Gallup polls, "nurses have been the mosttrusted profession in the U.S. since September 11th of 2001. Collectively, we are the largest health care profession with 3.3 million (and more than 200,000 NPs). We have the potential to educate legislators, policy-makers, and the general public on health care needs and reasonable solutions. It is time to 'find our voice.'"

Seminar Discussion Questions

1. What are the restrictions regarding prescribing medications that are applicable in your state?
2. Other than prescriptive authority, what are the key legislative issues that your state NP organization is currently working on?
3. Identify a health policy issue that you feel passionate about. Develop a 30-second elevator speech/sound bite that clearly articulates your position.
4. What topic would you be most comfortable discussing with a federal legislator? Why?
5. In the Health Policy Exemplars section of this chapter, Dr. Adams has noted that it is time for APRNs to "find our voice." What does that mean to you?

References

American Association of Nurse Practitioners. (2015a). *Issue briefs: Improve patient access to Medicare skilled nursing care.* Retrieved from https://www.aanp.org/images/documents/federal-legislation/issuebriefs/Issue%20Brief%20-%20Improve%20Patient%20Access%20to%20Medicare%20Skilled%20Nursing%20Care.pdf

American Association of Nurse Practitioners. (2015b). *Issue briefs: Remove barriers to nurse practitioners' ability to practice.* Retrieved from https://www.aanp.org/images/documents/federal-legislation/issuebriefs/Issue%20Brief%20-%20Removing%20Barriers.pdf

American Association of Nurse Practitioners. (2017a). *AANP celebrates 75,000 member milestone.* Retrieved from https://www.aanp.org/192-press-room/2017-press-releases/2082-aanp-celebrates-75-000-member-milestone

American Association of Nurse Practitioners. (2017b). *Nurse practitioners salute South Dakota for new health care law.* Retrieved from https://www.aanp.org/about-aanp/192-press-room/2017-press-releases/2063-nurse-practitioners-salute-south-dakota-for-new-health-care-law

American Association of Nurse Practitioners. (n.d.). *Historical timeline.* Retrieved from https://www.aanp.org/all-about-nps/historical-timeline

American Psychiatric Nurses Association. (2017). *APNA position statement: Whole health begins with mental health.* Retrieved from http://www.apna.org/files/public/Whole-Health-Begins-With-Mental-Health-Position-Paper.pdf

APRN Joint Dialogue Group. (2008). *Consensus model for APRN regulation: Licensure, accreditation, certification, & education.* Retrieved from http://www.aacn.nche.edu/education-resources/APRNReport.pdf

Association of American Medical Colleges. (2015, March 3). *New physician workforce projections show the doctor shortage remains significant.* Retrieved from https://www.aamc.org/newsroom/newsreleases/426166/20150303.html

Bartol, T. (2015). Nurse practitioners: Enhancing healthcare for 50 years. *Nurse Practitioner, 40*(6), 14–15.

Centers for Disease Control and Prevention. (2013). *The state of aging and health in America 2013.* Atlanta, GA: Author. Retrieved from https://www.cdc.gov/aging/pdf/State-Aging-Health-in-America-2013.pdf

Department of Veterans Affairs. (2016). *Advanced practice registered nurses: 81 FR 90198.* Retrieved from https://www.federalregister.gov/documents/2016/12/14/2016-29950/advanced-practice-registered-nurses

Institutes of Medicine. (1994). *Defining primary care: An interim report.* Washington, DC: National Academy Press. Retrieved from https://www.nap.edu/read/9153/chapter/2

Institute of Medicine of the National Academies. (2010). *The future of nursing: Leading change, advancing health.* Washington, DC: The National Academies Press. Retrieved from https://www.nap.edu/read/12956/chapter/1#ii

McDonald, L. (2006). *Florence Nightingale as a social reformer.* Retrieved from http://www.historytoday.com/lynn-mcdonald/florence-nightingale-social-reformer

National Center on Addiction and Substance Abuse. (2011). *Adolescent substance use: America's #1 public health problem.* Retrieved from https://www.centeronaddiction.org/addiction-research/reports/adolescent-substance-use-america%E2%80%99s-1-public-health-problem

National Organization of Nurse Practitioner Faculties. (2017). *Nurse practitioner core competencies content.* Retrieved from c.ymcdn.com/sites/ww.nonpf.org/resource/resmgr/competencies/2017_NPCoreComps_with_Curric.pdf

National Women's Hall of Fame. (2017). *Loretta C. Ford.* Retrieved from https://www.womenofthehall.org/inductee/loretta-c-ford/

Phillips, S. J. (2017). 29th annual APRN legislative update. *Nurse Practitioner, 42*(1), 18–46.

Robert Wood Johnson Foundation. (2017). *Charting nursing's future: Reports that can inform policy and practice.* Retrieved from http://www.rwjf.org/content/dam/farm/reports/issue_briefs/2017/rwjf435543

U.S. Department of Health and Human Services. (n.d.) *About HHS.* Retrieved from https://www.hhs.gov/about/index.html

U.S. Department of Health and Human Services. (2014). *Strategic plan: Introduction.* Retrieved from https://www.hhs.gov/about/strategic-plan/introduction/index.html

U.S. Department of Health and Human Services. (2015). *HHS strategic plan: Strategic plan FY 2014-2018.* Retrieved from https://www.hhs.gov/about/strategic-plan/index.html

White House President Obama Office of the Press Secretary. (2016). *Fact sheet: The Affordable Care Act: Healthy communities six years later.* Retrieved from https://obamawhitehouse.archives.gov/the-press-office/2016/03/02/fact-sheet-affordable-care-act-healthy-communities-six-years-later

CHAPTER 13

Quality, Safety, and Prescriptive Authority

Julie G. Stewart, Linda S. Morrow, and Tammy A. Testut

An Introduction to Quality

Healthcare quality and safety has taken major leaps in the past decade. Major stakeholders have set quality in health care as a priority in the fight for safe and quality patient care provision. Whether you practice in acute care or the community, quality measures are those benchmark criteria that set the standards for not only patient care but also for accreditation and payment. Gone are the days when quality was measured in days of stay or episodes of care. Quality care is a direct reflection of the patient-centered model of care. Patient outcomes are at the top of the list when it comes to validating or verifying the provision of care and overall prevention of illness.

Nightingale was likely the first quality improvement expert in the healthcare field. She tracked hospital death rates, which included a depiction of unnecessary military deaths caused by unsanitary conditions. Nightingale was an innovator in the collection, tabulation, interpretation, and graphical display of descriptive statistics (Riddle, 2010; Sheingold & Hahn, 2014). She was at the forefront of a specialty that once wasn't considered a major initiative in the overall provision of care.

Quality has been known by a multitude of terms since its inception in the 19th century. Many will reference quality initiatives as Quality Improvement (QI), Continuous Quality Improvement (CQI), and Quality Assurance (QA). There are notable differences among these various initiatives. The U.S. Department of Health and Human Services Health Resources and Services Administration (HRSA) defines each type of quality role:

> Quality Improvement (QI) refers to activities aimed at improving performance and is an approach to the continuous study and improvement of the processes of providing services to meet the needs of the individual and others.

> Continuous Quality Improvement (CQI) refers to an ongoing effort to increase an agency's approach to manage performance, motivate improvement, and capture lessons learned in areas that may or may not be measured as part of accreditation. It is an ongoing effort to improve the efficiency, effectiveness, quality, or performance of services, processes, capacities, and outcomes.
>
> Quality Assurance (QA) refers to a broad spectrum of evaluation activities aimed at ensuring compliance with minimum quality standards. The primary aim of quality assurance is to demonstrate that a service or product fulfills or meets a set of requirements or criteria. QA is identified as focusing on "outcomes," and CQI identified as focusing on "processes" as well as "outcomes." U. S. Department of Health and Human Services Health Resources and Services Administration [HRSA] 2011, p.2.

Today, quality and safety are the driving forces for improvement in all healthcare arenas. There is a current consensus that quality initiatives in any healthcare setting are crucial to the success and failure to its overall systems. The role of quality improvement in any healthcare setting has moved from a luxury to a necessity. This necessary component of healthcare allows the setting to develop systems to "monitor, quantify, and incentivize quality improvement in healthcare" (Marjoua & Bozic, 2012, abstract).

This chapter will briefly review quality and safety issues and initiatives, and conclude with an overview of safe prescribing.

Quality in Doctoral Education

Healthcare and educational standards both have an extreme focus on outcome measures to allow for a conscious awareness and act of qualifying and quantifying the provision of service. Within a doctoral education for Advanced Nursing Practice, essential elements and foundational outcome competencies are followed.

The Essentials of Doctoral Education for Advanced Nursing Practice delineate curricular elements and foundational outcome competencies. There are eight foundational competencies that are deemed essential for all DNP graduates regardless of whether they are preparing for a clinical, administrative, or academic role. The eight DNP Essentials are American Association Colleges of Nursing [AACN], 2006:

1. Scientific Underpinnings for Practice
2. Organization and Systems Leadership for Quality Improvement and Systems Thinking
3. Clinical Scholarship and Analytical Methods for Evidence-Based Practice
4. Information Systems/Technology and Patient Care Technology for the Improvement and Transformation of Health Care
5. Health Care Policy for Advocacy on Health Care
6. Interprofessional Collaboration for Improving Patient and Population Health Outcomes
7. Clinical Preventive and Population Health for Improving the Nation's Health
8. Advance Nursing Practice

Essential II focuses on organizational and systems leadership for quality improvement and systems thinking. This highlights the need for DNP graduates to "be proficient in quality improvement strategies and in creating and sustaining changes at the organizational and policy levels," to "ensure accountability for quality of health care and patient safety for populations with whom they work," and to be prepared to "lead quality improvement and patient safety initiatives in health-care systems" (AACN, 2006, p. 9).

U.S. Healthcare System

The U.S. healthcare system places a high priority on prevention of illness, early diagnosis, treatment of disease, and the use of advanced interventions to improve physical and mental health of its population (Agency for Healthcare Research and Quality [AHRQ], 2015). The Patient Protection and Affordable Care Act mandated the establishment of a National Strategy for Quality Improvement in Health Care (the National Quality Strategy, or NQS), as part of the goal of increasing access to high-quality, affordable health care for all Americans. Opportunities to improve healthcare services involve addressing the six dimensions of quality.

> The National Quality Strategy's six priorities address the range of quality concerns that affect most Americans: making care safer by reducing harm caused in the delivery of care; ensuring that each person and family are engaged as partners in their care; promoting effective communication and coordination of care; promoting the most effective prevention and treatment practices for the leading causes of mortality, starting with cardiovascular disease; working with communities to promote wide use of best practices to enable healthy living; and making quality care more affordable for individuals, families, employers, and governments by developing and spreading new health care delivery models. (AHRQ, 2015, p.13)
>
> Unfortunately, there have been inequalities in the access to care, poor communication, lack of patient–provider relationships, and/or low health literacy among U.S. residents.

The Agency for Healthcare Research and Quality (AHRQ) has devised three basic questions to guide Americans to improved health care:

1. What is the status of healthcare quality and disparities in the United States?
2. How have healthcare quality and disparities changed over time?
3. Where is the need to improve healthcare quality and reduce disparities greatest?

In the AHRQ 2015 National Healthcare Quality and Disparities Report, the number of Americans with access to health care has shown a dramatic improvement. Quality of health care shows a consistent level of improvement but varies across the National Quality Strategy (NQS) priorities. Areas such as effective treatment, patient safety, person-centered care, and healthy living indicate improvement overall with a continued focus on specific disparity reduction.

However, care coordination which is the process of promoting communication and coordination of care across the care continuum involving all stakeholders "measures have lagged behind other priorities in overall performance" (AHRQ, p.2).

Institute of Medicine Quality Reports

The three major reports related to healthcare quality include the Institutes of Medicine's (IOM's) National Roundtable on Health Care Quality report, *The Urgent Need to Improve Health Care Quality* (Chassin & Galvin, 1998); *To Err Is Human* (IOM, 2000);

and the IOM's *Crossing the Quality Chasm* (2001). In the IOM National Roundtable report, the contributors concluded that the U.S. healthcare system had serious and widespread issues affecting the delivery of quality care. It was noted that there was underuse, overuse, and misuse of healthcare practices which was stored under the umbrella of fraud and abuse. These three categories of use included various healthcare testing and interventions that were viewed, compared, and contrasted to quality and safety of patient care.

When *To Err Is Human* was published, it garnered the attention of healthcare providers and policy makers, as well as consumers (Ransom, Joshi, Nash, & Ransom, 2008; Taylor-Sullivan, 2013). Highlighted in the report were specific individual cases of preventable errors and startling statistics related to harm inflicted upon patients from the healthcare system's unacceptable, and often preventable, mistakes.

Shortly after *To Err Is Human* was published, *Crossing the Quality Chasm* was released by the IOM and contained a framework for improving the healthcare system. The six dimensions of quality health care are (IOM, 2000):

1. Safe—avoidance of injuries
2. Effective—provision of services based on scientific findings and abstinence of services to patients not likely to benefit
3. Efficient—avoidance of waste
4. Timely—reduction of delays for patients receiving care
5. Patient centered—provision of care based on patient needs, preferences, and value systems
6. Equitable—delivery of quality care irrespective of personal characteristics

Outcome measurements can indicate how well an organization or individual is doing in relation to these six dimensions. Examples of outcome measurements include percentages of adverse events, use of evidence-based practice guidelines, cost of care, wait times, patient satisfaction scores, and disparities in health care by gender or race (Ransom et al., 2008).

Attributes of quality care include (Ransom et al., 2008):

- Technical performance—The skill of medical providers in performing procedures and interventions
- Management of interpersonal relationships—Maintenance of a good patient–client relationship
- Amenities—Latest technology and equipment, wide range of services, best nurses and physicians, and most personalized care
- Access—Availability of necessary resources (e.g., prompt access to providers)
- Responsiveness to patient preferences—Respectful of complementary and alternative therapies and being culturally sensitive
- Equity—Provision of the same healthcare options to all individuals
- Efficiency—Wise use of resources
- Cost-effectiveness—Good value for the money; in other words, dollars spent enhance health outcomes

Professional Accountability and Teamwork

For quality initiatives to be successful, it is imperative to have leadership and all stakeholders promoting a culture of quality. Doctorally prepared NPs are poised to be in leadership roles either formally or informally; therefore, understanding the basic components of leadership and quality is essential. Scholtes, Joiner, and Streibel (2003) identified eight principles of quality leadership:

1. Having the customer as the focus of quality efforts
2. Exhibiting great passion for quality in the organization
3. Acknowledging and appreciating structure at work
4. Creating efficient work processes by reducing variation and instituting quality control measures
5. Fostering unity of purpose so all who work in an organization are clear about the vision
6. Examining systems for defects, and not placing blame on the individuals working within the confines of the system
7. Working collaboratively across disciplines
8. Offering initial training and continuing education to maintain the culture of quality in the organization

Leaders can also develop a culture of safety, or *just culture* in the work environment (AHRQ, n.d.). In a *just culture*, there is an understanding of the differences between human error, at-risk behaviors, and zero tolerance for reckless behaviors. This approach is viewed as being more balanced in that staff can be held accountable for errors in particular situations in the healthcare environment. Achieving a culture of safety needs to be a systemwide commitment, and the ability of the NP/DNP to foster collegial and collaborative teamwork is an asset to the culture of quality and safety.

In addition to putting the leadership quality principles into practice in the work environment, the NP/DNP should also evaluate his or her own practice outcomes. Outcome measurements as indicators of quality health care have largely been associated with medical interventions and treatments; however, nurse-sensitive patient outcomes have also been developed as indicators of quality associated with nursing care (Zaccagnini & White, 2011). The NP/DNP bases interventions on physiological, psychosocial, functional, behavioral, and knowledge-focused parameters (Zaccagnini & White, 2011). Numerous quality indicators can be used for outcome measurements including such indicators as total number of patients meeting standardized goals (e.g., HgA1C < 7.0, SBP mm Hg < 120, and DBP mm Hg < 80), patient satisfaction, patient adherence to treatment regimens, and immunization rates.

▸ Quality and Safety Education for Nurses

The Quality and Safety Education for Nurses (QSEN) initiative, funded by the Robert Wood Johnson Foundation, has resources for the practicing NP as well as NP nursing students (The Quality and Safety Education for Nurses [QSEN], 2012). The goal of QSEN is to develop curricula and competencies in patient-centered care, teamwork and collaboration, evidence-based practice, quality improvement, safety, and informatics in an effort to continuously improve the quality and safety of healthcare systems (QSEN, 2012).

The QSEN initiative aids in the NP's ability to analyze, synthesize, and use findings from credible evidence-based research to enhance one's own practice. The program meets the IOM challenge of preparing future nurses and fostering lifelong learning and advancement with the knowledge, skills, and attitudes to meet the ever-changing needs of health care (QSEN, 2012). The QSEN initiative has developed knowledge, skills, and attitudes for safety that are meant to minimize the risk of harm to patients and providers through both system effectiveness and individual performance (see **TABLE 13-1**).

TABLE 13-1 QSEN Knowledge, Skills, and Attitudes for Safety

Knowledge	Skills	Attitudes
Examine human factors and other basic safety design principles as well as commonly used unsafe practices (such as work-arounds and dangerous abbreviations) Describe the benefits and limitations of selected safety-enhancing technologies (such as barcodes, computer provider order entry, medication pumps, and automatic alerts/alarms) Discuss effective strategies to reduce reliance on memory	Demonstrate effective use of technology and standardized practices that support safety and quality Demonstrate effective use of strategies to reduce risk of harm to self or others Use appropriate strategies to reduce reliance on memory (such as forcing functions, checklists)	Value the contributions of standardization/reliability to safety Appreciate the cognitive and physical limits of human performance
Delineate general categories of errors and hazards in care Describe factors that create a culture of safety (such as open communication strategies and organizational error reporting systems)	Communicate observations or concerns related to hazards and errors to patients, families, and the healthcare team Use organizational error reporting systems for near miss and error reporting	Value own role in preventing errors
Describe processes used in understanding causes of error and allocation of responsibility and accountability (such as root cause analysis and failure mode effects analysis)	Participate appropriately in analyzing errors and designing system improvements Engage in root cause analysis rather than blaming when errors or near misses occur	Value vigilance and monitoring (even of own performance of care activities) by patients, families, and other members of the healthcare team
Discuss potential and actual effect of national patient safety resources, initiatives, and regulations	Use national patient safety resources for own professional development and to focus attention on safety in care settings	Value relationship between national safety campaigns and implementation in local practices and practice settings

QSEN, 2012. Reprinted with permission of Quality and Safety Education for Nurses Institute.

Patient-Centered Care

Patient-centered care focuses on the need for the provider to view patients as partners who have input into healthcare decisions. Knowledge and skills specific in this area include analyzing one's own and the healthcare team's limitations in providing culturally sensitive care, and collaborating and communicating as a team member to have successful patient outcomes. Value and respect are key components of the attitude aspect of patient-centered care. One of the key values can be related to the ability of the NP to use interprofessional consultations and referrals to obtain solutions for patients' issues, whether they are disease related or associated to psychosocial problems.

One of the well-known models in the acute care setting is the Planetree Model (Planetree Organization, 2012). This comprehensive approach to patient-centered care was founded in 1978 by Angelica Thieriot after she had experienced the depersonalized effects of being a patient as well as a care provider for her spouse and son. The model encompasses mind, body, and spirit for healing the patient. The focus of the health care in this model centers around the patient. Family members, caregivers, professionals—anyone in contact with the patient—must be sensitive to the patient's needs. Patient-centered care takes place in the office, clinic, and even during volunteer activities as described by Tracy, NP:

TRACY'S STORY

I used to volunteer in a community center in a low-income area in Queens, New York. The neighborhood population consisted of a significant number of elderly people who lived at or near the poverty level. While at the community center, I was asked by a concerned woman to "check in" on her neighbor. This neighbor was described as "all alone" and possibly incapable of properly caring for herself. Later that week, I knocked on the neighbor's door with the intention of inviting her to join our community center. I introduced myself, and the reason for my visit. While I was speaking to her about our center, I noted her apartment to be dark, cluttered, and dirty. She told me she lived alone with no family to speak of, had difficulty walking due to being overweight, and had tripped and fallen in her home a number of times. Additionally, she had difficulty seeing and hearing and was agoraphobic and thus, relied on neighbors to "pick up" groceries for her. She was scared every day of being without food or falling and not being able to get up again.

This elderly woman was identified as being socially isolated, at risk for falls, and unable to adequately care for herself as a result of limited resources (financial or otherwise). I spoke to her about going to the hospital, both for medical evaluation as well as for referral for needed services. She agreed. While hospitalized, it was determined she had hypothyroidism, contributing to her significant weight gain and loss of hearing. She was started on thyroid replacement. Her hearing eventually improved, and she lost weight, improving her mobility. She was also diagnosed with cataracts and has since undergone bilateral cataract surgeries, improving her vision. While hospitalized, she was deemed eligible for Medicaid and can now afford her medication and healthcare services. As a Medicaid recipient she is eligible for home care services. An aide visits 5 days a week and assists with cooking and ambulation outside the home. She has also started coming to our meetings at the community center. It was through identification of an individual in need and referral to appropriate services that we were able to create an improved quality (and safety) of life for this woman.

Communication and Care Coordination

Care coordination is a key concept that lays the foundation for successful care across the care continuum. As part of the healthcare team, NPs have a concerted responsibility to promote effective communication, to foster greater outcomes of care. According to the Institute for Healthcare Improvement (IHI), "Care coordination delivers health benefits to those with multiple needs, while improving their experience of the care system and driving down overall health care (and societal) costs" (Craig, Ebey, & Whittington, 2011, p. 2). Part of care coordination is the ability to communicate with multiple members of the team including the patient and family members.

Communication between the patient, healthcare providers, and members of the healthcare team is essential for obtaining excellent outcomes by allowing an interprofessional approach to caring for the patient. The Enhanced Calgary Cambridge Guide is one of the tools used in healthcare universities and colleges to enhance communication skills between providers and patients (Kurtz, Silverman, Benson, & Draper, 2003). Although this model was originally developed for medical students, it has been adapted for a variety of health-related professionals including veterinarians and pharmacists, and it is well suited to depict the communication used to develop the nurse practitioner–patient relationship. This type of communication encourages open discussion (led by the healthcare provider) that allows the patient to tell his or her story. Clarification occurs when the listener verifies any ambiguous areas of the story. Respect is paramount, and the listener is taught to use empathy and explore the patient's perspective and expectations. It will take time before the student or novice NP becomes proficient at integrating the physical examination and patient interview components into the full assessment.

An example of the integration of patient-centered care as part of NP practice is apparent in the following case, as explained by an experienced NP.

JANE'S STORY

I met Mr. L. in my heart failure clinic for the first time in January this year soon after he moved from Florida to live with his granddaughter (an RN at a nearby emergency department). He was 83 years old and had NYHA Class III heart failure symptoms. He had turned down any home care services because his granddaughter was able to take care of all his needs. We set him up for our telehealth service. On the third visit, I invited our palliative care APRN to a joint appointment to introduce him to the palliative care team. At that time he made it very clear that he wanted to die at home when the time comes. Our palliative care APRN provided whatever he needed to live independently at home—hospital bed, oxygen for prn use, and a "fat spoon" (because he had a hard time using utensils to feed himself from his rotator cuff injury that he suffered from a fall a year earlier). We helped him get hearing aids and determined what he needed in preparation to have globus. We also allowed the granddaughter to decide how much of his heart failure medicines to give him due to great fluctuation in his blood pressure.

During his last outpatient visit in early March he told me that he had fallen three times and no longer had enough energy to make his bed (according to his granddaughter, he was a very proper man and making the bed was a very important daily function that he insisted on doing). He also started choking when he ate. At this time, I had a very honest talk with him acknowledging that I knew he wanted to die at home, but I told him that it was no longer safe for him to stay at home during the day by himself (due to falling and choking). He clearly was in class IV HF. I told him that we could help make him comfortable and safe if he agreed to be admitted to the inpatient hospice service. To my surprise, it was almost a relief for him to hear that, and he instantly agreed. His granddaughter supported his decision. Since he had met with our palliative care team, they accepted him into our inpatient hospice unit directly from the outpatient clinic.

Mr. L. was a deeply religious person and he was happy to have a daily chaplain visit and repeatedly said to the chaplain that he had a good life and that he was at peace and ready to "go home" to see his wife and a deceased son. His sister visited from New Jersey, and his son came from Maine to be with him. I tried to go visit him daily, and he was always smiling and always had a relative by his bedside. Two weeks later he died peacefully with his family by his side. We respected his wishes, supported him, and transitioned him to an appropriate level of care when his health deteriorated. He trusted me and the palliative care APRN. With his cooperation, I think he received the most ideal end-of-life care. I still get choked up when I think of him. He was such a gentleman, and I was happy to be involved in his care.

Quality Improvement Planning

Although it may seem as though QI was introduced and perfected within the acute care hospital setting, it is as important in tertiary care sites as it is in outpatient clinics and private practices. The NP needs to acquire the specific skills to identify gaps in care and areas for improvement, recognize appropriate tools to use to measure variations, and collaborate to institute change based on the best practices found in the literature. Once change is implemented, it is vital to evaluate effectiveness and make alterations as necessary. The change process is seen along a continuum where checks and revisions are necessary for the improvement to stay viable.

The purpose of any QI initiative is to improve the performance of existing processes as well as to plan new ones. There are many ways to approach change within any organization whether the change is small or large in scale.

One common QI methodology is the Plan-Do-Study-Act (PDSA) framework. PDSA is an effective method for sustaining continuous change in an organization (Deming, 1986). W. Edwards Deming is known as the father of quality. Deming showed that by reducing waste, repetitive work, and staff turnover, organizations can improve quality and customer satisfaction. The PDSA process can be used to initiate a change in practice for ensuring quality. The key to this conceptual framework is to develop rapid cycles of change to sustain momentum in changing behaviors, procedures, and policies as quickly as possible. The four stages to a PDSA cycle are:

Plan: Plan the change to be tested or implemented.

Do: Carry out the test or implement change.

Study: Study data before and after the change, and reflect on what was learned.

Act: Plan the next change cycle or plan implementation.

A PDSA cycle involves testing the improvement ideas on a small scale before introducing the change on a large scale. By building on the learning from the test cycles in a structured and incremental way, a new idea can be implemented with greater chance of success. Barriers to change are often reduced when different people are involved in trying something out on a small scale before implementation on larger scale. The model is not meant to replace change models that organizations may already be using, but rather to accelerate improvement. This model can improve many different healthcare processes and outcomes, such as those related to health behavior and quality.

An example follows in the next case study.

QUALITY INITIATIVES

At our institution we use the Plan-Do-Study-Act (PDSA) method for quality improvement efforts. Our HIV clinic manager had identified opportunities for improvement in a few key areas of routine patient health maintenance. The healthcare providers and staff did not believe that the sample of charts reviewed were accurate. Once the top three quality indicators were identified that did not meet benchmark standards, a team meeting was held to discuss the current flow for patients in the clinic. Input was obtained as to where inconsistencies in care might be occurring along with suggestions for improvement.

Three separate quality efforts were developed to improve (1) the number of patients getting annual tuberculosis testing, (2) the number of females having gynecological examinations and PAP testing, and (3) the number of patients getting vaccinated for hepatitis B, if nonimmune. Each of these three indicators had a number of interventions that were agreed upon by the multidisciplinary team in an attempt to achieve 100% compliance.

Interestingly, there were multiple things that contributed to the top three problems. For instance, at the time of the chart reviews, there was no area to document if the patient had tested positive previously, thereby nullifying the need for further skin testing. This issue was easily remedied by revising the progress notes. Regarding the gynecological exams and PAP testing, we found that many of our patients did not visit our gynecology clinic and instead had their own provider outside of our institution, so we made note and started to get release forms to be able to share information with the outside provider. In addition, as the FNP, I had experience in basic gynecology and offered to do the PAPs and STD testing for anyone who needed it during their routine HIV care visit. As for the hepatitis B vaccinations, we instituted an alert in the patient's electronic health record that required the healthcare provider and follow-up RN to note that the patient was in need of a vaccination as well as an area to note if the patient had declined the vaccination for whatever reason.

This team approach worked well, not only for quality improvement but the unique contributions that make efforts really work well when there is interprofessional collaboration.

Safety

A basic concept such as safety initially may not appear to require much elaboration; however, when you consider the lack of standardization and monitoring in many practice settings, the need to continually work on safety issues is quite apparent. In 2002, The Joint Commission established its National Patient Safety Goals (NPSGs) program. The NPSGs were developed to assist accredited organizations focus on specific areas of concern in regard to patient safety. The Joint Commission is also responsible, with the help of the safety advisory board made up of multiple healthcare specialties, for determining the highest priority patient safety issues (The Joint Commission, 2016). The goal of patient safety is to avoid any harm or suffering as a result of any healthcare intervention (Ransom et al., 2008). Fortunately, errors do not always reach the patient, or they may not cause harm if they reach the patient. It is important to identify issues of concern, strive for transparency in reporting errors, and design and implement safety systems to prevent further errors.

An example of this is given by Nancy, FNP:

NANCY'S STORY

I remember sitting in the advanced health assessment course and listening to the professor discuss the significance of taking a good history from a patient. I distinctly remember her saying that a good history will give you most of the information you need. I have followed this advice in my practice, and it has proven to be invaluable, particularly in a situation where I treated a gentleman for diabetes.

The patient is a 68-year-old African American male with an extensive history including DM-2, HTN, CAD, hyperlipidemia, and CKD stage 2. His DM is well controlled with an A1C of 6.7 on a regimen of Januvia, Metformin, and bedtime Levemir. Generally he checks his BS 1–2 times a day and results range between 90 and 150. He is on many other medications for his CAD, HTN, and hyperlipidemia and is under the care of a cardiologist.

During a visit in March, the patient stated to me that he felt fine. In fact, that morning he had a visit with his cardiologist who also told the patient that he was doing well. The patient had not had any recent labs drawn, but he did have a log book of blood sugars that seemed to be fairly well controlled, albeit slightly higher than his previous averages. His blood pressure in the office was noted to be significantly lower than his norm. It was only after a period of time during our office visit (something that thankfully as a nurse practitioner I am allowed to have with my patients) that the patient mentioned that twice earlier in the week his legs had "given out" while he was walking. He insisted that he did not fall but rather "went down to his knees" and afterward was able to pull himself up. He also denied any change in LOC, speech, paresthesias, pain, or injury of any kind. His physical exam was unremarkable other than a lower than usual BP.

Still, it was not something that I was willing to let go of that easily. Despite the patient's insistence that he was fine and was not concerned, it bothered me. I told him that having his legs "give out" was not okay and that we had to get to the bottom of it. He had not checked his blood sugars at the time the events occurred, but he denied having any symptoms of hypoglycemia. We began to review all of his medications (an extensive list, definitely a case of polypharmacy), and he mentioned that he didn't feel that his blood sugars were as good since he had started taking the "white Januvia" which his wife (a certified nursing assistant) had reassured him was probably the generic form that had been substituted. As the prescriber, I was aware that there is no generic form of Januvia and that all Januvia would be described as pink, red, or brown. Thus, I asked the patient to return home and bring back the bottle of pills (he had a 3-month supply of these and had been taking them for the past 45 days). The patient returned with his bottle, and there was a pharmacy label clearly printed and marked as Januvia 100 mg that had been applied over each bottle of Losartan 100 mg. (He actually had three bottles all labeled

(continues)

the same way.) The patient was receiving an additional antihypertensive medication and he was already on a beta blocker, a thiazide diuretic, a calcium channel blocker, and an ACE inhibitor. I sent him for labs that afternoon and told him to stop his Metformin and hold on any (real) Januvia until I called him the next day. The next day the lab results confirmed an acute deterioration in his kidney function (with a GFR of 28 and creatinine of 2.7, most likely caused by hypoperfusion related to his hypotension).

I explained to the patient that this was most likely the reason for his leg weakness. He was instructed to keep himself well hydrated with water over the next few days and to refrain from taking the Metformin and Januvia until his kidney function tests returned to baseline. One week later I rechecked his kidney function, and it had returned to baseline. His medications were resumed; his blood sugars and blood pressure returned to baseline levels.

Later, when I discussed the case with the endocrinologist that I work for, she insisted that she would never have discovered the underlying reason for this man's leg weakness. I insisted that she would have, but she was emphatic about it. "No" she said, "I would never have been that thorough with his history."

I feel that it was because I had the time to spend with this patient that he had a successful outcome. I also felt that my professor's words of wisdom regarding a thorough history served as my "inner voice" that warranted delving further into this man's issue. I saw the patient a few weeks ago. He is doing great.

Informatics

An area of focus for quality and safety education for nurses is informatics. Electronic medical records (EMRs) or electronic health records (EHRs) are finally becoming the standard in many hospitals and practice sites; however, not all sites can afford to implement EMR/EHRs due to the costs associated with the initial purchase, implementation, and ongoing support and maintenance. Measures to quantify costs versus benefits can indicate a significant cost savings and error prevention related to implementation of EMRs. In fact, the Centers for Medicare and Medicaid Services (CMS) has an active program incentivizing providers to use EMR and electronic prescribing.

Another important area that relates to informatics is the vast amount of communication and education available to patients and healthcare providers who use technology. There are many evidence-based clinical decision support resources to aid healthcare practitioners in making the best decisions at the point of care. Certainly all of these avenues bring potential benefits to health care. It is important to always remember that strict measures need to be undertaken to safeguard patient privacy at all times.

Today, many health centers are connected to outpatient clinics and private provider practices. The benefit of access to electronic medical records is to be able to provide the best coordinated care to patients, without having to wait to obtain medical records and results from another department or site. The challenge is to ensure all safety measures are in place to prevent any lapse in patient privacy.

Team STEPPS

There are many tools for organizations to use to measure outcomes and develop methods to improve safety and quality. A comprehensive program has been developed by the AHRQ. This system for healthcare professionals is focused on developing a culture of safety. Team STEPPS is an evidence-based teamwork system to improve communication and teamwork skills among healthcare professionals. It is a source for ready-to-use materials and a training curriculum to successfully integrate teamwork principles into all areas of your healthcare system. Scientifically rooted in more than 20 years of research and lessons from the application of teamwork principles, Team STEPPS was developed by the Department of Defenses' Patient Safety Program in collaboration with the AHRQ.

This approach uses assessment and training tools to develop teams that work to improve patient outcomes. Clear roles and responsibilities are emphasized, as well as methods to improve communication, thereby reducing conflicts. Barriers to achieving and maintaining a culture of safety and quality are addressed. There are six regional training centers that provide intensive training to master trainers who can offer training to healthcare centers on Team STEPPS. Information can be found on the AHRQ Team STEPPS website.

Prescriptive Authority

Writing prescriptions safely is an important aspect of most NP practices. Prescriptive practice varies from state to state as well as from one practice setting to another. It is imperative that the NP is aware of what the state scope of practice and practice site allows and restricts. There are numerous states that have independent practice including full prescriptive authority and states that require some form of collaboration with or supervision by a physician (National Council of State Boards of Nursing [NCSBN], 2016).

The graduate NP needs to apply for a controlled substances registration if the state where he or she is employed requires registration. In addition, the NP needs to apply for registration with the Drug Enforcement Agency (DEA) in order to prescribe any controlled substances. It is easy to see how safety issues are concerning when there is not national legislation to standardize prescriptive authority. Many states have enacted Drug Prescription Monitoring Programs (DPMPs) which are electronic monitoring systems for tracking prescriptions of controlled substances (Centers for Disease Control and Prevention [CDC], 2017). Utilizing this form of tracking, the prescriber and pharmacist are able to review what prescriptions for controlled substances have been filled, when they were filled, and where. For the new NP, or for the NP who travels from state to state, keeping abreast of scope of practice guidelines and legislative issues is of paramount importance.

Writing a prescription is a process that not only requires considerable knowledge of pharmacology but also includes the need to have extensive knowledge about the pathophysiology of disease and comorbid conditions. How to properly order and interpret diagnostic testing related to illness and pharmacology, as well as apply knowledge about the patient's age, gender, and lifestyle, will affect outcomes of medication treatment, including adherence and management of side effects. Medication adherence is crucial for the patient as well as for the prescriber. Disease progression and exacerbations are directly correlated to many disease-specific medications such as long-acting bronchodilators for severe asthma and antiretrovirals for HIV infection. If a patient has been taking too little of the prescribed medication, drug toxicity can occur when the full dose is started, and conversely, medications can be discontinued needlessly if a patient was experiencing side effects that were related to overdosage.

Common errors can involve patient-related mistakes; pharmacy-related errors; look-alike drugs; and errors in dosage, strength, concentration, and misleading abbreviations, to name a few. The NP has to be aware of state Medicaid formularies and tiered medications; and be cognizant that if patients attempt to fill prescriptions out of state, they may experience difficulty as the state may not acknowledge prescriptions written by NP providers. Another consideration is that dispensing samples left by pharmaceutical representatives may not be allowed in a specific institution nor by the state licensing board. Again, NPs must know the rules and regulations in their state and institution. The NP is the expert in patient education, as well as goal setting in regard to compliance with treatment regimens.

All prescribers need to be aware of the guidelines issued by the U.S. Food and Drug Administration (FDA) that describe the acceptable relationship between pharmaceutical companies and their representatives with prescribers, including the types of gifts that can be given to prescribers that are not patient-care related items, and what type of interaction can occur when healthcare prescribers have continuing education events. There are codes and guidelines developed by the Pharmaceutical Research and Manufacturers of America (PhRMA) that address pharmaceutical companies' interactions with patient groups, healthcare centers, professionals, and direct-to-consumer advertising (PhRMA, n.d.). However, not all companies must comply with these guidelines; participation is voluntary.

The NP has responsibilities when writing prescriptions. These include:

- Generic versus brand name drugs: Know generic names of all the medications prescribed.
- When a drug is no longer on-label: Attend continuing education programs on medication updates, and subscribe to professional newsletters that provide updates on medications (SmartBrief, etc.).
- Formularies: Maintain a list of the most common formularies, as well as the list of low-cost pharmacies' generic medications.
- Failed therapies: Closely monitor all the medications the patient takes, as well as medications taken in the past, including when and why any have been discontinued.
- How stable is the patient on the currently prescribed regimen? Is the patient being adherent? Is the blood glucose or blood pressure under control?
- Food and Drug Administration position: It is your responsibility to stay abreast of the FDA's warnings, recalls, and pertinent information on medications you may prescribe.

In addition, prescribers should be aware of the official "Do Not Use" list developed by The Joint Commission regarding abbreviations that should not be used, to avoid medication errors (The Joint Commission, 2017). See **TABLE 13-2**.

Additionally, information regarding the dosage of the prescribed medication must be written out clearly for the pharmacist and/or nurse to read and dispense appropriately, as is shown here:

PATIENT PRESCRIPTION

Dosage:

1. Dose
2. Route
3. Frequency and times of administration
4. Duration of therapy
   - Patient errors
   - Pharmacy errors
   - Look-alike drugs
   - Errors in dosage, strength, and concentration
   - Misleading abbreviations
   - Patient alters the prescription

Other issues that prescribers need to be aware of:

- State Medicaid formularies
- Formularies vary and tiered medications
- Out-of-state prescriptions: May or may not take order from NP
- Telephone orders: Not for schedule I or II medications
- Dispensing samples
- Drug substitution; "Do not substitute" and "Dispense as written"

TABLE 13-2 Official "Do Not Use" List[1]

Do Not Use	Potential Problem	Use Instead
U, u (unit)	Mistaken for "0" (zero), the number "4" (four), or "cc"	Write "unit"
IU (International Unit)	Mistaken for "IV" (intravenous) or the number "10" (ten)	Write "International Unit"
Q.D., QD, q.d., qd (daily) Q.O.D., QOD, q.o.d., qod (every other day)	Mistaken for each other Period after the "Q" mistaken for "I" and the "O" mistaken for "I"	Write "daily" Write "every other day"
Trailing zero (X.0 mg)* Lack of leading zero (.X mg)	Decimal point is missed	Write "X mg" Write "0.X mg"
MS MSO_4 and $MgSO_4$	Can mean morphine sulfate or magnesium sulfate Confused for one another	Write "morphine sulfate" Write "magnesium sulfate"

[1]Applies to all orders and all medication-related documentation that is handwritten (including free-text computer entry) or on preprinted forms.

*Exception: A "trailing zero" may be used only where required to demonstrate the level of precision of the value being reported, such as for laboratory results, imaging studies that report size of lesions, or catheter/tube sizes. It may not be used in medication orders or other medication-related documentation.

Patient Adherence to Medication Treatment Plan

The definition of patient adherence to a medication treatment plan is the extent to which the patient continues the agreed-upon mode of treatment under limited supervision when faced with conflicting demands, as distinguished from compliance or maintenance.

Inadequate adherence to medications can cause inaccurate assessment of the drug's utility, toxicity when given incorrectly, disease exacerbations and progression, and increased acute care admissions. Methods to assess for compliance to the prescribed plan include:

1. Medications being refilled as prescribed
2. Patient self-report
3. Patient diaries
4. Patient contracts
5. Measurement of drug titers found in body fluids
6. Electronic medication monitors

The AHRQ encourages patients to ask their healthcare provider(s) questions if there are any concerns or doubts about the treatment plan, inquire about side effects, keep a medication list, bring a list of all medications currently being taken to all healthcare provider visits, and notify providers about medication allergies (AHRQ, n.d.).

Writing a Prescription: What Should It Include?

Following are all of the items that can be included on a prescription. Not all states will require all components (some may not require a DEA number on nonscheduled medication prescriptions):

- Patient's full name, address, date of birth
- Prescriber's full name and address
- Drug Enforcement Agency number
- Nurse practitioner license number
- Drug name
- Drug strength and dosage form
- Directions for use
- Quantity to be dispensed (written out long-hand if for narcotic)
- Refill instructions
- Substitution rights
- Signed and dated

FIGURE 13-1 shows a sample prescription.

In summary, the NP/DNP needs to be equipped to have the knowledge and skills to lead the way in supporting a culture of safety and quality in whatever type of healthcare setting she or he is practicing in. Understanding the tools and processes used for quality and safety improvement in order to use them to improve patient care is a vital component for the practice-based, doctorally prepared nurse practitioner.

▸ Seminar Discussion Questions

1. The mission of AHRQ is to improve the quality, safety, efficiency, and effectiveness of health care for Americans. Review the AHRQ website and examine current initiatives, research findings and reports, and funding for grants.

Juliana Butler, FNP-BC

License # ------

DEA# ---------

Practice Site Name, Address, and Phone Number

Patient Name: Jane Doe DOB: xx/xx/xx

Patient Address

℞: Amoxicillin 500 mg

Sig: 1 capsule every 8 hours × 10 days

Dispense: #30 caps

Refills: 0

Generic: yes signed: *Juliana Butler, FNP*

FIGURE 13-1 Prescription Example

2. Various quality improvement methodologies are used in clinical practice. Compare and contrast these methodologies.
3. Care coordination occurs throughout the span of the care continuum. Explore the concept of care coordination in your setting and beyond. Consider how you may enhance your NP role in care coordination.
4. Conduct a quality improvement project utilizing the PDSA methodology.
5. There are many patient safety organizations in existence. Explore these organizations and discuss their relevance for improving patient safety.
6. Consider how you can be a champion for patient safety in your organization.
7. Review the laws and regulations regarding nurse practitioners writing schedule II and III medications in your state.

References

Agency for Healthcare Research and Quality. (n.d.). *Patient safety network.* Retrieved from http://psnet.ahrq.gov

Agency for Healthcare Research and Quality. (2015). *National healthcare quality and disparities reports and 5th anniversary update on the national quality strategy.* Retrieved from http://www.ahrq.gov /research/findings/nhqrdr/nhqdr15/index.html

American Association of Colleges for Nursing. (2006). *The essentials of doctoral education for advanced nursing practice.* Washington, DC: Author.

Centers for Disease Control and Prevention. (2017). *Prescription drug monitoring systems.* Retrieved from https://www.cdc.gov/drugoverdose/pdmp/index.html

Chassin, M. R., & Galvin, R. W. (1998). The urgent need to improve health care quality. *Journal of the American Medical Association, 280*(11), 1000–1005.

Craig, C., Eby, D., & Whittington, J. (2011). *Care coordination model: Better care at lower cost for people with multiple health and social needs.* IHI Innovation Series white paper. Cambridge, MA: Institute for Healthcare Improvement.

Deming, W. E. (1986). *Out of the crisis.* Cambridge, MA: MIT.

HRSA 2011 Part 4. Retrieved from https://www.hrsa.gov/quality/toolbox/methodology/developingandimplementingaqiplan/part4.html

Institutes of Medicine. (2000). *To err is human: Building a safer health system.* Washington, DC: National Academy Press.

Institutes of Medicine. (2001). *Crossing the quality chasm: A new health system for the 21st century.* Washington, DC: National Academy Press.

Joint Commission (2017). *Facts about the official "do not use" list of abbreviations.* Retrieved from https://www.jointcommission.org/facts_about_do_not_use_list/

The Joint Commission. (2016). *Facts about the national patient safety goals.* Retrieved from https://www.jointcommission.org/facts_about_the_national_patient_safety_goals/

Kurtz, S. M., Silverman, J. D., Benson, J., & Draper, J. (2003). Marrying content and process in clinical method teaching: Enhancing the Calgary-Cambridge Guides. *Academic Medicine, 78*(8), 802–809.

Marjoua, Y., & Bozic, K. J. (2012). Brief history of quality movement in US healthcare. *Current Reviews in Musculoskeletal Medicine, 5*(4), 265–273. doi:10.1007/s12178-012-9137-8

National Council of State Boards of Nursing. (2016). *APRN consensus model: Can CNPs prescribe independently.* Retrieved from https://www.ncsbn.org/5411.htm

PhRMA. (n.d.). *Principles and guidelines.* Retrieved from http://www.phrma.org/about/principles-and-guidelines

Planetree Organization. (2012). *Planetree pioneers.* Retrieved from www.planetree.org

Quality and Safety Education for Nurses. (2012). *Graduate QSEN Competencies.* Retrieved from http://www.qsen.org/ksas_graduate.php

Ransom, E., Joshi, M., Nash, D., & Ransom, S. (2008). *The healthcare quality book: Vision, strategy, and tools* (2nd ed.). Chicago, IL: Foundation of the American College of Healthcare Executives.

Riddle, L. (2010). *Florence Nightingale by Cynthia Audain, 1998.* Retrieved from http://www.agnesscott.edu/lriddle/women/nitegale.htm

Scholtes, P., Joiner, B., & Streibel, B. (2003). *The TEAM handbook* (3rd ed.). Madison, WI: Oriel.

Sheingold, B., & Hahn, H. (2014). The history of healthcare quality: The first 100 years 1860–1960. *International Journal of Africa Nursing Sciences.* doi:10.1016/j.ijans.2014.05.002

Taylor-Sullivan, D. (2013). In S. DeNisco & A. Barker (Eds.), *Advanced practice nursing: Evolving roles for the transformation of the profession* (2nd ed.). Burlington, MA: Jones & Bartlett Learning.

US Department of Justice and Drug Enforcement Administration: Diversion Control Division (2016). *State prescription drug monitoring systems.* Retrieved from https://www.deadiversion.usdoj.gov/faq/rx_monitor.htm

Zaccagnini, M., & White, K. (2011). *The doctor of nursing practice essentials: A new model for advanced nursing practice.* Sudbury, MA: Jones and Bartlett.

CHAPTER 14

Mentoring

Julie G. Stewart

Historically, there has been a lack of emphasis in the nursing profession on being mentored or on mentoring others. As the business world has known for years, the benefits of mentoring for mentees include having a definitive career plan, increased job satisfaction, improved socialization to the role, higher levels of self-esteem and confidence, higher salaries, and more opportunity for advancement (Grindell, 2003; Harrington, 2011; Tracy, 2012).

Although new nursing professionals are often "precepted" by a more experienced nurse, these novice providers are frequently expected to practice on their own after the specified orientation period is over. Nurse practitioner graduates may or may not have a period of orientation with a preceptor, depending on the practice site. Various terms have been used to describe those who assist others as they develop and learn professionally. Common terms are *preceptor*, *teacher*, *educator*, *guide*, *coach*, *manager*, *role model*, and *mentor*. Oftentimes, these terms are used interchangeably, which adds to confusion about the roles. What defines these roles will be reviewed in this chapter with the focus on the mentor.

▶ Preceptor

A very common term in the nursing world is *preceptor*. The concept has been discussed in an earlier chapter; however, a short review is offered here. Prior to enrolling in a NP program, most nurses have been precepted by another nurse in a new clinical setting, and very often may have functioned in the preceptor role. A preceptor has been defined as "a teacher; in nursing, usually an experienced nurse who assumes responsibility for teaching a novice" (Chitty & Black, 2011, p. 460). Typically, NP students are assigned a preceptor for clinical experiences. In all of these scenarios, the preceptor has been assigned to the student or new graduate. The relationship is usually a prescribed length of time—typically a short duration—and the relationship is usually confined to the work environment.

Preceptors themselves should have at least 1 year of experience with a solid skill set in whatever clinical setting the experience will take place. Beyond their clinical expertise, the preceptor should have knowledge of the NP role in order to be a role model for the preceptee. For the NP student, the preceptor is not always another NP; the preceptor could be a physician's assistant, a certified nurse–midwife, or commonly, a physician.

The goals for the training period are prescribed by an organization such as the National Organization for Nurse Practitioner Faculty (NONPF) or an institution, such as an acute care hospital or university, and evaluation forms are used to ensure the preceptee has adequately met the goals upon completion of the predetermined time period. Obviously, the NP role cannot be role modeled by non-NP preceptors; however, they should be cognizant of what the role entails to provide some insight for direction and the skill set needed for practice. In addition, a non-NP preceptor most likely will have difficulty in discussing the scope of practice while training an NP student. However, the preceptor role is quite important, and a long-lasting relationship may occur with some preceptors and preceptees.

EXCERPT FROM A PRECEPTOR

Over the 18 years I have spent as an NP, I have precepted many students from a variety of universities, as well as precepted NPs new to the clinical practice I work in. Precepting NP students can be very challenging, as well as rewarding. I have learned it is imperative to be aware of where the student is in the program, and what didactic information has already been covered to avoid unrealistic expectations. In addition, I have usually not met the student in advance so that once we start working together we may discover personality differences that make the relationship strained. Successful strategies have included being open and honest with the student, but never in front of a patient, nor in front of other staff. Instead, spending 10–15 minutes in the morning reviewing the schedule, and going over appropriate patients and goals for the day is very helpful.

Spending time during the lunch break to check in and identify what went well and what could have been handled differently is beneficial. At the end of clinic, we touch base in this regard as well. Occasionally I end with assigning a little homework regarding a patient for the student to do prior to returning the following week. This is a similar approach to precepting novice NPs to the practice setting. There have been a few students and novice NPs who have maintained their relationship with me and are colleagues that I have become a mentor for.

Role Model

The definition of a role model is "an individual who serves as an example of desirable behavior for another person" (Chitty & Black, 2011, p. 462). Role models include those people in whom we find qualities that are admirable or appealing. We can choose one or more role models. There may not be a direct contact or a relationship with a role model. The role model could be a person who is from the same discipline, such as a current NP leader or faculty member, or the role model may not be from the same profession. NP students can identify what qualities they feel are important and would like to emulate. For instance, an altruistic NP may say that Mother Theresa is a role model because her qualities of selflessness, and working with the poor and needy are goals that the NP would like to work toward. Oftentimes students who spend clinical hours in a center providing health care for the indigent find a preceptor who goes above and beyond in caring about each patient, despite what his or her appearance or socioeconomic status may be. Having such a rewarding experience with a role model can set the NP student's professional self-expectations and goals.

Coach

Coaches, on the other hand, may be assigned, such as a sports team coach, or may be chosen, such as a writing or life coach. A coach is someone who helps move an individual forward to where he or she wants to be, whether this relates to a goal weight, becoming an expert swimmer, or writing an article for publication. Specific goals could be set by the coach, the individual, or mutually set depending on the context. Most often, the literature points to the individual's objectives and goals as the focus of the coaching relationship. The time limit of the relationship can be short term or long term, depending on the individual's desire to be coached and the setting. A preceptor can be viewed as a coach as he or she helps the NP student during the transition from RN to NP (Link, 2009). In this preceptor-as-coach role, NP students are coached to believe they are capable of meeting their goals.

Nurse practitioners are often taught during their role seminars that one of the functions of the NP is to be a coach for patients and families. In fact, coaching to assist the patient with positive behavior changes to improve health is a component of the standards set by NONPF (2012). A NP coach can be described as someone who encourages, inspires, and empowers patients to reach their maximum health potential. In this scenario, patients' desires and goals drive the coaching relationship. Many chronic diseases have shown improved health outcomes when NPs act as coaches. Today, there are NPs who are working as wellness coaches and holistic coaches. Two NPs who practice together as wellness coaches, Darlene Trandel, PhD, MSN, RN/FNP, and Eileen T. O'Grady, PhD, RN, NP, are very enthusiastic about this role. According to Trandel,

> The premise underlying health and wellness coaching is helping people define and design their personal health and wellness goals to create a lifestyle that is based on who they are. Many clients come to us to rev up their wellness status and live a more healthful lifestyle; some seek to prevent or reduce the risk of a chronic illness and to age with vitality; and still others want to better manage an existing condition. Wellness coaches help their clients develop a personal blueprint for their health and wellness, increase their awareness of barriers that impede their progress, and create strategies to overcome the impediments that prevent them from mastering and sustaining their goals in their everyday life. As wellness coaches, we leverage both the relationship and the process to raise self-confidence and self-esteem and encourage clients to feel empowered and in charge of their health. (Hanson, 2012)

Mentor

Although many people have written that the origin of the term *mentor* comes from Homer's *Odyssey*, written in approximately 700 BCE, the actual author and date of origin are debatable. In this epic poem, Odysseus provided Mentor, who was really the goddess of wisdom, Athena, as a protector for his son while he was away. In addition to protecting the prince, Mentor educated, coached, and guided Odysseus' son, Telemachus. Mentor was more than a teacher. He was half-god and half-human, half-male and half-female. Mentor was a representation of the merger of both goal and path, as well as the yin and yang of life. Mentors need to both push and pull their mentees at times, leading by guiding the interaction with the mentees—while always remaining supportive.

Grossman (2013) points out that a more modernized version has been identified, depicting the origination of the term as occurring in approximately 1699, by Fenelon. The definition of mentoring which is more applicable currently to NPs is a "voluntary, intense, committed, extended, dynamic, interactive, supportive, trusting relationship between two people, one experienced, and the other a newcomer, characterized by mutuality" (Hayes, 1998, p. 525).

A mentor may be a faculty person, a clinical preceptor, or a professional the graduate comes into contact with and identifies as a person that the graduate would like to engage in a supportive relationship for an extended period of time. Mentoring may be a formal relationship, where a mentor is assigned by an organization, or an informal agreement made between a mentor and mentee that have chosen each other; the relationship lasts for a mutually agreed upon time, typically long lasting. In the ideal mentoring relationship, both parties "develop personally and professionally within the auspices of a caring, collaborative, and respectful environment" (Grossman, 2013, p. 186). The mentor, then, is different from a preceptor or a coach, yet may function in those roles in addition, but a mentor encompasses much more. The differences between these roles are summarized in **TABLE 14-1**.

Kram (1986), an authority on mentoring, identified two components of this type of relationship: career and psychosocial. Within the career mentoring portion are activities such as sponsorship, networking, and coaching, while psychosocial aspects include helping the mentee to move forward in professional development, role modeling, and friendship. Even within an informal mentorship, there may be a

TABLE 14-1 Differences Among Mentor, Preceptor, and Coach

	Mentor	Preceptor	Coach
Match	By desire	Assigned	Either
Time	Longer term	Shorter term	Either
Goals	Set mutually	Prescribed	Either
Setting	Work/other	Work	Either

Reproduced with permission of Dori Taylor Sullivan.

contract or agreement to clarify goals and timelines. Mentors are inspirers, supporters, envisioners, sponsors, coaches, and role models.

Often there are not enough opportunities for nursing professionals to benefit from a formal mentoring relationship. However, nursing literature does provide evidence about the benefits of mentor–mentee relationships. Nurses who have been mentored reported the capability to model positive traits of their mentors, such as persistence, job dedication, honesty, and discipline (Carey & Campbell, 1994; Dyer, 2008). The mentor–mentee relationship was found to help the socialization of the mentored nurse into a specific nursing unit or nursing position (Dyer, 2008). In addition, nurses who have been mentored noted career advice, role modeling, education, and emotional support to be benefits of the relationship (Dyer, 2008).

A supportive environment for new graduates has been developed by Margaret Flinter, APRN, MSN (2005). This program is for novice NPs who aspire to work in the complex setting of a federally qualified health center (FQHC). The program is called a residency program, which Flinter has initiated in some community health centers in Connecticut. Flinter posits that NPs should have opportunity for training with the support of experienced healthcare providers in order to provide the comprehensive, complex care that most patients who use those types of health centers need. In this model, however, it may not be an NP who is formally provided as a mentor; it may be a physician.

The objective for this type of formal mentoring arrangement is to guide and assist these new NPs in a multi- and interdisciplinary setting in clinical decision making. The hope is that those who have intense support while learning their role in this type of setting will choose to continue working in the challenging FQHC arena. If this does become realized, there would be opportunity for more NP mentors who can truly speak to the role of the NP in this setting, and help to formulate and meet future professional goals including research, presenting, and publishing, in addition to becoming expert clinicians.

Few studies have been published regarding outcomes related to NPs and mentorship (Harrington, 2011). Hayes (1998) found a positive correlation between NP students' discernment of mentoring by their clinical preceptor and their own sense of self-efficacy. Brown and Olshansky (1997) found that productivity increased in the primary care setting when novice NPs had supportive work environments. Neal (2008) completed a study that examined NP students' perception of self-efficacy based upon whether the student had at least one preceptor identified as a mentor during clinical training. Neal found that predictors of self-efficacy included students' identification of a mentor and how the mentoring relationship facilitated the enhancement of skills needed to practice as an NP. In a survey seeking to identify the needs of APNs in a tertiary care center, findings were that both formal and informal mentoring would be useful, and that NPs should be matched with NPs (Doerksen, 2010). Also identified in this small survey were needs related to intellectual, financial, and administrative support, and that the needs for the mentee and mentor change over time.

For NP/DNP students, identifying a clinical mentor may be required by the university that encompasses more than the role of a clinical preceptor. Clinical mentors are academically and clinically qualified advanced practice nurses, physicians, faculty, nurse executives, and other healthcare professionals or health policy leaders who are able to facilitate and support the objectives of the student's clinical residency and DNP practice dissertation project.

Needs of the novice NP were identified in a think tank conducted by the American Academy of Nurse Practitioners (AANP, 2006). There were seven areas noted by these experienced NPs:

1. Caseload management
2. Time management and productivity
3. Developing clinical skills
4. Understanding the business component of practice
5. Overcoming fear and anxiety
6. Dealing with isolation
7. How to balance personal life and clinical practice effectively

The development of a mentorship program by the fellows of the AANP have identified the following important aspects of the relationship (AANP Fellows, 2006):

- Mutually benefit both the mentee and mentor
- Focus on helping and guiding toward professional goals
- Involve time, energy, initiative, and follow-through to be successful
- Involve mentors as generous learning brokers
- Involve mentees committed to achieving defined objectives

Various stages in the mentoring relationship are discussed, such as the ones listed in **BOX 14-1**.

In stage 1, initiation, the mentee and mentor are becoming acquainted. The experienced person believes that the novice can be successful and is willing to mentor the novice. The novice finds the mentor admirable and is willing to be guided and coached by the mentor. Mutual goals should be set in the cultivation stage. A contract clearly identifying what achievements are desired, and how the mentor will guide the mentee to reach those achievements, a note articulating the frequency and mode of meetings, as well as confidentiality, and a clause written about openness and conflict resolution should be included (see **FIGURE 14-1**).

At this time the mentee is becoming more confident that her or his professional and personal goals can be met. Dependence on the mentor can be strong during these early stages. In stage 4, the mentee has become self-confident and is not as dependent on the mentor, and will start the separation process. This time period can cause anxiety in the mentee (Grossman, 2013; Kram, 1986). As the relationship matures, the mentee and mentor have a more collegial relationship, and most likely, the mentee in turn has now become a mentor to a novice.

BOX 14-1 Stages of the Mentor Relationship

1. Initiation
2. Cultivation
3. Separation
4. Redefinition

Data from Kram, K. E. (1983, December). Phases of the mentor relationship. *Academy of Management Journal, 26*, 608–625.

We are voluntarily entering into a mentoring relationship from which we both expect to benefit. To this end, we have mutually agreed upon the terms and conditions of our relationship as outlined in this agreement.

Objectives/Goals

We hope to achieve:

Goal 1: ______________________________

Goal 2: ______________________________

Goal 3: ______________________________

Responsibilities of Mentor:

____

Responsibilities of Mentee:

____

Frequency of Meetings

We will attempt to meet at least __________ *[fill in amount]* times each month. If we cannot attend a scheduled meeting, we agree to be responsible and notify our partner, and make a specific plan to talk by phone, email, or text.

Duration

This mentoring relationship will continue as long as we both feel comfortable or until:

____

____

Confidentiality

Any sensitive issues that we discuss will be held in confidence. Issues that are off limits in this relationship include: ______________________________

No-Fault Termination

We are committed to open and honest communication in our relationship. We will discuss and attempt to resolve any conflicts as they arise. If, however, one of us needs to terminate the relationship for any reason, we agree to abide by the decision of our partner.

Mentor ______________________________ Date ______________

Mentee ______________________________ Date ______________

FIGURE 14-1 Sample Mentor and Mentee Agreement

Source: Modified from Brainard, S., Harkus, D., & George, M. (1998). *A Curriculum for Training Mentors and Mentees: Guide for Administration*. Seattle, WA: The Center for Workforce Development. (http://www.grad.washington.edu/mentoring/students/worksheet5.pdf). Reprinted by permission.

What should one look for when trying to find a mentor? In a study of 565 NPs, five aspects of a successful mentor were uncovered (Freeman, 2004). Components of these five aspects included (Grossman, 2013):

- Having a personal commitment to mentoring
- Having expertise in the field the mentoring occurs in
- Having the necessary qualities of counselor and educator
- Being prepared to be a sponsor
- Having an effective communication style

- Being respected in the profession
- Having good self-esteem
- Balancing work and personal life
- Willing to take on new challenges
- Being open to change

Four core competencies for effective mentoring developed by Bell (2002) form the acronym SAGE:

- Surrendering—leveling the learning field
- Accepting—creating a safe haven for risk taking
- Gifting—the main event
- Extending—nurturing protégé independence

In the surrendering component, all attempts to rid the relationship of the anxiety that can occur from the mentor's power and authority are embraced. Accepting the mentee as she or he is and providing a safe environment for learning and growth are vital to success. The value of being generous with useful advice, feedback, and opportunities without expecting anything in return is called gifting. Although we may think this is most beneficial to the mentee, anyone who has gifted in this manner knows that the equal, if not greater, gift is the satisfaction the mentor gets from watching the mentee flourish. Extending requires the mentor to be able to let go, to push the mentee beyond the boundaries of comfort, and to realize when to end the current relationship and allow the mentee to use alternate methods for future growth.

The Barker-Sullivan Model of Mentor Partnerships (DeNisco & Barker, 2013) begins with mutual attraction, which is based on congruency of values, and it is characterized by respect and trust. Honest, open, and discreet communications are emphasized in this model. The mentor, who has expertise that the mentee is seeking to learn from, has skills required by a mentor, and is a transformational leader in the role the mentee is involved with, or seeks to become expert in. The mentee needs to develop competence in the new role and in leadership skills. This type of mentoring relationship should encourage the mentee to be energized to engage in self-reflection, learn new skills and competencies, and take action to move forward.

Mentees can get the most of a mentoring relationship by recognizing that they have found someone who genuinely cares about them and their career. The following tips have been adapted for new NP/DNP graduates (Tracy, 2012; Zwilling, 2012):

- Set clear objectives for yourself in your career growth. Decide exactly what it is you need mentoring on before you start thinking of the ideal person to work with. This will help you to seek out the right person as mentor.
- Work to continually put the guidance into action. The best mentors are the most interested in helping someone who is willing to learn and grow; so take advantage by putting the suggestions and advice into action.
- Remember, the best mentors are busy people. When you meet, be prepared by having specific issues to discuss.
- Remember the difference between a mentor, a friend, and a coach. Expect a mentor to tell you what you need to hear, not like a friend who may tell you what you want to hear. A business coach is focused on helping you with generic skills, whereas a mentor's aim is to teach you based on specific situations.
- Send a note to communicate progress or touch base on a regular basis. A mentor is more likely to want to help you if you are making it clear that you are following through, and the relationship is helping you to reach your objectives and goals.

The mentor should use the following guidelines when working with a mentee:

- Advise the mentee about the duration of the meeting.
- Discuss the mentee's achievements, and give positive feedback.
- Be specific and kind when giving necessary constructive feedback that may not be what the mentee might want to hear.
- Be prepared to fill the meeting time with specific issues and objectives.
- Take every moment seriously.
- Reassure the mentee that trust, honesty, and confidentiality are of paramount importance to your relationship.

Peer mentoring is another format for a mentoring relationship that may be useful as the increased number of NP/DNP graduates seeking experienced NP/DNPs is mismatched. Identification of a peer mentor that can help in areas where she or he has expertise that the NP needs further growth in, and where the NP can offer her or his own expertise in an area the other person needs to grow in, can be a very rewarding experience. It can also be beneficial and practical to have a group of peer mentors that can offer a pool of expertise to help the NPs that form this group.

MY MENTOR

Feeling competent in my skills as a nurse practitioner, I realized that it was time to find a professional challenge in my career trajectory. I joined a few colleagues from a previous employment site who had contacted me to start a DNP cohort program that was going to begin in our area. Since I knew that my goal had never included a PhD in nursing because I did not want to focus solely on nursing research, I agreed the DNP was a great option.

We progressed through, sometimes loving the learning and networking this cohort afforded us, and sometimes moaning and groaning over the necessary research and writing of papers at such an advanced level. We were fortunate to have a senior faculty person discuss with us the need to seek mentors, and briefly cover the reason why we would need our own mentor. Another seasoned colleague spoke about her mentor, and how their relationship had been critical for her to meet her goals in her career. She also discussed how the time had come to part ways—when her mentor no longer seemed to be supporting her mentee's choices and current goals.

I realized I needed a mentor—but who? Who had been around a long enough time with a DNP and was an NP that could guide me? I also realized that I really wasn't sure what my goals were now. Accomplishing the completion of my research and publishing it were behind me now. What next?

After taking a full-time job in a university setting, having my clinical work each week, in addition to a full load of teaching and advising NP students, I quickly realized I needed a mentor to help me balance this juggling act. I was an expert clinician, and a good preceptor; however, my formal teaching abilities needed mentoring from someone who was doing both clinical and teaching, and had a family, and doing it all in a balanced manner. Not an easy bill to fill!

I am so fortunate to have found someone who is probably more of a peer mentor in some areas, but who has had many years of teaching and doing clinical, as well as an active family life. We both had obtained our DNPs doing classes and research together, so this new role was an area we agreed to work on together—finding ways to really help advance our careers and make a difference in our profession. Since these are early days for the NP/DNP, peer mentoring might be more accessible, and we suggest others consider that as an option.

Prior to graduating from NP programs, students should consider identifying a mentor and prepare to discuss the relationship with the person so there is more of a formal relationship for supporting the novice NP. Mentees should be prepared that down the road they should consider becoming mentors to others, whether peer mentors, or the more familiar relationship with a novice NP. The rewards are many for both.

Seminar Discussion Questions

1. How does a preceptor differ from a mentor?
2. Write down three professional or career objectives or goals that you want to work on.
3. Identify one or two people you consider as possible mentors to help reach those goals.
4. How will you discuss forming a mentor relationship with the person you think best suited to your goals and personality?

References

American Academy of Nurse Practitioners. (2006). *Mentoring assessment.* Retrieved from http://www.aanp.org

American Academy of Nurse Practitioners Fellows. (2006). *FAANP mentorship program.* Retrieved from http://www.aanp.org/fellows-program/faanp-mentorship-program

Bell, C. (2002). *Managers as mentors: Building partnerships for learning.* San Francisco, CA: Berrett Koehler.

Brainard, S., Harkus, D., & George, M. (1998). *A curriculum for training mentors and mentees: Guide for administration.* Seattle, WA: The Center for Workforce Development. Retrieved from http://www.grad.washington.edu/mentoring/students/worksheet5.pdf

Brown, M., & Olshansky, E. F. (1997). From limbo to legitimacy: A theoretical model of the transition to the primary care nurse practitioner role. *Nursing Research, 46*(1), 46–51.

Carey, S., & Campbell, S. (1994). Preceptor, mentor and sponsor roles: Creative strategies for nurse retention. *Journal of Nursing Administration, 24*(12), 39–48.

Chitty, K., & Black, B. (2011). *Professional nursing: Concepts and challenges.* Maryland Heights, MO: Saunders.

DeNisco, S., & Barker, A. M. (2013). *Advanced practice nursing: Evolving roles for the transformation of the profession.* Burlington, MA: Jones & Bartlett Learning.

Doerksen, K. (2010). What are the professional and mentorship needs of advanced practice nurses? *Journal of Professional Nursing, 26*(3), 141–151.

Dyer, L. (2008). The continuing need for mentors in nursing. *Journal for Nurses in Staff Development, 24*(2), 86–90.

Flinter, M. (2005). Residency programs for primary care nurse practitioners in federally qualified health centers: A service perspective. *Online Journal of Issues in Nursing, 10*(3). doi:10.3912/OJIN.Vol10No03Man05

Freeman, S. (2004). Effective mentoring skills for nurse practitioners. Lecture given at AANP Symposium. New Orleans, LA. June 12, 2004. Retrieved from http://66.219.50.180/NR/rdonlyres/e7pquryyesamqmduxs7dumbgai143wqbb45suegjn7nrtndoepkjjdz zhbr6gtqvzlno5oteja5ecmwi/4%252e3%252e12.pdf

Grindell, C. (2003). Mentoring managers. *Nephrology Nursing Journal, 30*(5), 517–522.

Grossman S. (2013). *Mentoring in nursing: A dynamic and collaborative process* (2nd ed.). New York, NY: Springer.

Hanson, D. (2012). Interview with nurse practitioner wellness coaches. *WebNPOnline.* Retrieved from http://www.webnponline.com/articles/article_details/interview-with-nurse-practitioner-wellness-coaches/

Harrington, S. (2011). Mentoring new nurse practitioners to accelerate their development as primary care providers: A literature review. *Journal of the American Academy of Nurse Practitioners, 23*(4), 168–174.

Hayes, E. (1998). Mentoring and self-efficacy for advanced practice: A philosophical approach for nurse practitioner preceptors. *Journal of the American Academy of Nurse Practitioners, 10*(2), 1–5.

Kram, K. (1986). Mentoring in the workplace. In D. Hall (Ed.), *Career development in organizations.* San Fransisco, CA: Jossey-Bass.

Kram, K.E. (1983). Phases of the Mentor Relationship. *The Academy of Management Journal, 26*(4), 608–625.

Link, D. (2009). The teaching-coaching role of the APN. *Journal of Perinatal and Neonatal Nursing, 23*(3), 279–283.

National Organization of Nurse Practitioner Faculties. (2012). *Domains and core competencies of nurse practitioner practice.* Washington, DC: Author.

Neal, T. I. (2008). *Mentoring, self-efficacy and nurse practitioner students: A modified replication.* Doctoral dissertation, Ball State University, Muncie, IN. Retrieved from Cumulative Index to Nursing and Allied Health Literature, 2010757741.

Tracy, B. (2012). *Earn what you're really worth: Maximize your income in any market at any time.* New York, NY: Vanguard Press.

Zwilling, M. (2012). How to make a business mentoring relationship work. *Forbes Online.* Retrieved from http://www.forbes.com/sites/martinzwilling/2012/03/20/effective-business-mentoring-is-a-relationship

CHAPTER 15

Reimbursement for Nurse Practitioner Services

Lynn Rapsilber

Introduction

Greater availability of primary and preventative healthcare services has been tied to cost savings and improved patient care outcomes. Nurse practitioners (NPs) have been shown to provide cost-effective care compared to their physician colleagues; therefore, reimbursement for healthcare services is the fiscal responsibility of every nurse practitioner. The 1997 Balanced Budget Act authorized specialists to bill directly for their professional services and be reimbursed at 85% of the physician rate for services provided to a patient (Department of Health and Human Services [DHHS], 2007). The rise in healthcare costs and the inability for the nursing profession to show cost savings has been an obstacle to obtaining direct payment for services (Stanley, 2010). The majority of patients, unless uninsured, will have a third-party insurance participant involved in setting fee schedules and reimbursement criteria.

Understanding proper medical record documentation and billing procedures for an office visit can maximize reimbursement for services affecting both the practice and the nurse practitioner's bottom line. This chapter will inform the nurse practitioner of the tools for reimbursement and how to use the key components of evaluation and management to select the most appropriate code for the service provided and recognize audit triggers. Lastly, "incident to" billing will be reviewed so the nurse practitioner will be able to identify and protect him- or herself from unintentional fraudulent billing and legal issues, as the NP is accountable for all the services billed by a practice.

Important Steps in Reimbursement Eligibility

Nurse practitioners have been providing safe, cost-effective, quality health care for years and graduate with the competencies needed to provide excellent patient care at the point of service. While NPs are making strides in understanding the business of health care, they still lack the reimbursement knowledge and skills needed to be key players in the healthcare arena. Aside from the educational, board certification, and licensure requirements, the nurse practitioner must obtain several other identifiers to be eligible for reimbursement by a third-party payor. Obtaining a national provider number and employer number, and being credentialed by private and public insurers, will be described in the following sections.

National Provider Number

Nurse practitioners, physician assistants, and physicians can be reimbursed for the provision of healthcare services. For a nurse practitioner to be eligible for reimbursement, he or she must hold a minimum of a master's degree in nursing and successfully pass the national certification exam given by the American Association of Nurse Practitioners (AANP) or the American Nurses Credentialing Center (ANCC). The Health Insurance Portability and Accountability Act of 1996 (HIPAA) mandated the adoption of a standard unique identifier for healthcare providers. In 2004, the Centers for Medicare and Medicaid Services (CMS) adopted the national provider number as the standard unique identifier number for all healthcare providers to use when filing and processing healthcare claims (Stanley, 2010). All NPs are required to apply for a national provider number and be assigned only one number that will follow the NP wherever he or she practices. The application must be completed by the nurse practitioner to avoid any potential error that could delay billing and reimbursement (National Plan and Provider Enumeration System, 2012).

Employer Provider Number

Whether employed by a practice or as a practice owner, the nurse practitioner will be assigned a provider number reflecting where the services will be provided to a patient. If the medical practice has two office locations, there will be a different provider number for both practice settings. Before billing a third-party payor, whether Medicare, Medicaid, or private insurer, the patient service must have the national provider number of who provided the service and the provider number where the service occurred in order to bill.

Third-Party Credentialing

Lastly, the nurse practitioner must receive credentialing by the third-party payor in order to bill insurance companies for his or her services. While this is usually completed by the practice manager, the nurse practitioner should become familiar with the rules and policies of the third-party payor. A provider application form is filled out, which is also known as the "credentialing form." The nurse practitioner will be required to complete an attestation form to verify that the information submitted is correct. The nurse practitioner must make sure the information is correct. Any errors may delay the application process. Once the nurse practitioner has obtained a national provider number, employer provider number, and third-party credentialing or insurance company membership, then he or she is ready to begin billing for services.

Practice Authority

The nurse practitioner practice authority is determined by the state. The level of practice authority is defined by the American Association of Nurse Practitioners as full, reduced, or restricted practice as determined by the ability to assess, diagnose, treat, and prescribe. Reduced practice authority requires a collaborative agreement with an outside "like-minded" healthcare discipline to provide patient care. Some states allow a physician or a nurse practitioner to be a collaborator. Restricted practice requires supervision, delegation, or team management by an outside health discipline in order for the nurse practitioner to provide patient care. Consult the AANP website (www.aanp.org) for the latest state practice map.

▸ Coding and Billing Resources

Before billing for services rendered, the nurse practitioner needs to identify appropriate diagnoses for the patient, the type of patient encounter (for example, new or established visit), and what procedures were performed during the patient encounter. Other reportable, billable services would include medications administered, if any, and what supplies were used to provide care. Lastly, the nurse practitioner must provide clear and accurate documentation validating the reported diagnoses and procedural codes reported for billing purposes. An understanding of medical coding and resources to support these activities are the responsibility of the nurse practitioner.

Definition of Medical Coding

Medical coding is best defined as the translation of the original medical record documentation regarding patient diagnoses and procedures into a series of code numbers that describe the information in a standard manner. Coded medical information is used for patient care, research, reimbursement, and evaluation of services (Aalseth, 2006). International Classification of Diseases (ICD) codes, developed by the World Health Organization, are used to identify the patient's diagnoses or reasons for seeking care. These codes cover specific illnesses or diseases as well as signs and symptoms resulting in the patient encounter (Centers for Disease Control and Prevention [CDC], 2011). ICD codes are also useful for classifying morbidity and mortality data from inpatient and outpatient records and most National Center for Health Statistics (NCHS) surveys.

Another component of medical billing is the *Current Procedural Terminology* (CPT), which describes the services and/or procedures for which reimbursement is sought. The American Medical Association publishes the CPT. This publication was initiated in 1966 as a way of standardizing terms for medical procedures used for documentation purposes (Phillipsen, 2008). CPT codes are used for specific types of patient encounters and innumerable procedures and diagnostic studies that will be described in more detail later in this chapter.

The CPT and ICD-10 Books

There are several resources the nurse practitioner needs to be aware of regarding medical coding and billing for services. As previously mentioned, one such publication is the CPT. This book is updated annually providing coding additions and deletions. Only nurse practitioners, physician assistants, and physicians can use these codes. CPT reflects "what was done," such as types of visits, consultations, referrals, procedures, diagnostic studies, and treatment regimens. Obtaining a copy of the CPT is very important, as the information presented in this chapter is found in the beginning sections of the book.

Another necessary reference book is the *International Classification of Diseases, Tenth Edition*, or ICD-10. This reflects "why it was done." This book classifies diseases, symptoms, injuries, and accidents with numeric codes. The NP must select a code for the disease or symptom by "what you know," being as specific as possible. If you have not yet determined or confirmed the patient's diagnosis, then you should list or code for the presenting symptoms. For example, if the patient has "heartburn" and you have not completed your evaluation, do not choose the ICD-10 code for gastroesophageal reflux with esophagitis (K 21.0). Instead, designate heartburn as the diagnostic code (R 12.0) until you have results of an endoscopic testing.

The ICD-10 classification system is widely used in Europe and adapted in the United States on October 1, 2015 (National Center for Health Statistics, 2012).

Medical Necessity

When you have the "what was done" with the "why it was done," this equals medical necessity: CPT + ICD-10 = medical necessity. Medical necessity is defined as medical items and services that are "reasonable and necessary" for a variety of purposes. By statute, Medicare may only pay for items and services that are "reasonable and necessary for the diagnosis or treatment of illness or injury or to improve the functioning of a malformed body member," unless there is another statutory authorization for payment. Determination of medical necessity involves comparing the procedure being billed to the diagnosis being submitted. Determining medical necessity does not necessarily guarantee payment. If the NP receives a denial notification from the payor for a particular procedure, it means that the payor does not think the procedure was justified for the diagnosis given (Aalseth, 2006).

There is an additional resource called the Healthcare Common Procedure Coding System, or HCPCS. For Medicare and other health insurance programs to ensure that healthcare claims are processed in an orderly and consistent manner, standardized coding systems are essential. The HCPCS Level II code set is one of the standard code sets used by medical coders and billers for services such as medical supplies, durable medical goods, non-physician services, and services not represented in the Level I code set determined by the CPT (e.g., ambulance, prosthetics, orthotics) (American Association of Professional Coders [AAPC], 2012). With the utilization of the electronic health record, all these codes are recorded and the information is submitted electronically to the insurance payer for reimbursement (**EXHIBIT 15-1**).

EXHIBIT 15-1 Sample Encounter Form

Date of service:		Insurance:		Account #:	
Patient name:		Subscriber name:		Physician/NP name:	
Address:		Group #:		Physician/NP signature:	
Phone:		Copay:			
DOB:		Age:		Sex:	

Procedure Codes												
	Labs	CPT		Office Procedures	CPT		Immunizations and Injections	CPT		Office Visit	CPT New	CPT Est
	Blood draw	36415		Anoscopy	46600		Allergen, one	95115		Minimal		99211
	CT/DNA probe	87490		Audiometry	92551		Allergen, multiple	95117		Problem focused	99201	

(continues)

EXHIBIT 15-1 Sample Encounter Form *(continued)*

	GC/DNA probe	87590		Cerumen removal	69210		Imm admin, one	90471		Expanded problem focused		
	Glucose	82948		Colposcopy	57452		Imm admin, each add'l	90472		Detailed		
	Hem occult	82270		Colposcopy w/ biopsy	57455		Imm admin, intranasal, one	90473		Comprehensive		
	HGB	83068		ECG, w/ interpretation	93000		Imm admin, intranasal, each add'l	90474		Comprehensive (new pt.)		
	KDH prep	87220		ECG, rhythm strip	93040		Injection, joint, small	20600		Significant, separate service		
	Pap smear	88150		Endometrial biopsy	58100		Injection, joint, intermediate	20605		**Well Visit**	**New**	**Est**
	Sed rate	85651		Flexible sigmoidoscopy	45330		Injection, joint, major	20610		< 1 y	99381	99391

EXHIBIT 15-1 Sample Encounter Form *(continued)*

Strep screen	86403	Flexible sigmoidoscopy w/biopsy	45331	Injection, ther/proph/diag	90772	1–4 y	99382	99392
Urinalysis (dipstick)	81005	Fracture care, cast/splint Site: ________	29___	Injection, trigger point	20552	5–11 y	99383	99393
Urine pregnancy test	81025	Nebulizer	94640	**Vaccines**	**CPT**	12–17 y	99384	99394
Wet mount	87210	Nebulizer demo	94664	DT, < 7 y	90702	18–39 y	99385	99395
Dressings	**CPT**	Spirometry	94010	DTP	90701	40–64 y	99386	99396
Ace wrap/elastic		Spirometry pre & post	94060	DTaP, < 7 y	90700	65 y +	99387	99397
Bandage (amt ________)	A4460	Tympanometry	92567	Flu, 6–35 mos	90657	**Medicare Preventive Services**		**CPT**
Casting tape	A4590	Vasectomy	55250	Flu, 3 y +	90658	Pap		Q0091

(continues)

EXHIBIT 15-1 Sample Encounter Form *(continued)*

Foam dressing	A6209	**Skin Procedures**	**CPT**	Hep A, adult	90632	Pelvic & breast	G0101
Irrigation solution	A4323	Burn care, initial	16000	Hep A, ped/adol, 2 dose	90633	Prostate/PSA	G0103
Nonsterile gauze	A6216	Foreign body, skin, simple	10120	Hep B, adult	90746	Tobacco counseling/3–10 min	99406
Skin sealants	A6250	Foreign body, skin, complex		Hep B, ped/adol, 3 dose	90744	Tobacco counseling/> 10 min	99407
Tapes (all types)	A6265	I&D, abscess		Hep B-Hib	90748	Welcome to Medicare exam	G0344
Other Services	**CPT**	I&D, hematoma/seroma		Hib, 4 dose	90645	ECG w/Welcome to Medicare exam	G0366
After posted hours	99050	Laceration repair, simple Site: __________ Size: ____		HPV	90649	Flexible sigmoidoscopy	G0104

EXHIBIT 15-1 Sample Encounter Form *(continued)*

	Evening/ weekend appointment	99051		Laceration repair, layered Site: __________ Size: ___		IPV	90713		Hemoccult, guaiac	G0107
	Home health certification	G0180		Lesion, biopsy, one		MMR	90707		Flu shot	G0008
	Home health recertification	G0179		Lesion, biopsy, each add'l		Pneumonia, > 2 y	90732		Pneumonia shot	G0009
	Post-op follow-up	99024		Lesion, destruct., benign, 1–14		Pneumonia conjugate, < 5 y	90669		**Consultation/Pre-op Clearance**	**CPT**
	Prolonged/30–74 min	99354		Lesion, destruct., premal, single		Td, > 7 y	90718		Expanded problem focused	99242
	Special reports/forms	99080		Lesion, destruct., premal, each add'l		Varicella	90716		Detailed	99243
	Disability/ workers' comp	99455		Lesion, excision, benign Site: __________ Size: ___		**Misc. Procedures**	**CPT**		Comprehensive/mod complexity	99244

(continues)

EXHIBIT 15-1 Sample Encounter Form

(continued)

	Miscellaneous	CPT								
				Lesion, excision, malig. Site: __________ Size: ___		Pulse oximetry	94762		Comprehensive/high complexity	99245
				Lesion, paring/cutting, one		Vision test	92583		**Radiology**	**CPT**
				Lesion, paring/cutting, 2–4		O^2 treatment	94760			
				Lesion, shave Site: __________ Size: ___		Burn treatment	16020			
				Nail removal, partial		Cast removal	29705		**Diagnoses**	
				Nail removal, w/matrix		Peak flow	94735	1		
				Skin tag, 1–15		EKG		2		

	Current	30 Days	60 Days	90 Days	120+ Days	Total
Pt. balance						
Ins. balance						

Medical Record Documentation

The medical record is the most important document in the reimbursement process. Any information provided to the patient on a particular date of service must be recorded in the record. **If it was not documented, it was not done.** The medical record clearly should state what was done and why it was done. CMS has specific documentation criteria. The medical record should be complete and legible. It should include a chief complaint, why the patient presents to the office or management of chronic disease(s), relevant history, assessment, physical exam, diagnostic testing, and treatment plan. It must be signed by the provider of record (the one who performed the service). Rationale for testing must be apparent. Health risks must be identified. Responses to treatment and follow-up must be clear. CPT and ICD-10 must be supported in the documentation. The data must be sequential. If something is inadvertently omitted from a previous date of service (DOS), it can be entered using today's date and stated as an "addenda to DOS on date" and added the omitted information. If something is erroneously entered, an addendum to the health record is made detailing the reason for the error and the correction. CMS recognizes the electronic health record should not replace the need for good documentation by the nurse practitioner. A summary of CMS documentation criteria is represented in **FIGURE 15-1**.

Payment for Services

The current system for reimbursement is based upon the resourced-based relative value scale (RBRVS). This system replaced the fee for service. The system was developed based upon data acquired by Dr. Hsaio and a multidisciplinary team of researchers from Harvard University in 1988 (Goodson, 2007). Three separate factors were used to calculate physician value: (1) work effort (52%), (2) practice expense (44%), and (3) malpractice expense (4%). Provider work effort is defined by a relative value unit (see **BOX 15-1**). The Geographic Practice Cost Index (GPCI) refers to the cost of service applied to geographic

CMS medical record documentation criteria

- The medical record should be complete and legible
- Reason for the encounter and relevant history, physical examination findings, and prior diagnostic test results
- Assessment, clinical impression, or diagnosis
- Plan for care
- If not documented, the rationale for ordering diagnostic and other ancillary services should be easily inferred
- Past and present diagnoses should be accessible to the treating and/or consulting physician
- Appropriate health risk factors should be identified
- The patient's progress, response to and changes in treatment, and revision of diagnosis should be documented
- The CPT and ICD-10 codes reported on the health insurance claim form or billing statement should be supported by the documentation in the medical record

FIGURE 15-1 CMS Medical Record Documentation Criteria

BOX 15-1 Resourced Based Relative Value Scale (RBRVS)

Converting an RBRVS to a Dollar Amount

(Work RVU X Work GPCI) + (Practice Expense RVU XPractice Expense GPCI) + (Malpractice RVU XMalpractice GPCI) X Conversion Factor X Practitioner Payment Rate = Allowed Amount

RVU = relative value unit

GPCI = geographic practice cost indices

locations within the country. In New York and California, it costs more to deliver care than in Tennessee or Mississippi. The conversion factor is the variable that changes from year to year. Medicare reimburses the nurse practitioner at 85% of the physician rate. Other insurance payors reimbursement fees can and should be negotiated.

Evaluation and Management Documentation Guidelines

Evaluation and management documentation guidelines are the foundation of fiscal responsibility and were developed by the American Medical Association and the Health Care Financing Administration (HCFA) (Aalseth, 2006), which is now the Centers for Medicare and Medicaid Services (CMS). Understanding this system will ensure proper coding of visits and maximize reimbursement; these guidelines are used by Medicare and other third-party payors when making reimbursement decisions. There are three key components to evaluation and management documentation: (1) history, (2) examination, and (3) medical decision making. These variables get broken down into their own set of levels. This will be discussed further in the key components section of this chapter.

Additionally, the NP needs to identify who is a new patient versus an established patient. A new patient is defined as an individual new to the practice (seeing any provider in the practice for the first time) or has not been seen in 3 years. The new patient can also be a hospital patient who is being referred for care and not previously seen by any provider in the practice. An established patient is one who has an ongoing relationship with a practice. The hospital patient can be an established patient if a provider from the practice has seen the patient in the hospital and is returning for a follow-up visit. Contained within the CPT book is a decision tree that helps a provider identify the difference. A specialty provider for this discussion will be defined as a healthcare provider and as part of a group and is considered a specialist; the provider must have received special training and be board certified in that specialty.

General Coding Guidelines

The next step is to know which ICD-10 codes you will use to bill for the office visit. Coding takes the words the NP used as the diagnosis or symptom and converts them into a category code. Codes for valid diagnoses may have seven digits. Codes that describe symptoms as opposed to diagnoses are acceptable if the NP has not yet established a diagnosis responsible for the symptomatology of the patient.

Structure of the ICD-10 Diagnoses Codes

The diagnosis system is contained in three volumes: Tabular List, Instruction Manual, and Alphabetical Index accounting for 64,000 codes.

1. Tabular List: Diseases and health-related problems containing 22 chapters. Within each of these chapters are categories logically sequenced by body system, site, or etiology. Combination codes are available for certain diseases. The use of "other" NOS (not otherwise specified) or NEC (not elsewhere classified) is no longer permitted in ICD-10.
2. Instruction Manual provides data for morbidity (hospital statistics) and mortality (causes of death).
3. The Alphabetical Index contains diseases and nature of injury, external causes of injury, and table of drugs and chemicals.

Submission electronically allows unlimited number of diagnostic codes to be used, each is linked to a CPT or procedural code. A word of caution: Use only the codes you intend to do something about or have a correlation to the patient's treatment plan, otherwise it can trigger an audit.

Structure of the CPT Procedure Codes

CPT codes are categorized into six main sections with five numbers representing a service:

1. Anesthesia (00100–01999)
2. Surgery (10021–69990)
3. Radiology (70010–79999)
4. Pathology and Laboratory (80300–8939)
5. Medicine (90281–99607)
6. Evaluation and Management (99201–99499)

The categories of the codes do not mean that a primary care provider cannot use a code in the surgery section; for example, CPT code 10060—Incision and Drainage of Abscess (cutaneous or subcutaneous abscess, cyst, or paronychia) may be used by the NP in the outpatient setting. The categorization of the codes is set up for the expediency of the provider, and billing personnel may also use the index to look up specific items.

Location of Patient Encounter

Know where your feet are planted and that specific patient encounter locations will result in a different code for billing purposes. If the NP is in the office, the following CPT codes will be used: (1) new patient codes 99201–99205, and (2) established patient codes 99211–99215. Care may be provided in the inpatient or outpatient settings or in the home or extended care facility. See **BOX 15-2** for codes corresponding to the geographic location of care. Consult the CPT book for specific criteria for each code.

BOX 15-2 Geographic Location of Care

Common Codes

Office or outpatient

New patient: 99201, 99202, 99203, 99204, 99205

Established patient: 99211, 99212, 99213, 99214, 99215

Hospital inpatient

Initial: 99221, 99222, 99223

Subsequent: 99231, 99232, 99233

Discharge: 99238, 99239

Nursing facility

Comprehensive assessment: 99301, 99302, 99303

Subsequent: 99311, 99312, 99313

Discharge: 99315, 99316

Home services

New patient: 99341, 99342, 99343, 99344, 99345

Established: 99347, 99348, 99349, 99350

Used with author permission.

Levels of Patient Encounter

The NP will bill for level of office visit based upon the amount of work involved with history, examination, and medical decision making. There are five levels of codes to bill for new and established office patients. The level 1 visit code is for a nurse visit and is not listed in the discussion. Problem focused is a level 2. Expanded problem focused is a level 3. Detailed is a level 4. Comprehensive is a level 5. Billing a higher-level office visit requires more documentation of history, examination, and medical decision making. This will be discussed in an upcoming section.

Key Components of Reimbursement

The history, physical examination, and medical decision-making level are the key components determining reimbursement for the patient encounter. Counseling, coordination of care, nature of presenting problem, and time also weigh into the evaluation of a patient visit.

The History and Reimbursement Decisions

The history is the first key component of the reimbursement process. There are four components of the history that are considered in determining the level of the visit:

1. The history includes the chief complaint: what brought the patient to the office that day. It can also include chronic disease management and follow-up care.

TABLE 15-1 Components of History

History of Present Illness (HPI)	Review of Systems (ROS)	Past, Family, and/or Social History (PFSH)	Type of History (number equals level of history)
Brief	n/a	n/a	Problem focused (2)
Brief	Problem pertinent	n/a	Expanded problem focused (3)
Extended	Extended	Pertinent	Detailed (4)
Extended	Complete	Complete	Comprehensive (5)

Used with author permission.

2. The nurse practitioner gathers the history of present illness (HPI). This includes location, quality, severity and timing, context, modifying factors, and associated signs and symptoms.
3. The review of systems (ROS) is performed, which is conducted systematically to gather information including constitutional signs such as weight loss and overall condition, as well as ears, eyes, nose, mouth, throat, respiratory, cardiovascular, gastrointestinal, genitourinary, musculoskeletal, skin, neurological, psychiatric, hematologic and lymphatic, and immune and allergy.
4. The last component—past family and social history (PFSH)—is considered. Past medical history includes illnesses, surgeries, injuries, treatment, and current medications. Family history includes hereditary diseases that increase the patient's risk factors for those conditions. Social history should include military service. The components of history are placed into a table by the amount of work done by the provider.

Problem focused is a level 2, which includes only a brief HPI. Expanded problem focused is a level 3, which includes a brief HPI, and problem focused ROS but no PFSH is done. Detailed visits are coded at level 4, which includes an extensive HPI, ROS, and pertinent PFSH. Comprehensive visits are coded at level 5 and include comprehensive histories, extended HPI, extended ROS, complete ROS, and complete PFHS (see **TABLE 15-1**).

The Physical Examination and Reimbursement Decisions

The next key component is the physical examination. There are four levels of physical examination:

- Level 2 problem focused (brief or perform and document one to five elements identified by a bullet)
- Level 3 expanded problem (focused and brief or perform and document at least six elements identified by a bullet)

- Level 4 detailed (perform and document at least two elements identified by a bullet from six areas/systems or at least twelve elements identified by a bullet in two or more areas/systems)
- Level 5 comprehensive (perform all elements identified by a bullet and document at least two elements identified by a bullet from nine areas/systems)

There are specific documentation guidelines created by the American Medical Association and CMS. There are two sets of documentation guidelines: those published in 1995 and those published in 1997. The 1995 guidelines are body system focused, and the 1997 is system area focused (Medicare Learning Network, 2010).

The documentation guidelines determine the level of physical exam to be performed. There is a general multisystem examination and several specialty examination options. The specialty examinations include cardiology; hematology/oncology; musculoskeletal; neurology; ear, nose, and throat; genitourinary; psychiatry; respiratory; and skin. The NP should select the examination appropriate for the patient population. **TABLE 15-2** lists the differences between the 1995 and 1997 guidelines for physical examination.

TABLE 15-2 Documentation Guidelines for Physical Examinations

Exam Description	1995 Guidelines	1997 Guidelines	Type of Exam
Limited to affected body area of organ system	1 body area or organ system	1, 2, 3, 4, 5 bulleted items	Problem focused (2)
Affected body area/organ system and other symptomatic or related organ system	2, 3, 4, 5, 6, 7 body areas or organ systems	6, 7, 8, 9, 10, 11, or more bulleted areas	Expanded problem focused (3)
Extended exam of affected area/organ system and other related symptomatic or related organ systems	2, 3, 4, 5, 6, 7 body areas or organ systems	12, 13, 14, 15, 16, 17, or more for 2 or more systems	Detailed (4)
General multisystem	≥ 8 body areas or organ systems	18 or more for 9 or more systems	Comprehensive (5)
Complete single organ system	n/a	See the specific criteria for each	Comprehensive (5)

Used with author permission.

If the provider documents an abnormal finding, an accompanying explanation is required. Normal and negative examination results must be listed by organ or body system. Subjective results without any documentation cannot be counted.

Medical Decision Making and Reimbursement

Medical decision making is the last key component. It takes into account the diagnosis, the information required to make the diagnosis, and risks and complications associated with the diagnosis. This is where the NP obtains credit for the decision regarding diagnosing and treatment options. The evaluation and management documentation guidelines describe four levels of medical decision making:

- Level 2 straightforward
- Level 3 low complexity
- Level 4 moderate complexity
- Level 5 high complexity

Factors such as number of diagnoses, comorbid conditions, data to be reviewed, number of management options, and risk of morbidity and mortality are considered in the level of medical decision making selected. The more risk involved in the patient's care, the greater the level of medical decision making. **TABLE 15-3** details what is included in a low, moderate, and high complexity level.

TABLE 15-3 Risks Associated with Complexity Level of Visit

Level of Risk	Presenting Problem	Diagnostic Procedures Ordered	Management Options Selected
Minimal	One self-limited or minor problem (e.g., rash or oral ulcers, cold, insect bites)	Lab tests requiring venipuncture Chest x-rays EKG/ECG UA Ultrasound	Rest Splints Superficial dressings
Low	Two or more self-limited or minor problems or symptoms One stable chronic illness (e.g., well-controlled HTN or NIDDM, BPH) Acute uncomplicated illness (e.g., cystitis, allergic rhinitis, simple sprain)	MRI/CT, PFTs Superficial needle biopsies Clinical lab test requiring arterial puncture Skin biopsies	OTC drugs Minor surgery with no identified risk factors PT/OT IV fluids without additives

(continues)

TABLE 15-3 Risks Associated with Complexity Level of Visit *(continued)*

Moderate	One or more chronic illnesses with mild exacerbation, progression, or side effect of treatment Acute illness systemic symptoms (e.g., pyelonephritis, pneumonitis) Two or more stable chronic illnesses Acute complicated injury (e.g., vertebral compression fracture, head injury with brief LOC) Undiagnosed new problem with uncertain prognosis (e.g., lump in breast)	Diagnostic endoscopies with no identified risk factors Cardiovascular imaging studies with contrast, no risk factors (e.g., arteriogram) Arthrocentesis, LP Physiologic tests under stress test (e.g., cardiac stress test) Deep needle or incisional biopsy	Prescription drug management Minor surgery with identified risk factors IV fluids with additives Therapeutic nuclear medicine Elective major surgery (open, percutaneous, or endoscopic) with no identified risk factors Closed treatment of fracture or dislocation without manipulation
High	One or more chronic illnesses with severe exacerbation, progression, or side effects of treatment Acute or chronic illness that may pose a threat to life or bodily function (e.g., progressive severe RA, multiple trauma, acute myeloid leukemia, PE, severe respiratory distress, psych illness with threat to self or others, acute renal failure) An abrupt change in neurological status (e.g., seizure, TIA, weakness, or sensory loss)	Cardiac EP tests Cardiovascular imaging studies with contrast, with identified risk factors Diagnostic endoscopies with identified risk factors Discography	Elective major surgery with risk factors Emergency major surgery Administration of parenteral controlled substances Drug therapy requiring intensive monitoring for toxicity Decision not to resuscitate or to de-escalate care because of poor prognosis

BPN = benign prostatic hyperplasia; CT = computed tomography; EKG/ECG = electrocardiography; EP = electrophysiology; HTN = hypertension; IV = intravenous; LOC = loss of consciousness; LP = lumbar puncture; MRI = magnetic resonance imaging; NIDDM = noninsulin-dependent diabetes mellitus; OT = occupational therapy; OTC = over the counter; PE = pulmonary embolism; PFT = pulmonary function test; PT = physical therapy; RA = rheumatoid arthritis; TIA = transient ischemic attack; UA = urinalysis

Used with author permission.

How to Bill for a Visit

To bill for a visit, you must know what ICD-10 and CPT codes to use. In review, know where your feet are planted, and use the specific location codes for where the care is provided. Decide if the patient is a new or established patient. Evaluate the level of history, physical examination, and medical decision making performed, and you will have the tools to establish the codes for the visit. A new patient requires the level for patient history, physical examination, and diagnoses to be weighted equally. For example, if you have documented a level 4 history, level 2 examination, and level 3 complexity, the visit is coded as a level 4 (99204). If this were an established patient, the highest two components out of the three would be weighted for the visit. In the scenario just described, the level 4 history and level 3 medical decision making would be considered for billing purposes. The physical exam would be dropped. The visit would be coded as a level 3 (99213).

TABLE 15-4 is a tool to assist the NP in accurately coding a visit by circling the amount of history, examination, and medical decision making performed for the visit. Documentation begins at the farthest right column. Once all columns are filled, the visit can be billed. If it is a new patient, the history, exam, and medical decision making are weighted equally. Look for the column where you have to the circle the item to the farthest left. That is the level of service billed. If you have an established patient, the lowest level is thrown out, and you bill to the next circled item to the farthest left. This becomes the billed visit code.

Coding Conundrums

There are coding situations that can be a challenge or a benefit if you know what they are and how to use them effectively. Coding by time, evaluation and management plus procedure, modifiers, shared evaluation and management, and "incident to" are examples described in greater detail. Understanding these situations can make a difference in revenue for the practice as well as avoiding legal pitfalls.

Coding by time is used when greater than 50% of the face-to-face time is spent discussing options with a patient, family member, or legal guardian. Little if any physical exam is performed. The visit is based upon the time spent with the patient, family member, or legal guardian. Nurse practitioners spend time teaching their patients about their disease or how to stay healthy or show them how to perform a task. All these can fall under coding by time. Documentation must support the time spent listed as a fraction (i.e., 35/40) and what was discussed. The amount of time corresponds to the code billed. Established patient code 99213 equals 15 minutes, 99214 equals 25 minutes, and 99215 equals 40 minutes.

Evaluation and management plus a procedure occur when the same provider performs the evaluation and management plus the procedure on the same patient on the same day. A diabetic patient comes into the office for a follow-up visit (evaluation and management) and asks about a warty growth on his or her shoulder. It is a seborrheic keratosis, and the NP performs cryosurgery (procedure) on the lesion. The nurse practitioner bills a 99214 for the diabetic visit and codes for the cryosurgery one lesion (17000). Since there is duplicity in work effort, there will be a modifier (25) placed on the office visit, and the value will be decreased but the

TABLE 15-4 Documentation Grid for Patients

New/ Established	99211	99201/99212	99202*/99213	99203/99214	99204** 99205/99215
		Problem Focused	Expanded Problem Focused	Detailed	Comprehensive
History	minimal	HPI 1–3 ROS none PFSH none	HP 1–3 ROS 1 system PFSH none	HPI 4+ ROS 2-9 systems PFSH 1+	**HPI 4+ ROS 10+ PFSH 3+
Physical Exam	minimal	1–5 bullets	6–12 bullets	12–18 bullets 2 or more body systems or 2 bullets from 6 body systems	18 bullets 9+ organ systems
Decision Making	minimal	Straight-forward	*Moderate Comp Low Complexity 2+ minor or 1 stable + 1 acute OTC TX	Moderate complexity 1+ chronic + exacerb or 2+ stable + 1 new RX mgmnt low risk surg	** Moderate Comp High Complexity 1+ chronic + severe exacer Acute or chronic abrupt chg RX inc surg risk
Time	EP 5 min	EP 10 min	NP20/EP15 min	NP30/EP25 min	204NP45/205NP60/EP40
For New Patient: all three history, exam and medical decision making					
For Established: Need two or three components to base level of visit					
How to Code: Take credit for information documented in HX.PE and Med-Dec to the farthest right Code the visit to the farthest left If a new patient, all three weigh the same and use the circle to the farthest left b. If an established patient, cross out the lowest, then take the next lowest unless they are both in the same column.					

© 2017, Rapsilber. Adapted from CMS 1997 Documentation Guidelines.

procedure will be reimbursed at the highest rate. Be aware a preventative visit and a same-day evaluation and management pose a problem. The patient has no copay associated with a preventative visit and will needed to pay a copay for the evaluation and management part of the visit. This should be disclosed to the patient prior to the preventative visit.

Modifiers are a way to show the evaluation and management code has changed. The service or procedure is altered. Modifiers can increase or decrease a value. It can indicate bilateral or multiple procedures. It can indicate additional work was performed in rendering the service. The two-digit modifier is always attached to the evaluation and management code. Most modifiers are used in the surgical arena.

Shared evaluation and management occurs when the nurse practitioner sees a patient in the hospital and documents the visit in the medical record. Later, the physician sees the patient and further documents in the medical record. The visit from both providers can be billed as a shared visit and billed under the physician's national provider number. There must be clear, separate documentation in the patient medical record. It does not mean the physician has to cosign the nurse practitioner's note. This is used for hospital billing and reimbursement purposes. This is different than "incident to" billing.

"Incident to" billing has been used in the care of Medicare patients. The term "incident to" has been used by physicians to bill for various services provided in the office by healthcare personnel that are performed in "relation to" or "incident to" the care the physician provides (Goolsby, 2002). In this situation, the nurse practitioner bills for her services with the physician's national provider number. The visit is reimbursed at 100%. This is problematic in that the NP is not visible in this method of billing and cannot show the income he or she is generating for the practice.

There are three major criteria that must be met by the practice before "incident to" billing can occur. The first criterion is that the nurse practitioner must be employed and directly supervised by the physician. This is problematic for in most states, nurse practitioners either practice autonomously or in collaboration with a physician. This stipulation means the physician must be available onsite to provide consultation to the NP. The physician cannot be in the hospital, on vacation, or out of the office. It does not mean the physician has to see the patient, but the physician must be available for questions if the need arises. The second criterion for "incident to" billing to occur is that the physician must see the patient for the initial visit and develop the treatment plan. The nurse practitioner cannot see any new Medicare patients under the current guidelines. The last criterion is that the physician must have ongoing participation in the patient's care. The patient cannot have a new problem when they see the nurse practitioner. The physician cannot cosign the nurse practitioner's documentation in this situation but must actually see the patient and modify the treatment plan, or otherwise bill the service under the nurse practitioner's NPI number.

There are numerous problems with this type of billing for a nurse practitioner. The Office of Inspector General is looking at the use of "incident to" billing and checking to see the rules are being followed. Significant monetary penalties are being levied and the potential removal as a Medicare provider for violation of the rules. In addition, there are considerations subjecting the practice to an audit. Audit triggers include billing noncovered services as covered, double billing, coding all visits at the same level, coding that does not meet medical necessity, "incident to" billing when the physician is not present in the office, waiving of copays, and documentation not supportive of

BOX 15-3 Basic Components of a Compliance Plan

Internal auditing system
Policies and procedures specific to the practice
Compliance officer in the practice to oversee and enforce the plan
Education of all employees about the plan
Prompt responses to any errors or offenses with corrective action
Open communication

Used with author permission.

the level billed. NPs should check their state nurse practice acts for reasons for loss of professional licensure such as false reports, willful misrepresentation, submitting false statements, or other unprofessional conduct (Phillipsen, 2008). **BOX 15-3** shows basic components of a compliance plan that should be instituted in each practice setting.

Changes to Reimbursement

There is a significant change to reimbursement with attention to quality (outcomes) versus quality (procedures). The Quality Payment Program (QPP) established by Medicare as part of the 2015 Medicare Access and CHIP Reauthorization Act (MACRA), seeks to improve quality of care to keep patients healthier. Nurse practitioner participation is imperative. There are two ways one can enter this program: through MIPS (Merit-based Incentive Payment System) or APM (Advanced Alternative Payment Model). Both programs offer participants incentives for providing quality care. Failure to participate will result in a reduction in payments or penalty. Nurse practitioners who see greater than 100 Medicare patient and bill more than $30,000 in Part B services should participate. Participation can be checked by entering a National Provider Number (NPI) into the QPP (www.QPP cms.gov) database. There is a timeline for participation. In 2017, registration occurs and data will be submitted on selected quality measures through a certified electronic health record. This data will be collected until March 31, 2018, and reviewed throughout 2018. In 2019, payment adjustments in the form of an incentive (positive payment adjustment) or penalty (negative payment adjustment) will be rendered yielding plus or minus 4%. As the programs progresses, the adjustments will be more significant.

The nurse practitioner is responsible for what is billed during the patient encounter. The practice, physician, and billing staff is not. It is imperative the nurse practitioner understand the method to code and bill for a patient visit properly to avoid an audit and to avoid fraudulent activity. With the changes to reimbursement under MACRA, reimbursement will be affected. Nurse practitioner care allows the opportunity for success in this program. Education and participation are crucial. It is fiscally prudent to have an understanding of this process.

Seminar Discussion Questions

Two case studies are presented. Read the following the case studies, and answer the questions that follow.

CASE STUDY ONE

Jenna Ward is a 19-year-old female who presents to the clinic with a chief complaint of 2-day history of burning with urination and vaginal discharge. The discharge is foul smelling. She has tried OTC vaginal treatment without improvement. She has been sexually active with several partners. She is G1, P0, A1. She takes oral contraceptives and menses are regular. She denies any cramping, abdominal pain, or unusual vaginal bleeding. No fever or chills. No routine medications. NKDA.

Past Medical History: Appendectomy age 16
Family History: M 32 A&W F 33 IDDM, B 22 asthma
Smokes ½ PPD, denies alcohol or drug use
She is 5'4" in height and weighs 137 lbs. Her blood pressure is 120/62, P 76. NAD, afebrile, abdomen soft, +BS, tender in suprapubic area. GU: external genitalia WNL with thick white vaginal discharge noted. No bleeding noted, Cervix pink, no CMT, GC & Chlamydia cultures taken, wet mount obtained, PAP smear performed, bimanual examination WNL no adnexal masses or tenderness.
Labs: UA 20-30 WBCs per HPF/C&S sent, wet mount: + whiff test, + clue cells

1. What are the potential ICD-10 codes in this case?
2. How can the NP determine if this patient is a new patient versus an established patient at the clinic?
3. What components of care will be used for reimbursement decisions for Ms. Ward?
4. What type of physical examination level best fits what was performed on Ms. Ward?
5. If you were coding the visit for Ms. Ward, how would you determine what decision-making level you would choose? Provide your rationale, and be specific.

CASE STUDY TWO

Robert Jones is a 45-year-old male who presents for diabetes. He has been struggling with blood sugar control. He travels for his job and eats out most days. He walks or goes to the gym when he can at least once a week. Takes metformin but forgets to take the second dose. AM BS 200-300, PM BS 300-400. Did not go to diabetic education classes. "I could not fit them in to my busy schedule."

Past Medical History:
Back surgery for "protruding lumbar disc" 5 years ago
Depression
Allergies:
Codeine; rash
Medications:
Zoloft 100 mg QD
Metformin BID
Family History:
Osteoarthritis, DM, HTN; mother 75 y.o. Cerebral vascular accident; father deceased age 60 y.o.
Social History:
Happily married to an attorney for 15 years, works in sales
Nonsmoker
No children
< 3 alcoholic drinks weekly

(continues)

CASE STUDY TWO

(continued)

Review of Systems:
General: Denies fever, weight loss, actually gained 10 lbs, night sweats
Respiratory: Denies difficulties
Cardiac: No CP or palpitations
Gastrointestinal: Appetite good, denies problems
GU: Denies urinary frequency, no nocturia
Musculoskeletal: Denies numbness, weakness, or sensation of pain in the upper extremities.
Physical Examination:
General: NAD. HT 5′9″, WT 285 lb, BP 130/80, P-76, R-18.
Cardiac RRR, S1,S2 no S3,S4, 3/6 SEM throughout precordium (new finding), Lungs CTA, Abd: soft, +BS no HSM, extremities no edema noted

1. What are the potential ICD-10 codes in this case?
2. How can the NP determine if this patient is a new patient versus an established patient at the clinic?
3. What components of care will be used for reimbursement decisions for Mr. Jones?
4. What type of physical examination best fits what was performed on Mr. Jones?
5. If you were coding the visit for Mr. Jones, how would you determine what decision-making level you would choose? Provide your rationale, and be specific.

References

Aalseth, P. (2006). *Medical coding: What it is and how it works.* Sudbury, MA: Jones & Bartlett.

American Association of Professional Coders. (2017). *What is HCPCS?* Retrieved from http://www.aapc.com/resources/medical-coding/hcpcs.aspx

Centers for Medicare and Medicaid. (2015). *Quality payment program.* Retrieved from https://qpp.cms.gov/

Contexo Media. (2015). Procedural coding expert ultimate guide to CPT coding. *Contexo Media,* 1–33.

Department of Health and Human Services. (2007). *Direct billing and payment for non-physician practitioner services.* Baltimore, MD: Centers for Medicare & Medicaid Service. Retrieved from https://www.cms.gov/Outreach-and-Education/Medicare-Learning-Network-MLN/MLNMattersArticles/downloads/MM5221.pdf

Federal Register. (2015). *Public Law 114-10: Medicare Access and CHIP Reauthorization Act.* Retrieved from https://www.congress.gov/114/plaws/publ10/PLAW-114publ10.pdf

Goodson, J. (2007). Unintended consequences of resource-based relative value scale reimbursement. *Journal of American Medical Association, 298*(19), 2308–2310.

Goolsby, M. (2002). *Nurse practitioner secrets: Questions and answers to reveal the secrets to successful NP practice.* Philadelphia, PA: Hanley & Belfus.

MedLearn Network. (2010). *Evaluation and management services guide.* CMS. Retrieved from https://www.cms.gov/Outreach-and-Education/Medicare-Learning-Network-MLN/MLNProducts/Downloads/eval-mgmt-serv-guide-ICN006764.pdf

National Center for Health Statistics. (2012). *Classification of diseases, functioning, and disability: International classification of diseases* (10th rev. ed., Clinical Modification [ICD-10-CM]). Retrieved from http://www.cdc.gov/nchs/icd/icd10cm.htm

National Plan and Provider Enumeration System. (2012). *National provider identifier.* Retrieved from https://nppes.cms.hhs.gov/NPPES/StaticForward.do?forward=static.npistart

Phillipsen, P. S. (2008). The most costly billing practices ever. *Journal for Nurse Practitioners, 4*(10), 761–765.

Rapsilber, L. M., & Anderson, E. H. (2000). Understanding the reimbursement process. *Nurse Practitioner, 25*(5), 36–56.

Stanley, J. (2010). *Advanced practice nursing: Emphasizing common roles* (3rd ed.). Philadelphia, PA: F.A. Davis.

CHAPTER 16

Professional Employment

Julie G. Stewart and Susan M. DeNisco

Nurse Practitioner Certification

National board certification in your specialty area is a mark of excellence and establishes that a new graduate NP has met the educational criteria and clinical competencies to work as a safe and prudent clinician. This chapter will help the new graduate understand the steps necessary to take as you prepare for certification and state licensure. There is much confusion among healthcare providers, insurance companies, and consumers regarding the role of the NP and rigorous practice requirements needed to attain and maintain certification and licensure.

Preparing for Graduation

It is an exciting time for the NP student when getting ready to graduate and start in a new professional role. The process of certification and advanced practice licensure can be quite confusing, and the student needs to develop a timeline for this at least 3 months prior to graduation. It is very easy to procrastinate as one is busy completing didactic and clinical requirements, but there is paperwork that the NP graduate and the academic institution need to complete prior to the NP taking the national certification examination.

A signature from the NP academic program director may be needed for verification of the advanced pharmacology requirements and certain national certification examination applications. Official academic institution transcripts need to be sent to the state department for advanced practice licensure as well as the national certification body the graduate will be applying to. Staying organized is key to completing the appropriate paperwork on a timely basis to ensure early certification and licensure. Employers typically require that the NP be legally ready to practice and have the ability to go through the credentialing process required by many institutions and insurance companies.

National Certification

Upon completion of the graduation requirements, the NP should apply for national board certification from either the American Academy of Nurse Practitioners (AANP) or the American Nurses Credentialing Center (ANCC). Graduates of women's health or neonatal NP programs should apply to the National Certification Corporation for the obstetric, gynecologic, and neonatal nursing specialties. Candidates for the pediatric NP examination should apply to the Pediatric Nursing Certification Board.

The candidate should check with the board of nursing for the state in which he or she plans to practice to see which certifications are acceptable for licensure application. All states require an NP to be board certified in order to practice, except for California. New York does not require it if the graduate attended the NP program in NYS. In recent years, there have been efforts to allow multistate compacts so NPs can legally practice in more than one state with one license.

What to Expect on the Certification Examination

Most certification examinations allot at least 3 hours, except for the ANCC, which allows 4 hours for the examination. The candidate must go to the website of the chosen organization to review the domains that will be covered in the examination. The ANCC Family Nurse Practitioner Examination covers the following content domains:

- Foundations for Advanced Practice
- Professional Practice
- Independent Practice

Detailed test content information can be found on the ANCC website that outlines specific topics for each domain. The examination contains 200 questions, of which 175 questions will be scored. Once the eligibility requirements to take the certification examination are completed and the NP has successfully passed the exam, the credential is awarded: family nurse practitioner–board certified (FNP-BC) by the National Commission for Certifying Agencies. The Accreditation Board for Specialty Nursing Certification accredits this ANCC certification. Certification is awarded for a 5-year time period.

AANP National Certification Examinations are entry-level, competency-based examinations for nurse practitioners reflective of nurse practitioner knowledge and expertise for each of the following specialties: adult-gerontology, family nurse practitioner, and a new emergency nurse practitioner specialty for family nurse practitioners. The AANP examinations have four knowledge areas:

- Assessment
- Diagnosis
- Plan
- Evaluation

Go to the website to review the updated domains for testing to familiarize yourself with them and to choose which examination may be best suited for you as well as acceptable to your state and potential practice site(s).

Practice, practice, practice before taking the board certification examination. Since all the certification examinations are multiple choice, the applicant should practice taking test questions answering one per minute. Both the AANP and ANCC offer a multiple-choice practice examination for the FNP certification candidates to identify areas in which further study may be needed in anticipation of taking an official competency-based examination. This is highly recommended—practice makes perfect. It is wise to study with a partner or in small groups. Preparation for taking the certification examination should start months before graduation; attending a review course or purchasing review CDs is a wise way to become familiar with the material covered in the certification examinations. Many successful certified NPs listened to the review CDs to and from class and work for weeks or even months preparing for the examination. Remember that the exams are developed for entry-level NPs, and extremely complex questions will not be on the test.

Nurse Practitioner Licensure for Prescription Privileges

Currently nurse practitioners must be licensed in the state where they plan to practice, to have prescriptive authority. They prescribe medications, including controlled medication with varying levels of restriction and should be checked in the state practice act. Variation exists among states in the area of authorization to prescribe controlled medications and the relationship, if any, that must be maintained with a physician. Nurse practitioners should refer to the Drug Enforcement Agency website to clarify what the controlled substances prescriptive authority is in each state.

Advanced Practice State Licensure

Once the certification exam has been passed successfully, the graduate sends required documentation to the state in which she or he is applying to practice in for advanced practice nurse licensure. Most states require successfully completing 30 hours of education in pharmacology for advanced nursing practice, as well as holding a master's degree in nursing or in a related field recognized for certification as a nurse practitioner, such as a clinical nurse specialist or a nurse anesthetist recognized by one of the certifying bodies. Most states will want the application to be notarized and have photo identification.

The American Association of Nurse Practitioners has detailed, updated information on state practice acts as well as prescriptive authority. In addition, the *Pearson Report* is an excellent reference for all nurse practitioners; it provides an annual state-by-state national overview of nurse practitioner legislation and healthcare issues. It is very important that the NP understand the specific functions included in his or her state's definition of NP scope of practice related to diagnosing, treatment, prescribing practices, hospital admission privileges, referrals, education, and ordering diagnosis tests (Buppert, 2018). Each state's scope of practice delineates what the legal role and requirements are of physician involvement in the NP practice. Language such as *collaboration*, *supervision*, *independent practice*, and *consultation* are examples of varying forms of physician involvement with the NP.

Drug Enforcement Agency (DEA) Licensure

In addition, the NP must apply for the state-controlled substances licensure and the DEA (U.S. Drug Enforcement Administration) licensure. Through the Department of Justice and DEA, the NP must apply for a DEA number pursuant to Title 21, Code of Federal Regulations, Section 1300.01(b28), which states

> The term *mid-level practitioner* means an individual practitioner, other than a physician, dentist, veterinarian, or podiatrist, who is licensed, registered, or otherwise permitted by the United States or the jurisdiction in which he/she practices, to dispense a controlled substance in the course of professional practice. (U.S. Drug Enforcement Administration, 2017)

Examples of midlevel practitioners include, but are not limited to, healthcare providers such as nurse practitioners, nurse midwives, nurse anesthetists, clinical nurse specialists, and physician assistants, who are authorized to dispense controlled substances by the state in which they practice.

National Provider Identification (NPI)

The Health Insurance Portability and Accountability Act of 1996 (HIPAA) mandated the adoption of a standard unique identifier for healthcare providers. This is particularly important for reimbursement of healthcare services that the NP provides. In 2004, the Centers for Medicare and Medicaid Services (CMS) adopted the National Provider Identifier (NPI) as the standard unique identifier number for all healthcare providers to use when filing and processing healthcare claims (Stanley, 2010). All NPs are required to apply for a national provider number and are assigned only one number that will follow the NP wherever she or he practices. The application must be completed by the nurse practitioner to avoid any potential error that could delay billing and reimbursement (National Plan and Provider Enumeration System, 2012).

Malpractice Insurance

Professional liability is a recognized risk for nurse practitioners and advanced practice clinicians. With increased autonomy and responsibility at the point of care comes increased risk for errors and omissions that can result in harm to the patient. It is your professional responsibility to understand the current care practice environment and understand methods of risk reduction. It is important to remember to change the malpractice insurance policy from student NP and RN to NP malpractice insurance, even if the workplace offers to put the NP under its umbrella. While you may be an employee of a hospital, physician office, or other healthcare organization and are considered to be covered under the employer's malpractice program, it behooves the NP to carry individual malpractice insurance to avoid conflicted interests of the employer (Joel, 2013). Check with state and federal regulations to see what may affect malpractice insurance and what the advisable amounts of coverage are. Additionally, it is the NP's responsibility to minimize risk of being sued by maintaining current clinical skills and knowledge, clearly documenting all ordered or refused diagnostic testing and treatments, and careful evaluation of the patient's response to treatment.

Résumé vs. Curriculum Vitae Development for Nurse Practitioners

The current job market for nurse practitioners is highly competitive. Some experts recommend that nurse practitioners use curricula vitae as opposed to résumés

(Beauvais, 2016). Although the two documents are similar, there are some significant differences. A résumé is typically an abbreviated document that gives an overview of education, employment history, and achievements in one to two pages. Curricula vitae, on the other hand, are typically longer and more detailed. Curricula vitae are used when seeking positions in an academic setting, but often nursing professionals will use them if seeking a leadership role in the healthcare field.

As a new graduate you will want to highlight your clinical education and hours spent in each specialty area because you have no formal work experience as an NP (Dahring, 2012). Whether you use a résumé or a curriculum vitae, the NP must have a well-organized and coherent document that highlights the individual's abilities, skills, and accomplishments to promote his or her career. **BOX 16-1** provides an outline of a résumé for a new graduate nurse practitioner.

Dos and Don'ts of Résumé Writing

The résumé is the nurse practitioner's first introduction to a potential employer, making it imperative that the NP use this opportunity to make a positive impression with the goal of being invited to a first interview. However, a résumé can quickly leave a negative connotation if it contains errors such as misspellings, typos, and poor grammar. If the employer receives a document that is poorly constructed, this will likely give the impression that the NP is inattentive to detail and perhaps is unprofessional. Recent studies have stated that over 75% of organization leaders interviewed indicated that only one or two typos in a curriculum vitae would eliminate the candidate from consideration for the position (Hosking, 2010).

Print your résumé on high-quality paper using a professional font such as 10–12 point Times New Roman, as it is easy to read (Beauvais, 2016). Be sure your email address is professional sounding, and avoid using your current employer's email address or telephone number. Account for all gaps in your employment history, and do not list nonmedical employment history. Include a cover letter explaining how your skills and talents can provide immediate benefits to the organization (Beauvais, 2016).

BOX 16-1 Graduate Nurse Practitioner Résumé Outline

- Summary of Qualifications
- Education
- Clinical Rotations:
    - Name and type of clinical facility
    - Population focus of the rotation
    - Number of clinical hours
    - Number of patients seen daily
    - Level of autonomy
    - Procedures mastered
- Work History
- Certifications and Licensure
- Awards and Honors
- Activities
- Languages
- References Available on Request

▶ Job Satisfaction

As the NP student prepares for graduation, or for the NP considering workplace change, it is imperative to consider factors that enhance the work environment to be able to choose a successful practice option. The initial transitional year of professional practice is thought to provide the critical foundation on which new professionals build their knowledge and expertise. Having a supportive workplace environment has been shown to improve work effectiveness, enhance the ability to provide high-quality patient care, contribute to cost effectiveness, and promote the retention of NPs in successful collaborative practices in a variety of healthcare settings (DeNisco & Barker, 2016).

Job satisfaction has proven to decrease absenteeism, improve employee retention, improve productivity, and enhance job performance (Kacel, Miller, & Norris, 2005). In a study looking at factors leading to job satisfaction and dissatisfaction in NPs from the Midwest, the Misener Nurse Practitioner Job Satisfaction Scale (MNPJSS) was used. The MNPJSS consists of 44 items grouped into six categories: intrapractice partnership/collegiality; challenge/autonomy; professional, social, and community interaction; professional growth; time; and benefits. The factors that received the highest ratings for satisfaction were sense of accomplishment, challenge in work, and level of autonomy.

Job satisfaction has been linked to autonomy and is important in attracting and retaining NPs in the workplace, in addition to greater outpatient clinical productivity (Chumbler, Geller, & Weier, 2000; Schiestel, 2007). Clearly, autonomy is an important factor to consider when selecting a practice site.

Nurse practitioners working in nurse-managed health centers (NMHCs) have been shown to be accessible to their clients and provide health care that is at the least equitable to, and has been shown to be better than, in some cases, other providers (Pron, 2012). Nurse practitioners who work in this type of setting are the main healthcare providers but frequently have to deal with the numerous barriers to practice related to recognition by insurers and adequate resources. In a study published by Pron (2012), the majority of NPs working in NMHCs were found to perceive themselves as autonomous and had good job satisfaction as it related to the concept of autonomy. A sense of accomplishment was noted to be very high in this group of NPs, with the suggestion that this is related to the ability to provide improvement in the health care of the vulnerable patients that use NMHCs.

Successful practice for NPs has been linked to intrinsic factors such as challenge, sense of accomplishment, ability to deliver quality care, and level of autonomy (Kacel et al., 2005; Pron, 2012). The NP/DNP has much to offer in providing health care to the vulnerable and underserved populations needing improved health. In any case, the graduating NP/DNP should consider the various options and the pros and cons of the various practice settings that will provide job satisfaction.

▶ Collaboration

Although the topic of collaboration has been discussed earlier in this book, the relationship between collaboration and job satisfaction, as well as success, will be reviewed. Relational theory suggests that fostering collaborative relationships within the workplace can enhance empowerment and increase job effectiveness. Collaboration is an important component for NP practice, and one that is inherent to nursing in general. Collaborative care may be defined as "an arrangement whereby an NP and a physician provide primary health care to a group of patients, with the professionals sharing authority for providing care within their scope of practice" (Bellini & Shea, 2006, p. 233). Resnick and Bonner (2003) defined collaboration as "a joint and cooperative enterprise that integrates the individual perspectives and expertise of various team members" (p. 344), and they identified collaboration as a foundation for successful practice.

Collaboration has been associated with improvements in patient outcomes, healthcare costs, decision making, and as part of a response to the current nursing shortage (Hojat et al., 2003).

Nurse practitioners perceive that they collaborate well with physicians (Maylone, Ranieri, Quinn Griffin, McNulty, & Fitzpatrick, 2011), but some physicians may not understand what NPs' roles are. Bellini and Shea (2006) assessed medical residents' perceptions of nurse practitioners who worked in a collaborative model with assessments before and 1 year after implementation of the model. The majority of medical residents had a positive view of NPs prior to the collaborative model implementation; yet 1 year after the implementation, results indicated that more medical residents viewed NPs as colleagues and appreciated NPs' clinical judgment.

Successful collaborative practices need an orientation to the process of collaboration, education to the NP role and scope of practice to prevent underutilization of NPs, and promotion of effective collaborative care (Bailey, Jones, & Way, 2006). Trust, mutual respect, and open communication are critical components of a collaborative practice (Hallas, Butz, & Gitterman, 2004).

Empowerment

Empowerment—it sounds important, but what exactly is it? Power has been defined as "the ability to get things done, to mobilize resources, to get and use whatever it is that a person needs for the goals he or she is attempting to meet" (Kanter, 1993, p. 166). Empowerment has been said to be a central component of advanced practice nursing (Ackerman, Norsen, Martin, Wiedrich, & Kitzman, 1996). There are two perspectives of empowerment within the work environment: structural and psychological. Laschinger's (Almost & Laschinger, 2002; Laschinger, Finegan, Shamian, & Wilk, 2004) and Spreitzer's (1995, 2007) studies suggest that there are at least two components of empowerment, structural and psychological, that are separate from each other, although a positive relationship appears to exist between them.

Structural empowerment occurs when nurse practitioners have access to "information, support, resources, and opportunities to learn and grow" (Laschinger et al., 2004, p. 528). Psychological empowerment is a process that occurs when one has a sense of motivation in relation to the workplace environment (Manojlovich, 2007; Manojlovich & Laschinger, 2007).

When NPs' values, beliefs, and behaviors are congruent with workplace requirement's one finds meaning to professional practice (Stewart, 2008). Findings from these studies suggest that workplace environments that foster collegiality, provide support and access to resources, afford opportunities for professional growth, and permit visibility can enhance job satisfaction.

Psychological empowerment is felt to be a motivator for people and has been associated with an increased sense of self-efficacy and increased self-determination, which can encourage involvement and commitment by these individuals (Knol & Van Linge, 2009; Laschinger, Purdy, & Almost, 2007; MacPhee, Skelton-Green, Bouthillette, & Suryaprakash, 2011; Spreitzer & Doneson, 2005).

Interviewing Skills

Going on a job interview may seem intimidating to the newly minted nurse practitioner, but honing interview skills can help transform the experience into a stepping-stone to a new career. The interview process is competitive given the influx of primary care providers, so the NP needs to set him or herself above the rest. CMS maintains the National Provider Identifier (NPI) dataset, which lists approximately 106,000 practicing nurse practitioners and 70,000 practicing physician assistants in 2010. This estimate represents approximately 10,000 more nurse practitioners that report having NP in their title in a 2008 national survey (Agency for Health Care Research & Quality, 2011).

The Interview Process

For many candidates, the first step in the interview process may be a telephone interview. The telephone interview is used as a mechanism to screen candidates in order to decide if they warrant a face-to-face interview. The NP should not take a casual approach to the telephone interview, and should be prepared with questions as if he or she were in an in-person interview; some experts believe that standing while being interviewed will make you stronger and increase your confidence. NPs that make it past the initial telephone interview should not assume that they have the position (Kess, 2011).

If called in for a face-to-face interview, the NP must prepare by dressing professionally, having several copies of his or her resume in hand, and have a list of questions for the employer. Doing research on the company's mission and goals shows interest and initiative on the part of the NP. **BOX 16-2** shows discussion items that the NP should be prepared to answer during an interview for a clinical position.

Questions for the Employer

Too often nurse practitioners will ask about salary and benefits on the first interview. While compensation packages are important, this should be reserved for the second interview, as finding a position that is a "good fit" for your skills, talents, and personal needs should be

BOX 16-2 Potential Discussion Items for the Interview

What key tasks do you see yourself doing as a nurse practitioner?
What are the most important knowledge and skills that you bring to the NP role?
What do you know about this organization?
Describe two major trends in your profession.
What nonclinical qualifications do you bring to your role as a NP?
What are your strengths and weaknesses?
Where do you see yourself in 5 years?
When will you receive certification and licensure?

BOX 16-3 Questions to Ask a Potential Employer

What is the expected patient volume?
Expected hours/day/week?
Weekend hours?
"On call" expectations?
"Moonlighting" allowed?
Number of days/hours for orientation?
Peer review process and timeline?
Orientation to policies and procedures?
Offsite facilities?
Physician support?
Nursing support staff?
Community education program attendance?
Provider mix: NPs, PAs, MDs?
Billing for services?

of upmost importance. The NP should be prepared to ask a myriad of questions regarding practice issues, employer contract, and credentialing, which will be discussed later in this chapter. Other important questions will pertain to the patient population, practice hours, and facility setup, such as exam rooms and equipment. Very often, job satisfaction is dependent on the availability of a strong support team that helps make the practice as efficiently productive as possible. Ask about the number of patients you will be expected to see per day.

New graduate NPs often start out at between 8 and 12 patients a day, while experienced NPs usually see between 18 and 22 patients a day (Tumolo, 2005). Higher patient numbers may increase job pressure, but again, if your salary is productivity based, it could increase your bottom line (Tumolo, 2005). **BOX 16-3** lists important questions the NP should ask a potential employer.

Negotiating an Employment Contract

Every employment agreement or contract is unique, and various factors should be addressed before negotiation. The NP must determine his or her needs while assessing the potential employer's needs. Reflecting on and balancing your needs and your family's needs is paramount before accepting a position and negotiating your contract. Understand what aspects of the position are desired, negotiable, and non-negotiable. In the previous section compensation package, job obligations, and practice issues were areas of negotiable elements. The process of negotiating a contract should include preparation, bargaining, and finalizing (Chien, 2002).

Preparation

Do your research ahead of time and be able to clearly articulate what you know about local and national compensation patterns. The NP should have a reference range for both annual and hourly wages for similar positions and write down what the bottom line is for both earnings and benefits. The NP should also be prepared to understand the potential offers in regard to the reimbursement system for the office or organization. The NP should research and find out if it is a fee-for-service practice or a capitated practice. Ask the employer if there are bonus opportunities as well as rewards for productivity and effort.

Bargaining

The NP must market him or herself as a high-quality, cost-effective healthcare provider. Highlight your previous contributions to nursing and as an NP. Familiarize yourself with the business of medicine. Savvy negotiators will calculate the NP's potential revenue for the practice. Be flexible, and listen to the employer's perspective; gaining the trust of the employer will facilitate the negotiating process.

Finalizing

Once an agreement is reached, it is important for the NP to finalize the contract with a written agreement. There are varying opinions on whether or not a formal contract is needed for an NP and the employer. There are many advantages of a written employment contract:

- Increased job security and control over professional practice
- Legal protection in relation to finances and job responsibilities
- Upfront agreement on potential problems and professional issues
- Protection from termination

NPs should secure an attorney familiar with NP law and business contracts. If any employer has a well-established, profitable practice, the NP should expect to be rewarded well under the employment agreement. If the practice is losing money, the NP will find it difficult under the best circumstances to negotiate an acceptable agreement, no matter what the skill set and experience the NP has (Buppert, 2018).

Credentialing

The public has the right to safe, quality health care delivered by healthcare professionals with the appropriate education, training, and experience. The Joint Commission, the Accreditation Association for Ambulatory Healthcare, and managed care organizations take this commitment very seriously (Magdic, Hravnak, & McCartney, 2005). One mechanism required by these agencies to ensure patient safety is the process of credentialing and delineation of clinical privileges for medical staff, including nurse practitioners. Obtaining clinical privileges was once reserved for physicians, but as nurse practitioners have integrated themselves as equal partners in the healthcare delivery system, credentialing and obtaining clinical privileges to practice is commonplace. Nurse practitioners must become familiar with the regulations that impact and guide the process of credentialing and obtaining clinical privileges.

Credentialing and clinical privileging follows licensure and is the process through which a provider obtains authorization to practice in a select healthcare or hospital setting. Typically the credentialing process involves verification of education, licensure, certification, health requirements, and reference checks. Ongoing clinical privileges are contingent on maintaining skills and board certification. Clinical privileges are a specifically delineated list or description of the privileges granted within your scope of practice. For example, standard clinical privileges for a nurse practitioner would include obtaining a history and physical examination and ordering and interpreting diagnostic tests. A peer review process is a usual part of maintaining the privileges, which are reviewed by your employer periodically.

Collaborative Agreements

The nurse practitioner must be familiar with the legal scope of practice in the state she or he wishes to practice in. Each state has regulations that define the scope of practice; some statutes are governed by state legislature and other states give the board of nursing the authority to enforce the scope of practice law (Buppert, 2018). Each state must define the legal requirement for physician involvement in the nurse practitioner's practice. This involvement, if any, is depicted as "supervision" or "collaboration" and further explains the details of the terms of the involvement. Some state laws give tremendous detail in regard to the specifics of the level of involvement, ranging from prescribing controlled substances to establishing a referral and consultation arrangement between the physician and NP. When entering an employment contract in a state where the scope of practice statute mandates a "collaborative" agreement between an advanced practice nurse and a physician, it is important to draft a mutually agreeable collaborative practice agreement that will support the scope of practice law in your state. **TABLE 16-1** is a sample collaborative practice agreement that details prescriptive authority, systems for peer review, coverage in the absence of the clinician, and referral and consultation arrangements.

TABLE 16-1 Collaborative Practice Agreement for Advanced Practice Nurses Requesting Prescriptive Authority

1. Complete names, home and business addresses, zip codes, and telephone numbers of the licensed practitioner and the advanced practice nurse:	
Licensed Practitioner: Licensed practitioner name and license number Street address of home City, state, & zip of home Home phone number Business street address City, state, & zip of business Business phone number	*Advanced Practice Nurse:* Advanced practice nurse name and license number Street address of home City, state, & zip of home Home phone number Business street address City, state, & zip of business Business phone number
2. List of all locations where prescriptive authority is authorized by this agreement.	
Business street address City, state, & zip of business Business phone number	Business street address City, state, & zip of business Business phone number
3. List all specialty or board certifications of the licensed practitioner and the advanced practice nurse. Licensed practitioner is board certified in a medical practice specialty in. The advanced practice nurse is a nurse practitioner, clinical nurse specialist, certified nurse midwife, etc., with a specialized certification as a family nurse practitioner, etc.	

(continues)

TABLE 16-1 Collaborative Practice Agreement for Advanced Practice Nurses Requesting Prescriptive Authority *(continued)*

4. Briefly describe the specific manner of collaboration between the licensed practitioner and advance practice nurse. *Specifically, how they will work together, how they will share practice trends and responsibilities, how they will maintain geographic proximity, and how they will provide coverage during an absence, incapacity, infirmity, or emergency by the licensed practitioner.*

How they will work together:
The licensed practitioner and advanced practice nurse shall collaborate on a continual basis, etc.
How they will share practice trends and responsibilities:
The advanced practice nurse shall make rounds at the request of the licensed practitioner and consult with the license practitioner as needed, etc.
How they will maintain geographic proximity:
The licensed practitioner will maintain a physical presence within a reasonable geographic proximity to the advanced practice nurse's practice location.
How they will provide coverage during absence, incapacity, infirmity, or emergency by the license practitioner:
In the case of the absence, incapacity, or unavailability of the licensed practitioner, coverage and consultation will be coordinated and maintained by another licensed practitioner as arranged in advance by the licensed practitioner and the advanced practice nurse.

5. Provide a description of limitations, if any, the licensed practitioner has placed on the advanced practice nurse's prescriptive authority.

There are no additional limitations on the advanced practice nurse or there are the following limitations on the advanced practice nurse, etc.

6. Provide a description of the time and manner of the licensed practitioner's review of the advanced practice nurse's prescribing practices. Specifically, the description should include provisions that the advanced practice nurse must submit documentation of prescribing practices to the licensed practitioner within 7 days. Documentation of prescribing practices shall include, but not be limited to, at least a 5% random sampling of the charts and medications prescribed for patients.

The advanced practice nurse must submit documentation of the advance practice nurse's prescribing practices within 7 days to the licensed practitioner for review. The documentation of prescribing practices shall include at least a 5% random sampling of the charts and medications prescribed for patients.

7. Provide a list of all other written practice agreements of the licensed practitioner and advanced practice nurse.

There are no other practice agreements, or list all other practice agreements, etc.

8. Provide the duration of the written practice agreement between the licensed practitioner and advanced practice nurse.

Either party may terminate this practice agreement without cause at any time, effective immediately upon notice to the other party, etc.

Signature of licensed practitioner: **Date:**	***Signature of advanced practice nurse:*** **Date:**

▸ The Consensus Model—Stay Tuned!

Licensure, accreditation, certification, and education is the collaborative work of the APRN Consensus Work Group and National Council of State Boards of Nursing (NCSBN) APRN Advisory Committee. The Consensus Model was intended to ease the confusion surrounding advanced practice nursing. It clarifies the population foci for APNs and scope of practice issues (NCSBN, 2009). After receiving critical input from NP educators and practicing APNs, some changes related to the overlap that occurs between acute care and primary care APNs were suggested. The goal remains for all NPs to have a DNP as entry level into practice; however, due to the myriad of state licensing regulations, it is difficult to expect that to be mandated anytime soon. As shown in many research studies, NPs have been providing high-quality, cost-effective health care with master's level education for years.

The addition of doctoral education is a goal to have parity with our colleagues, such as physicians, physical therapists, psychologists, and pharmacists. Having additional preparation to improve the NP's ability to expand leadership initiatives in individual, community, and global health is the direction we need to be heading in these tumultuous times in our current healthcare system. Kudos to those of you who are reaching that goal, and we encourage those of you obtaining MSNs to seriously consider continuing on with your education to obtain a DNP. Either way, we know you will connect with your patients, and make a difference in their lives.

▸ Seminar Discussion Questions

1. Discuss the elements that are important to you when seeking a place of employment. What is negotiable and what is non-negotiable?
2. Share your résumé with a peer. Discuss strengths and weaknesses of your peer's current résumé and offer suggestions for improvement.
3. Discuss the process of certification and licensure, and list what steps need to be taken to become gainfully employed after graduation.
4. What resources are available to the NP in understanding the state-by-state NP scope-of-practice laws?
5. Identify the benefits of formal employment.

References

Ackerman, M. H., Norsen, L., Martin, B., Wiedrich, J., & Kitzman, H. J. (1996). Development of a model of advanced practice. *American Journal of Critical Care, 5*(1), 68–73.

Agency for Health Care Research & Quality. (2011). *Primary care workforce: Facts and stats No. 2: The number of nurse practitioners and physician assistants practicing primary care in the United States*. Retrieved from http://www.ahrq.gov/research/pcwork2.htm

Almost, J., & Laschinger, H. S. (2002). Workplace empowerment, collaborative work relationships, and job strain in nurse practitioners. *Journal of the American Academy of Nurse Practitioners, 14*(9), 408–420.

Bailey, P., Jones, L., & Way, D. (2006). Family physician/nurse practitioner: Stories of collaboration. *Journal of Advanced Nursing, 53*(4), 381–391.

Beauvais, B. (2016). Role transition: Strategies for success in the marketplace. In S. DeNisco & A. Barker (Eds.), *Advanced practice nursing: Evolving roles for the transformation of the profession* (pp. 763–783). Burlington, MA: Jones & Bartlett Learning.

Bellini, L. M., & Shea, J. A. (2006). Improvement of resident perceptions of nurse practitioners after the introduction of a collaborative care model: A benefit of work hour reform? *Teaching and Learning in Medicine, 18*(3), 233–236.

Buppert, C. (2018). *Nurse practitioners' business practice and legal guide* (6th ed.). Sudbury, MA: Jones & Bartlett Learning.

Chien, A. (2002). Negotiating a contract. In M. Goolsby, *Nurse practitioner secrets: Questions and answers to reveal the secrets to successful NP practice* (pp. 1–4). Philadelphia, PA: Hanley & Belfus.

Chumbler, N. R., Geller, J. M., & Weier, A. W. (2000). The effects of clinical decision making on nurse practitioners' clinical productivity. *Evaluation & the Health Professions, 23*(3), 284–304.

Dahring, R. (2012). *Nurse practitioner job search.* Retrieved from http://www.nursepractitionerjobsearch.com/nurse-practitioner-resume.html

DeNisco, S., & Barker, A. (2016). *Advanced practice nursing: Evolving roles for the transformation of the profession* (3rd ed.). Burlington, MA: Jones & Bartlett Learning.

Hallas, D. M., Butz, A., & Gitterman, B. (2004). Attitudes and beliefs for effective pediatric nurse practitioner and physician collaboration. *Journal of Pediatric Health Care, 18*(2), 77–86.

Hojat, M., Gonnella, J. S., Nasac, T. J., Fields, S. K., Cicchetti, A., Lo Scalzo, A., . . . Torres-Ruiz, A. (2003). Comparisons of American, Israeli, Italian, and Mexican physicians and nurses on the total and factor scores of the Jefferson scale of attitudes toward physician-nurse collaborative relationships. *International Journal of Nursing Studies, 40,* 427–435.

Hosking, R. (2010). Top 10 tips for job seekers. *OfficePro, 70*(2), 5.

Joel, L. A. (2013). *Advanced practice nursing: Essentials for role development* (3rd ed.). Philadelphia, PA: F.A. Davis.

Kacel, B., Miller, M., & Norris, D. (2005). Measurement of nurse practitioner job satisfaction in a midwestern state. *Journal of the American Academy of Nurse Practitioners, 17*(1), 27–32.

Kanter, R. M. (1993). *Men and women of the corporation* (2nd ed.). New York, NY: Basic Books.

Kess, S. (2011). *Clinical advisor.* Retrieved from http://www.clinicaladvisor.com/job-interview-tips-for-physician-assistants-and-nurse-practitioners/article/197218

Knol, J., & Van Linge, R. (2009). Innovative behavior: The effect of structural and psychological empowerment on nurses. *Journal of Advanced Nursing, 65*(2), 359–370.

Laschinger, H. K., Finegan, J. E., Shamian, J., & Wilk, P. (2004). A longitudinal analysis of the impact of workplace empowerment on work satisfaction. *Journal of Organizational Behavior, 25,* 527–545.

Laschinger, H. K., Purdy, N., & Almost, J. (2007). The impact of leader-member exchange quality, empowerment, and core self-evaluation on nurse manager's job satisfaction. *Journal of Nursing Administration, 37*(5), 221–229.

MacPhee, M., Skelton-Green, J., Bouthillette, F., & Suryaprakash, N. (2011). An empowerment framework for nursing leadership in development: Supporting evidence. *Journal of Advanced Nursing, 68*(1), 159–169.

Magdic, K. S., Hravnak, M., & McCartney, S. (2005). Credentialing for nurse practitioners: An update. *American Association of Critical Care Nurses Clinical Issues, 16*(1), 16–22.

Manojlovich, M. (2007). Power and empowerment in nursing: Looking backward to inform the future. *Online Journal Issues of Nursing, 12*(1). Retrieved from http://www.medscape.com/viewarticle/553403

Manojlovich, M., & Laschinger, H. (2007). The nursing worklife model: Extending and refining a new theory. *Journal of Nursing Management, 15,* 256–263.

Maylone, M., Ranieri, L., Quinn Griffin, M., McNulty, R., & Fitzpatrick, J. (2011). Collaboration and autonomy: Perceptions among nurse practitioners. *Journal of the American Academy of Nurse Practitioners, 23*(1), 51–57.

National Council of State Boards of Nursing. (2009). *Consensus model for APRN regulation: Licensure, accreditation, certification & education.* Retrieved from http://www.nonpf.com/displaycommon.cfm?an=1&subarticlenbr=26

National Plan and Provider Enumeration System. (2012). *National provider identifier.* Retrieved from https://nppes.cms.hhs.gov/NPPES/StaticForward.do?forward=static.npistart

Pearson, L. (2012). The Pearson report. *American Journal for Nurse Practitioners.* Retrieved from http://www.pearsonreport.com

Pron, L. (2012). Job satisfaction and perceived autonomy for nurse practitioners working in nurse-managed health centers. *Journal of the American Academy of Nurse Practitioners, 25*(4), 213–221.

Resnick, B., & Bonner, A. (2003). Collaboration: Foundation for a successful practice. *Journal of the American Medical Directors Association,* 344–349.

Schiestel, C. (2007). Job satisfaction among Arizona adult nurse practitioners. *Journal of the American Academy of Nurse Practitioners, 19,* 30–34.

Spreitzer, G. (1995). Psychological empowerment in the workplace: Dimensions, measurement, and validation. *Academy of Management Journal, 38*(5), 1442–1465.

Spreitzer, G. (2007). Toward the integration of two perspectives: A review of social-structural and psychological empowerment at work. In C. Cooper & J. Barling (Eds.), *The handbook of organizational behavior.* Thousand Oaks, CA: Sage.

Spreitzer, G., & Doneson, D. (2005). Musings on the past and future of employee empowerment. Forthcoming in T. Cummings (Ed.), *Handbook of organizational development.* Thousand Oaks, CA: Sage.

Stanley, J. (2010). *Advanced practice nursing: Emphasizing common roles* (2nd ed.). Philadelphia, PA: F.A. Davis.

Stewart, J. (2008). Psychological empowerment, structural empowerment, and collaboration among nurse practitioners (doctoral dissertation). Cleveland, OH: Case Western Reserve University.

Tumolo, J. (2005). *Advance for NPs & PAs.* Retrieved from http://nurse-practitioners-and-physician-assistants.advanceweb.com/Article/Question-Authority-2.aspx

U.S. Drug Enforcement Administration. (2012). *Mid-level practitioners authorization by state.* Retrieved from http://www.deadiversion.usdoj.gov/drugreg/practioners/index.html

Index

Note: Page numbers followed by *e*, *f*, *t*, *b* indicates exhibits, figures, tables and boxes respectively

A

B

C

D

E

F

G

H

I

J

K

L

M

N

O

P

Q

R

S

T

U

V

W